PRAISE FOR PSYCHOSIS, PSYCHIATRY AND PSYCHOSPIRITUAL CONSIDERATIONS

"As a consultant clinical psychologist and sangoma (South African shaman) with a PhD on sangoma trance states, my clinical work within indigenous communities often directly challenges me in regard to the complex relationship of psychosis and psychospiritual states. In that spirit, I appreciate how Brian Spittles not only dismantles epistemological definitions of psychosis, but also, with subtle finesse, elucidates the dynamics of psychospiritual approaches. For example, his work on Tibetan Buddhist spirit possession is exquisite. And don't skip the appendices, as they hold scintillating treasures. Such a rich contribution, worth savouring, if this topic is meaningful to you."

—**Dr Ingo Lambrecht** is a Consultant Clinical Psychologist,
and author of *Sangoma Trance States* (2014)

"Fearlessly, and with the authority that comes from an impeccable, thoughtful literature review, Dr. Spittles challenges psychiatry to accept a broader view of human experience. He reflects on ancient wisdom traditions that describe, validate, and draw benefit from extraordinary states of consciousness. He makes the case that psychiatry must open its doors and accept this wisdom. In many circumstances, what has been categorically perceived as psychosis can be understand as a beneficial psychospiritual transformation that needs to be nurtured, and not medicated or labelled as mental illness."

—**Dr Emma Bragdon** is a transpersonal psychologist,
founder and Executive Director of Integrative Mental Health for You,
and the author of *A Sourcebook for Helping People in Spiritual Emergency* (2006)

"This timely, progressive book questions the validity of psychiatry's materialistic concept of 'psychosis' and raises the pertinent issue of what it means to be 'fully human'. Could interventions based on dominant psychiatric assumptions that underpin current conceptualisations be limiting a natural healing process which is trying to emerge? Spittles' suggested feasibility of psychospiritual research in psychiatry establishes a broader investigative scope, inclusive of metaphysical and cross-cultural lenses, and offers a more productive approach than psychiatry's claim that psychosis is essentially incomprehensible. This book opens the way for further investigative research and proposes a hopeful and much needed new paradigm of 'medical holism'."

—**Katie Mottram** is an author, Campaign Founder, and Inaugural Director of the International Spiritual Emergence Network

"Like a skilful conductor leading a very large orchestra, the author has done a masterful job drawing together and harmonizing a vast range of at times seemingly incompatible information and concepts with engaging, informative, and enlightening results. I heartily endorse his key assertion: psychiatry must transcend its current fixation with biology and pathology and rebuild itself upon bona fide, rigorously researched psychospiritual foundations if it is to ever justify calling itself a profession of "soul doctors". The challenges this book articulates so well not only invite but should command the attention of everyone with a serious interest in these issues."

—**John Watkins** is a mental health counsellor, researcher, and educator, and is the author of *Hearing Voices* (1998), *Healing Schizophrenia* (2006), and *Unshrinking Psychosis* (2010)

"This book is a deep dive into what Foucault called the "Reason-Madness nexus", which constitutes a core dialogical dimension of the originality of western culture as reflected in its art and its spirituality. However, this creativity wellspring of active dialogue has been drying up since the Age of Reason. Even in the mental health field, where diagnosis and treatment of psychosis directly confronts the psychiatrist with complex issues, the language of psychiatry has been reduced to a monologue of reason about madness. In this light, Dr. Spittles' book offers a reservoir of mental health vitality to those who are restricted by routine rationalism."

—**Professor David Lukoff** is a licensed psychologist, author of 80 articles, and co-author of the DSM-4 and DSM-5 'Religious or Spiritual Problem' category

"Dr Spittles has made an indispensable contribution to a broader understanding of the perennial experience of extreme states/psychosis/madness. His book shows how the psychiatric disease model has failed in its mission to provide an honest theoretical grasp of, or humane response to, the timeless human nature of madness. It also offers a necessary broader vision of madness that embraces the true depth of the mythic and archetypal forces that drive extreme emotional upheavals and potential transformations. His book is encyclopaedic in the best sense of the word—of leaving no stone unturned. It is truly unsurpassed in its bold and comprehensive scholarship."

—**Dr Michael Cornwall, PhD** is editor of the 2 volume *Journal of Humanistic Psychology* special issue on extreme states, an Esalen Institute conference leader on alternative approaches to psychosis, and has published follow-up research on the Jungian Diabasis House psychosis program

"*Psychosis, Psychiatry and Psychospiritual Considerations* offers a comprehensive examination of the interface between psychotic and spiritual experience and distress. Exploring a neglected area in the psychiatric literature, this important book illuminates the history of the development of psychiatric classification in North America, how the meaning of psychotic experiences has become ignored, and how spiritual understandings in psychiatric practice have been side-lined. It includes a fascinating overview of a wide range of models designed to help mental health professionals assist the people they work with in discerning psychospiritual experiences from psychopathology."

—**Dr Allister Bush** is a Consultant Psychiatrist at Te Whare Marie, Māorii Mental Health service, Porirua New Zealand, and co-author of *Collaborative and Indigenous Mental Health Therapy: Tātaihono- Stories of Māori Healing and Psychiatry*

PSYCHOSIS, PSYCHIATRY AND PSYCHOSPIRITUAL CONSIDERATIONS

PSYCHOSIS, PSYCHIATRY AND PSYCHOSPIRITUAL CONSIDERATIONS
Engaging and Better Understanding the Madness and Spiritual Emergence Nexus

Brian Spittles

AEON

First edition published in 2022 by
Aeon Books

British Library Cataloguing in Publication Data

A C.I.P. for this book is available from the British Library

ISBN-13: 978-1-80152-015-7

Typeset by Medlar Publishing Solutions Pvt Ltd, India

www.aeonbooks.co.uk

I dedicate this book to all of us who navigate the vicissitudes of life as best we can.

The world is no more the alien terror that was taught me.
Spurning the cloud-grimed and still sultry battlements
whence so lately Jehovan thunders boomed,
my gray gull lifts her wing against the nightfall,
and takes the dim leagues with a fearless eye.

—Benjamin Paul Blood, 1874.

CONTENTS

FOCAL SETTING THREE:
UNDERSTANDING PSYCHOSIS:
DISCERNING PSYCHOSPIRITUAL FROM PSYCHOPATHOLOGICAL

FOCAL SETTING FOUR:
UNDERSTANDING PSYCHOSIS: PSYCHOSPIRITUAL
AND PSYCHOPATHOLOGICAL AS INDISTINGUISHABLE

APPENDICES

TABLES AND FIGURES

.

Figures

ACRONYMS

AMPA	American Metapsychiatric Association
APA	American Psychiatric Association
ASC	Altered States of Consciousness
DSM	Diagnostic and Statistical Manual of Mental Disorders
GAP	Group for the Advancement of Psychiatry
HVN	Hearing Voices Network
ICD	International Classification of Diseases
IASP	International Association for Spiritual Psychiatry
MEPF	Mystical Experiences with Psychotic Features
PDMF	Psychotic Disorders with Mystical Features
PMA	Primordial Mental Activity
RCP	Royal College of Psychiatrists
RIST	Regression in the Service of Transcendence
SE	Spiritual Emergence or Spiritual Emergency
SEN	Spiritual Emergence Network
SPSIG	Spirituality and Psychiatry Special Interest Group
WHO	World Health Organisation

FOREWORD

In this remarkable, enjoyable, and eye-opening book, Dr. Brian Spittles elucidates the history of how the psychiatric diagnostic criteria for psychosis were formulated, who helped create them, the cultural backgrounds in which they arose, the influence of various factions and industries that shaped them, and how we ended up in our current highly suboptimal situation of reductionist diagnostics. He then critiques the key psychosis diagnostic criteria, demonstrating how each are part of the global range of human spiritual experience and provides a range of other possible spiritual and pragmatic interpretative frameworks from various traditions and cultures that might lead to vastly more satisfying outcomes for patients, providers, healthcare systems, societies, and humanity.

When I first studied mental health diagnosis in medical school, circa 2000, diagnostic categories were presented to us with a sense of extremely confident and unquestioned solidity, along the lines of, "These are the criteria for psychosis. These are the criteria for schizophrenia. These are the criteria for schizotypal personality disorder. These are the criteria for bipolar disorder". They were presented as if timeless Platonic Universals, in the same sense as, "This is a femur fracture, this is a bacterial infection, this is a stroke". I am certain that most of my classmates took these mental health diagnoses at face value, memorizing their signs and symptoms like everything else we learned for our bi-weekly exams and later national medical exams. Recent conversations with those currently undergoing medical training show that little has changed as to how mental health diagnosis is taught.

However, a few of my classmates and I had a very different relationship to the specifics of these mental health diagnostic criteria, as we had each had experiences sufficient to place us in one or more of those categories, at least temporarily, and simply had the very good sense not to have told a healthcare professional. These experiences had arisen from a complex mix of various life experiences, meditative and other spiritual practices, psychedelic use, and sometimes without obvious causes. Many had been very carefully and diligently sought out and cultivated, sometimes at great expense, often in the form of personal meditation retreats at spiritual centres around the world, and through other time-consuming practices.

Many of these experiences and longer-lasting consciousness transformations were among the most treasured of our lives, yet we found ourselves given no diagnostic options, billing codes, explanatory models, acceptable medical language, nor other conceptual paradigms in which to place these profound and life-enhancing treasures should we encounter a patient having them, or if we ourselves wished to have an honest conversation about them with a healthcare provider.

The established criteria for psychosis, schizophrenia, schizotypal personality disorder, and bipolar disorder were being taught without any sense of the fascinating histories, the remarkable personalities and debates that underlay them, the complex politics, other possible ways to conceptualize them, the cultural wars, nor the countries and the times in which they arose to become established as our current mainstream clinical options. Instead, they were presented as simple biological facts typically requiring specific medications, often for the rest of patients' lives, end of story.

Yet, those of us in the class who, through accident or intent, had plunged various depths of what turns out to be the normal, expected range of human experiences and mental states (as described by the likes of Dr. William James, the Harvard psychiatrist, in 1902), knew directly for ourselves that there were positive ways to relate to at least some of the range of what was being called psychosis, schizophrenia, schizotypy, and bipolar disorders. We knew that such experiences were often potentially healing, profoundly transformative, and vastly more nuanced and workable than what we were being told. Thus began our compartmentalized careers practising in a system we knew from first-hand experience to be profoundly flawed.

I believe that this book is essential foundational reading for anyone wishing to understand how we got here and how various attempts to make things better have failed. It also offers, in part, a clearer picture of the challenging puzzle of how to successfully remake the current global mental healthcare system into one that is vastly more nuanced in its diagnostic options. This includes an improved focus on pragmatic outcomes, function, and adding value to care, instead of needlessly and harmfully pathologizing potentially and profoundly transformative instances of human experience and spiritual development.

I hope you enjoy reading it as much as I did.

Dr. Daniel M. Ingram, MD MSPH

CHAPTER 1

Introduction

1.0 Introduction

Psychosis, and psychotic-like experience, has occurred within all cultures through-out recorded human history in apparently mad and mystic forms. Over time, different and divergent views concerning the nature and cause of such experiences have been proffered within various cultural frameworks of understanding. Western psychiatry has traditionally viewed psychosis as a psychopathological and innately incomprehensible mental disorder of probable biological aetiology. Throughout this book I argue that such a view is limited and limiting, and that a better understanding of the nature and determinants of psychosis can be gleaned through investigating psychospiritual considerations.[1] Indeed, in other conceptual and cultural frameworks of understanding, psychotic-like experiences are seen to be of a psychospiritual nature and cause. Therefore, this book undertakes a process of creating a provisional conceptual bridge between physical and metaphysical worldviews in order to better understand both psychotic and psychospiritual human experiences. Accordingly, I use an open-ended heuristic approach[2] that enables the systematic examination and critical appraisal of views on psychosis across the materialist-to-metaphysical spectrum.

My aim throughout this book is not to negate the discipline of psychiatry, but to demonstrate the viability and efficacy of incorporating psychospiritual considerations

---

[1] A definition and explication of the term 'psychospiritual' is provided in Chapter Two, Section 2.1 and Appendix One.
[2] See Section 1.2 below and Appendix 9 for further details on my heuristic approach.

1

into psychosis research. Additionally, the aim here is not to ascertain what psychosis *is* per se, but to systematically extend the scope of exploration to glean a better, or broader, understanding of psychotic and psychotic-like experience, beyond the traditional psychiatric picture. My investigative process therefore challenges several foundational psychiatric beliefs and calls for the discipline to extend its investigative parameters beyond the limited epistemological bounds of materialism. Overall, this book demonstrates the importance and validity of incorporating psychospiritual knowledge into conventional psychiatric thinking and practice, while challenging the view that psychosis is a biogenic and incomprehensible form of psychopathology characterised by specific diagnostic criteria. This challenge suggests the necessity for fundamental changes to psychiatric thinking and practice in order to foster a better understanding of psychosis. While recognising that psychoses, or psychotic-like events, are often distressing and socially disabling, I contend that examining psychospiritual factors and realities can open pathways to comprehend such anomalous human experiences more fully.

1.1 Explicating the challenge to psychiatry

A baseline proposition driving this book is that the word 'psychosis' represents an anomalous and enigmatic phenomenon which is poorly understood by Western psychiatry.[3] Indeed, *Campbell's Psychiatric Dictionary* states that the term 'psychosis' "has been anything but precise and definite ... As a result of conflicting usage, there is no single acceptable definition of what psychosis is" (Campbell, 2009, p. 812). I substantiate the veracity of this statement throughout the ensuing chapters, wherein I argue that such paucity of understanding is essentially due to psychiatry being governed by the principles of medical materialism, which work to restrict its conceptual and investigative scope. This has resulted in a predominantly biogenic understanding of psychosis by psychiatry. Indeed, the 2005 American Psychiatric Association (APA) president Steven Sharfstein (2005) acknowledges that "we have allowed the biopsychosocial model to become the bio-bio-bio model". As a consequence of this prominent focus on a biological model of understanding, the consideration of psychospiritual matters is all but absent from psychiatric epistemology and psychosis research. Yet, Andreasen (2005) has proposed that "it's useful for psychiatrists to remember that the word [psychiatry] comes from the Greek psyche, which means breath, life,

---

[3] Throughout this book various adjectives are used in reference to psychiatry (e.g. Western, medical, biomedical, biogenic, mainstream, traditional, conventional, categorical, etc.). Such terms basically infer a psychiatric model that understands the aetiology of psychopathology to be anatomical. It also refers to a reductive model of psychiatry which seeks to concretise anomalous human experiences into discrete diagnostic categories. This includes psychoanalytic psychiatry, for while it does not subscribe to a biomedical understanding of psychopathology, it does employ a categorical diagnostic approach. Also, my frequent anthropomorphic use of the word 'psychiatry' (i.e. speaking of psychiatry as if a person) is a matter of expediency. It is a shorthand and convenient inference to the general thinking of psychiatrists within the discipline of psychiatry.

animating principle or spirit … Literally, a psychiatrist is a healer of the spirit, not of the mind or brain". How, then, might a psychiatrist as healer of the spirit understand and therapeutically respond to the phenomenon and experience of psychosis? Prospective answers to this question are revealed throughout my unfolding investigative process which, in its quest to better understand psychosis, examines psychotic-like phenomena within both materialist and metaphysical contexts.

In terms of my challenge to psychiatry, I adopt a heuristic approach to demonstrate systematically the validity and value of incorporating psychospiritual considerations into the quest for a better understanding of psychosis. The open-ended nature of this investigative approach leads beyond the limited scope of simply studying psychopathology, into a deeper conceptual and phenomenological exploration of the subliminal depths of being human. Indeed, Bentall (2004, p. xiv) states that "I do not think it is an exaggeration to say that the study of psychosis amounts to the study of human nature". My research leads me to concur with this view. Hence, my overall challenge is composed of three key interrelated foci:

1. a challenge to psychiatry to extend beyond the materialist assumptions that govern its thinking and practice and include psychospiritual considerations within its epistemological remit;
2. a challenge to the subsequent psychiatric construal of psychosis as a biogenic and discrete form of psychopathology that can be clinically identified via certain characteristic diagnostic criteria; and
3. a challenge to the psychiatric idea that psychotic experiences are fundamentally incomprehensible.

I propose that, if psychiatry is to consider and accept the feasibility of this composite challenge, it will be better able to understand and therapeutically respond to anomalous human experiences within the psychotic-psychospiritual nexus. The signs of psychosis which appear incomprehensible from a materialist perspective become increasingly comprehensible when considered from other paradigms of understanding. Hence, it appears that the perceived incomprehensibility of psychosis is more a reflection of inherent limitations to psychiatry's worldview, than of the nature of psychosis per se.

Overall, then, I maintain that a psychospiritual investigation of the anomalous state of consciousness called 'psychosis' leads beyond the limited materialist parameters of medical psychiatric thinking to afford an enhanced understanding of the nature, and numerous possible determinants, of this phenomenon. As suggested by Winship (2014, p. xix),

> a theory of spiritual crisis in psychosis, rather than an approach which begins by assuming biological imbalance, tracks one of many new directions and gives an intriguing vista for debates … The challenge of working with people with psychosis can shift with new insights.

This approach challenges some of the fundamental tenets underpinning psychiatric thinking and practice. For instance, the notion of psychopathology, upon which the existence of psychiatry depends, is shown to be ambiguous when examined in light of psychospiritual considerations. Concomitantly, conventional psychiatric understandings of psychosis become questionable and contestable. Whereas the traditional psychopathology-seeking approach is largely prescriptive and restricted to identifying presumed forms of mental illness, a heuristic approach engages enigmatic states of consciousness in an open-ended process of investigation, that aims to glean new knowledge as to their physical, psychological, socio-cultural, and psychospiritual natures. My investigative approach throughout this book endeavours to exemplify the latter approach.

1.2 Methodological approaches and processes

Throughout this book I utilise three methodological approaches[4] to facilitate the joint task of drawing on psychospiritual considerations to challenge medical psychiatry while concurrently working to glean a better understanding of psychosis. As mentioned already, my primary approach is heuristic, which Douglass & Moustakas (1985, p. 44) describe as a research modality that operates "free from external methodological structures that limit awareness or channel it". Therefore, as an open-ended and unbounded research medium it enables me to examine a variety of perspectives on psychotic and psychotic-like experiences across the physical-metaphysical spectrum.[5] Accordingly, my endeavour is driven by the research question: Can, and how can, psychosis be better understood by employing a heuristic approach which includes psychospiritual considerations within its investigative ambit?

Second, my overall heuristic initiative is orchestrated through the use of four focal settings that sequentially examine the construal of psychosis within different paradigms of psychospiritual understanding. This is a methodology of my own invention. It enables me provisionally to span the materialist-metaphysical divide and gradually take the reader into deeper domains of psychospiritual investigation and understanding. Focal Setting One provides a historical overview of evolving understandings of psychosis within the tradition of psychiatry, in which psychospiritual matters are generally not considered. Focal Setting Two aims to demonstrate

---

[4] For readers interested in a fuller explication on my heuristic and focal settings approaches, see Appendix Nine.

[5] Further to my heuristic approach, I endorse a *phenomenological approach* in the latter chapters of this book. By this I mean a particular modality of non-reductive and non-prescriptive observation that open-endedly allows any given phenomenon (in this instance, psychosis) to reveal its nature, as free as possible from predetermined ideas and expectations. Owen (1994, p. 261) describes this approach as a "reliable and accurate basis for building an acausal, non-reductionistic and non-reifying philosophical psychology for understanding human nature". To me, 'heuristic' and 'phenomenological' are concomitant aspects of the same investigative approach (i.e. heuristic-phenomenological). In terms of operating together, the former is the open-ended act of 'journeying' while the latter is the open-minded act of 'perceiving'. Together they enable the research of phenomena to go evermore deeper into understanding.

that, although psychiatry has traditionally eschewed psychospiritual considerations, such investigation is possible. Focal Setting Three critically investigates the problem of discerning psychotic from non-psychopathological psychotic-like psychospiritual experiences. Finally, Focal Setting Four argues that, in the absence of deep metaphysical knowledge, it is ultimately impossible to discern culturally normative psychotic-like experiences from psychotic instances.

Third, in Chapter Nine, I conduct a comprehensive critical content analysis of literature wherein commentators have sought to differentiate psychotic from non-psychotic psychospiritual experiences. This undertaking is loosely based on de Menezes Junior & Moreira-Almeida's (2009) meta-analysis which similarly identifies the top nine differentiation criteria identified by authors. However, whereas their study aimed only to formulate a prospective list of differential diagnostic criteria, mine goes a step further to critically appraise and contest the psychopathological validity of each identified criterion. Doing so challenges the assumption that diagnostically categorising signs of psychopathology is an effective model for construing and better understanding psychosis.

As a final heuristic exercise, my investigation of spirit possession serves to demonstrate the considerable degree to which understanding can be advanced through the close examination of any given psychospiritual phenomenon. Choosing this over other psychospiritual phenomena is deliberate because spirit possession is recognised by psychiatry as a culturally normative occurrence. However, whereas psychiatry's understanding of such phenomena, and their possible nature in psychosis, goes little beyond a culturally sensitive nod of diagnostic acknowledgement, my detailed exploration in Chapters Twelve and Thirteen illustrates the validity and potential value of deeper research into cross-cultural and psychospiritual matters. Showing just how much can be learned from a depth examination of psychosis in light of spirit possession acts as a challenge for psychiatry to do likewise with all so-called 'culture-bound' beliefs. That which may appear to be of marginal diagnostic interest from a traditional psychiatric perspective can, if examined more closely, open to vast realms of potential new knowledge and understanding about the nature of reality, psychosis, and the illimitable mysteries of being human.

1.3 Original aspects of my research

Throughout this book I add to the existing literature regarding psychotic and psychotic-like psychospiritual human experiences in various ways. In general, I:

- proffer a challenge to mainstream psychiatry through a psychospiritual lens;
- comprehensively elucidate the psychospiritual-psychosis nexus within a psychiatric context, and within interdisciplinary and cross-cultural views beyond this;
- create a heuristic investigative structure, comprised of four focal settings, which enables the systematic examination of how psychospiritual matters can be considered in better understanding psychosis;

- propose that a heuristic-phenomenological and non-psychopathological investigative approach may lead to better understanding both psychosis and the psychospiritual domain of being human.

More specifically, I:

- provide an in-depth critical appraisal of the third edition of the American Psychiatric Association's *Diagnostic and Statistical Manual of Mental Disorders* (DSM-III)[6] to demonstrate the degree to which social, economic and political factors have shaped this key psychiatric manual and its depictions of psychosis (see Chapter Five, Section 5.3 and Appendix Two);
- elucidate and critically appraise psychiatrist Stanley Dean's unique work on 'ultra-consciousness' and 'metapsychiatry' (see Chapter Six, Section 6.2);
- undertake a detailed examination and critical review of Lukoff and company's research venture, which resulted in a 'Religious or spiritual problem' V-Code category being introduced into the DSM-IV manual (see Chapter Seven, Section 7.1);
- conduct a comprehensive content analysis and critical review of literature on discerning psychospiritual from psychotic experiences. However, contrary to standard practice whereby researchers strive to formulate a list of differential diagnostic criteria, I analyse and challenge the differentiation validity of each criterion (see Chapter Nine);
- propose and demonstrate that psychospiritual and psychotic experiences are ultimately indistinguishable (see Focal Setting Four);
- demonstrate how psychospiritual investigation can work to gain a deeper understanding of psychosis by undertaking an in-depth investigation of spirits and spirit possession within various cultural and conceptual frameworks (see Chapter Twelve, Section 12.4; Chapter Thirteen; and Appendices Seven and Eight).

Combined, these endeavours constitute a significant contribution to the psychosis-psychospiritual field of study, set the stage for further such research, and challenge psychiatry to participate in this. While the multidimensional and multidisciplinary breadth of this undertaking is valuable in having elicited a comprehensive body of views about psychosis for appraisal, this book ideally could have included more first-person input from people about their views and experiences of psychosis, psychiatry, and psychospiritual realities. I did consider the potential merit of conducting such research, but decided it was apposite to first undertake the formidable task of spanning the materialist-metaphysical divide in my critical investigation of psychosis and psychiatric practices. Having done so sets the epistemological ground from which further investigation in a first-person experiential context can be undertaken.

---

[6] The acronym 'DSM' refers to the *Diagnostic and Statistical Manual of Mental Disorders*. DSM-III is the third manual in this series.

CHAPTER 2

Scoping the psychospiritual
challenge to psychiatry

2.0 Introduction

This chapter sets the stage for my systematic investigation of psychosis. Here, I define and explain my reasons for adopting the key notion of 'psychospiritual' and then scope my challenge by elucidating how psychiatry's materialist and psychopathological approaches inherently limit a better understanding of psychosis.

2.1 Explaining the psychospiritual domain

Throughout this book the term 'psychospiritual' is used synonymously with other terms such as 'spiritual', 'metaphysical', 'transpersonal', and 'mystical'. This is because such terms are difficult to define separately, as their domains of meaning overlap. Hence, for the purpose of simplification, I use these terms interchangeably to connote, and encompass, a vast spectrum of phenomena, experiences, and states of consciousness or being, that exist beyond the normal limits of human cognitive and sensory capacity. This spectrum ranges from the more common human experiences of dreaming, intuition, and myth-making, through the various modes of extrasensory perception, to the myriad aspects and experiences of a more classically spiritual nature. Accordingly, this includes phenomena, experiences, and states of consciousness that are generally beyond the ken of Western knowledge systems, yet are known and named by other cultures. Generically, these constitute what I refer to as 'the psychospiritual domain'.[7]

---

[7] Appendix One proffers a historical overview of uses of the term 'psychospiritual' from its inception to present date. This illustrates the historical significance and substance of the term and gives weight to the definition provided in this section and to my use of it throughout this book.

Importantly, I also use the term 'psychospiritual' because it intrinsically characterises the idea that a synthesis exists between the psychological and spiritual self. In this context, it connotes the psychological and spiritual nexus of human life, where it is impossible to identify the end of 'psychological' and the beginning of 'spiritual'. It is understood here that both are intrinsically merged domains of human consciousness. This reflects Gleig's (2010, p. 738) explanation that "the term psychospiritual has entered psychological and religious discourse as a loose designation for the integration of the psychological and the spiritual", and Wilber's (1975, p. 113) view that states of human consciousness "infinitely shade into one another". From this perspective, it is impossible to identify a discrete border between the end of 'psychological' and the beginning of 'spiritual' because the two interpenetrate.

2.2 Psychospiritual as psychopathological

Within the history of mainstream psychiatry, psychospiritual considerations have largely been ignored and psychospiritual experiences have often been construed as evidencing psychopathology. The psychiatric literature clearly demonstrates the discipline's discomfort with, or antipathy towards, matters pertaining to psychospiritual phenomena and knowledge. This is particularly evident in instances whereby psychiatrists have depicted psychospiritual experiences as intrinsically psychopathological and/or psychotic.

A marked example of such depiction occurred in the early twentieth century when "the historical Jesus was subjected to post mortem psychiatric examination" (Peavy, 1974, p. 154, fn. 14). This 'post mortem' was conducted in books published by three psychiatrists: one German (George de Loosten (1905), *Jesus Christus von Standpunkte des Psychiaters (Jesus Christ from the Standpoint of the Psychiatrist)*); one French (Charles Binet-Sanglé (1910–1915), *La Folie de Jésus (The Dementia of Jesus)*); and one American (William Hirsch (1912), *Religion and Civilization: The Conclusions of a Psychiatrist)*.

First, De Loosten's view concerning the insanity of Jesus was unequivocal. For instance, he interpreted Jesus' seemingly atypical behaviour as indicative of a "fixed delusional system" (de Loosten in Havis, 2001), spoke of the "pathological elements in his nature", and concluded that "Jesus was regarded by many of his contemporaries as actually insane and that from this fact certain conclusions can be drawn regarding the personal impressions made by him" (de Loosten in Bundy, 1922, pp. 75, 78). Binet-Sanglé also used psychiatric terminology to describe Jesus' behaviour. For example, he identified him as a sick individual who suffered hallucinations and "religious paranoia" (Binet-Sanglé in Havis, 2001). He also described him as a fanatic who made declarations which were "identically that of the megalomaniacs in our present day asylums", and as a "psychic degenerate" who exhibited a "purely pathological process" that ultimately delivered him "into the ranks of the incurables" (Binet-Sanglé in Bundy, 2001, pp. 106, 92, 94, 97). After five years of research and deliberation he concluded in the fourth and final edition of his study that, "I believe that I can say for the alienists, medical men, for all learned and sincere persons, the insanity of the founder of the Christian religion is a demonstrated truth" (ibid., p. 107). Finally, Hirsch (1912, p. 99) invested his views about Jesus with putative empirical validity by asserting "all his manifestations can be explained entirely satisfactorily by purely scientific facts". According to his evaluation, "Christ belongs to those cases of paranoia in which the patients are quiet and self-engrossed during their youth" (ibid., p. 103). In sum, he deduced that "such a course of the disease, a transition from the latent to the active state of paranoia, is altogether characteristic of this psychosis" (p. 106). All three men, therefore, adopted and transposed the tenets of scientific materialism to make a psychiatric assessment of Jesus' sanity, whereby the consideration of valid cultural and psychospiritual matters were eclipsed. Here, psychospiritual is seemingly analogous to psychopathological.

Unsurprisingly, some commentators have challenged the veracity of the controversial assessments made by De Loosen, Binet-Sanglé, and Hirsch. For instance, the German physician Albert Schweitzer (1948 (1913)) conducted an appraisal of these three works in his medical dissertation titled *The Psychiatric Study of Jesus*. He concluded that, although Jesus' experiences and behaviours personified an extreme expression of the religious and cultural beliefs of Judaism at the time, "the exaggeration of an idea does not in itself justify our considering it the manifestation of a psychosis" (ibid., pp. 63–64). In closing, and in light of psychiatric theory at the time, he determined that the findings of De Loosen, Binet-Sanglé, and Hirsch were, by-and-large, a mix of "false preconceptions" and "entirely hypothetical symptoms" (p. 72). In his view, then, they were more the product of subjective bias and confabulation than of objective medical science. A later assessment by psychiatrist Walter Bundy (1922, p. 268) likewise concluded that De Loosen, Binet-Sanglé, and Hirsch had failed to consider cultural dynamics in their assessments and that their works constituted "an amateur application of the principles of the science of psychiatry". Also, Jung (1966, p. 45) described these psychiatrists as exemplifying "how irresponsibly a psychologizing doctor can falsify his subject through narrow, pseudo-scientific prejudice". These commentators clearly question the veracity of using materialist thinking to guide diagnostic practice and repudiate the consequent depiction of psychospiritual experiences as being intrinsically psychopathological.

Far from being extreme examples, it appears that the views of De Loosen, Binet-Sanglé, and Hirsch represent a general bias within mainstream psychiatry against recognising the legitimacy of psychospiritual realities. Since the inception of psychiatry as a discipline, personal reports of psychospiritual experiences have commonly been viewed by clinicians as possible, or definite, signifiers of psychosis and psychopathology. For instance, Harrowes (1929, p. 17) held that any "mystic" interests of a patient are "an example of imperfect reality contacts", Alexander (1931, p. 130) claimed that Buddhist spiritual practices were a "training in catatonia" and "a sort of artificial schizophrenia", and Devereux (1956, p. 29) maintained that, despite the cultural acceptance of shamanic beliefs and practices, they were essentially psychopathological ("ego dystonic"). More recently, in their clinical analysis of some key religious figures, Murray et al. (2012, p. 410) concluded that "Abraham, Moses, Jesus, and St. Paul … had experiences that resemble those now defined as psychotic symptoms, suggesting that their experiences may have been manifestations of primary or mood disorder-associated psychotic disorders". Such clinicians plainly equate psychospiritual experiences with psychopathology.

The main task here has been to demonstrate the existence of an inclination within traditional psychiatry to view mystical or paranormal experiences as forms of psychopathology. Although psychiatric diagnostics over the past two decades have seen a growing trend toward the inclusion of cultural matters, and a tentative acceptance of religious and psychospiritual concerns, there still remains a general disinclination by clinicians to consider the veracity of reported psychospiritual experiences. Rather, personal reports of psychospiritual experiences by patients are routinely viewed as signifiers of psychosis and psychopathology. This view seems unlikely to change in the near future, for the predominant focus in contemporary medical psychiatry is to discover the biological cause of psychosis; a venture strongly influenced by pharmaceutical companies who have considerable vested interests in the biological treatments of psychosis (Frances, 2013a, pp. 89–97). Yet, while the core psychiatric notion of psychopathology is accepted as fact, its precise nature remains undefined.[8] Frances (ibid., p. 117) consequently acknowledges that "in evaluating any given person, we lack a general definition of mental disorder to help us decide whether he is normal or a patient". This ambiguity of definition arguably creates the conceptual space for questioning whether various psychotic-like experiences are psychopathological or psychospiritual in nature.

2.3 Challenging the medical psychiatry and materialism nexus

The quest of science is fundamentally one of investigating and better understanding the nature of reality. Ideally, this is an open-ended process of interplay between observation, theory, and knowledge formulation, in relation to the multifarious objective and subjective phenomena that constitute reality. However, many commentators maintain that the materialist view of science is outdated and represents a poor grasp of the nature of reality, in that it operates by a set of reductive theoretical assumptions which limit the scope of investigation to physical reality only, thus ignoring other domains of investigation that may advance understanding about the nature of life and human experience. This is particularly so in the field of quantum physics where theorists have long questioned the universal application of materialism's key tenets (Beauregard, 2012, p. 228). For instance, Jeans (1984, p. 44) proffers the broad view that "every conclusion that has been tentatively put forward [by materialist science], is quite frankly speculative and uncertain". In the context of understanding human

---

[8] As discussed in Chapter Five and Appendix Two, psychiatrists have unsuccessfully wrestled with the core task of defining mental illness since the formulation of DSM-III.

nature, Peierls (2000, p. 75) argues that "the premise that you can describe in terms of physics the whole function of a human being … including its knowledge, and its consciousness, is untenable". Indeed, Laszlo (2003, p. 1) envisions an emergent scientific paradigm shift whereby conventional mechanistic science will be superseded by integral quantum science. Whereas the former views reality as atomistic, the latter proposes "an integrated unified vision of living and non-living systems" that will "give us the coherent universe, where all things are intrinsically connected" (ibid., pp. 20, 101). Furthermore, from the field of neuroscience, Beauregard (2012, p. 6) takes a more radical stance in expressing his "vehemently" held view that "*the materialist framework is not science*" because it operates according to a set of "*beliefs without proof*" (italics in original).[9] He envisions an "expanded model of reality" whereby "scientists, free of the materialist box, are … invited to embark on research into the whole gamut of psi phenomena, expanded and altered consciousness, and spiritual experiences" (ibid., pp. 212–214). These are but a few of many examples whereby scientists have challenged the veracity of strict scientific materialism.

Similar views have been proffered from within the mental health field. For instance, Boyle (2002, p. 316) refers to the materialist scientific approach as "squeezing data into existing belief systems rather than changing theory in line with data". In the context of understanding psychosis, she further maintains that scientific materialism shows "a striking lack of a reflective approach to the production of knowledge about psychotic behaviour and experience" (ibid.). Likewise, in his early psychiatric career, Jung (1960) maintained that a better understanding of the psyche, mental disorders, and particularly psychoses, required extending the scope of conventional scientific investigation to include the immediacy and depths of subjective experience. In fact, the term 'scientistic' has been coined "in ironic contrast to 'scientific'" (Gallagher et al., 2002, p. 701), to denote the traditional reductive approach to scientific inquiry whereby the scope of investigation is limited to exclude, or dismiss, phenomena that apparently exist beyond the epistemic bounds of strict materialism. Maritain (1964, p. 264) defines 'scientistic' simply as "secularized positivism", while Phillips (2009, p. 175) proffers the more pejorative explanation that "the term 'scientistic' evolved to cover cases where there was exaggerated respect for, and a narrow and illiberal account of, the 'scientific method'". Regarding the impact of 'scientistic' thinking in psychiatry, Szasz (1991, p. 6) argues that "like all ideologies, the ideology of insanity—communicated through the scientistic jargon of psychiatric 'diagnoses', 'prognoses', and 'treatments' … finds its characteristic expression in what it opposes: commitment to an officially forbidden image or definition of 'reality'". This goes to the heart of the issue of understanding psychosis, for materialist assumptions not only determine what reality *is*, but also what reality *is not*, and therefore, which phenomena are, and are not, worthy of serious clinical investigation. Extending this into psychiatric practice

---

[9] Henceforth, text quoted in italics appears as such in the original. In instances where I add italics to quotes for emphasis, I include the notation '(italics added)'.

results in the occlusion of subjective and psychospiritual experience from the process of trying to understand psychosis.

It is therefore apparent that much of the understanding, or misunderstanding, of psychosis stems directly from the transferral of limited materialist assumptions into medical science, and subsequently, into medical psychiatry. These assumptions are used to dictate what is real, and thus normal, and what is unreal, and thus deviant, and to then assert a clinical boundary that separates normality from mental illness. This is evident below in Table 1, which lists the foremost "axiomatic assumptions" of materialism (Kimura, 2008, p. 11) alongside the neo-Kraepelinian credo which, according to Klerman (1978, p. 104), consists of nine tenets that guided "psychiatry towards greater integration with medicine" during the formation of DSM-III.[10] As shown below, the latter are clearly reflective of the former.

In cross-referencing these two lists it is apparent that materialist theory has fundamentally shaped the worldview and practice of medical psychiatry. For instance, in the neo-Kraepelinian credo, psychiatry is unequivocally identified as a branch of medicine that exemplifies scientific methodologies and knowledge. Hence, the materialist presumption that physical reality is the only 'real' reality is reflected in the assertion that psychiatry's predominant focus should be on 'the biological aspects of illness'. The related materialist idea that consciousness is epiphenomenal to the brain is a root idea governing the theory, research, and practice of medical psychiatry. This generally results in psychiatry disregarding subjective reality. As Beauregard (2012, pp. 211–212) claims, materialist theory compels scientific investigators "to neglect the subjective dimension of human experience and downplay the importance of mind and consciousness. In so doing, they create a severely distorted and impoverished understanding of human beings and reality". Hence, understanding has become impoverished to the point that any altered state of consciousness is viewed as psychopathologically suspect. Furthermore, the materialist theory of an atomistic reality composed of discrete physical entities is reflected in psychiatry's notion that a boundary exists between normal and pathological, and also fuels its penchant for the categorisation of distinct diagnostic criteria.

The above critical appraisal of the conceptual and investigative limitations of a psychiatric model based on the tenets of medical materialism sets the stage for my ensuing psychospiritual challenge to medical psychiatry. This challenge unfolds by systematically demonstrating, via an engagement with psychospiritual considerations, that it is not only possible to comprehend reality beyond the epistemological parameters of materialism, but it is preferable, if not necessary, for psychiatry to do so in order to better understand psychosis.

---

[10] The term 'neo-Kraepelinian' refers to a group of American biomedical psychiatrists who, during the 1960s and 1970s, played a key role in changing the DSM from a psychoanalytic model to a medical model. DSM refers to the American Psychiatric Association's *Diagnostic and Statistical Manual of Mental Disorders*. Both the neo-Kraepelinian phenomenon and the evolving editions of the DSM manuals are further examined in Chapter Five and a critical analysis of DSM-III is provided in Appendix Two.

Table 1. A comparison of key materialist assumptions with key tenets of medical psychiatry.

Key materialist assumptions (Kimura, 2008, p. 11)	Key tenets of medical psychiatry (Klerman, 1978, pp. 104–105)
1. Physical reality as such is reality; there is no reality other than physical reality. 2. No phenomenon is a phenomenon in reality, unless it is observed, or in theory observable, through the senses and its mechanical extensions (such as telescopes). 3. Reality exists independent of consciousness. 4. Reality exists in objective (i.e. objectively measurable) space-time. 5. Reality consists of fundamental (or subatomic) particles in motion in space. 6. Reality in its base-state is a non-living and non-conscious (or unconscious) process. 7. Life emerged from and through non-living processes not by necessity but by chance. 8. Consciousness is an epiphenomenon of the unconscious brain activities and processes. 9. The scientific method is the only valid method for achieving objective knowledge. 10. All valid scientific knowledge is reducible to mathematical equations or other logical formulations such that the sequential train of inferences therefrom shall at some stage suggest an empirically possible experiment or observation that can verify or falsify the inference. 11. Objective scientific knowledge thus achieved is the only valid knowledge of reality.	1. Psychiatry is a branch of medicine. 2. Psychiatry should utilize modern scientific methodologies and base its practice on scientific knowledge. 3. Psychiatry treats people who are sick and who require treatment for mental illnesses. 4. There is a boundary between the normal and the sick. 5. There are discrete mental illnesses. Mental illnesses are not myths. There is not one but many mental illnesses. It is the task of scientific psychiatry, as of other medical specialities to investigate the causes, diagnosis, and treatment of these mental illnesses. 6. The focus of psychiatric physicians should be particularly on the biological aspects of illness. 7. There should be an explicit and intentional concern with diagnosis and classification. 8. Diagnostic criteria should be codified, and a legitimate and valued area of research should be to validate such criteria by various techniques. Further, departments of psychiatry in medical schools should teach these criteria and not depreciate them, as has been the case for many years. 9. In research efforts directed at improving reliability and validity of diagnosis and classification, statistical techniques should be utilized.

2.4 Challenging the assumed incomprehensibility of psychosis

A fundamental notion in the psychiatric construal of psychosis is that it is, by nature, an enigmatic phenomenon that is ultimately impervious to comprehension. This idea stems from the work of German psychiatrist Karl Jaspers (1997 v2, p. 577), who maintained that psychotic experience is essentially "ununderstandable".[11] Indeed, many commentators have identified incomprehensibility as a defining feature of psychotic disorders. For instance, Henriksen (2013, p. 106) contends that "incomprehensibility is considered the hallmark of schizophrenia", while Heinimaa (2008, p. 26) holds that, from a Jaspersian perspective, "incomprehensibility was conceived of as constitutive" of psychotic disorders, and that, subsequently, "the field of psychoses came to be structured primarily in terms of the degree to which they appeared as 'ununderstandable'". Hence, in the context of psychiatric practice, the notion of incomprehensibility essentially acts to discern non-psychotic from psychotic disorders.

In drawing on psychospiritual considerations to glean a better understanding of psychosis, this book intrinsically challenges the psychiatric assumption that psychotic experiences are unfathomable. This idea represents a key obstacle in the quest to better understand psychosis, for if something cannot be understood, then why attempt to understand it? However, delineating that which is comprehensible from that which is not, is relative to the observer's axiomatic assumptions. For instance, in operating by the materialist assumption that reality is primarily physical and that psychic life (including psychosis) is an epiphenomenal reality, it is logical for psychiatry to assume that the form and content of psychotic experience is ultimately impervious to comprehension. From this perspective, the definitive truth as to the cause of psychosis can only be explained in biological terms, with psychosocial and psychospiritual considerations being of secondary or no importance. This book's heuristic approach of examining psychosis within various psychospiritual contexts, works to challenge the notion that psychosis is incomprehensible. As the investigative process unfolds from one focal setting to the next, it systematically demonstrates that examining psychosis and psychotic symptomatology through the lens of psychospiritual considerations opens to vistas of understanding that are invisible and seemingly impossible from a materialist perspective.

2.5 Challenging the assumed psychopathology of psychosis

For psychiatry, psychosis is synonymous with psychopathology. Therefore, psychiatric research into psychosis is driven by the unquestionable assumption that psychotic experiences are intrinsically psychopathological. I critically examine and challenge this basic psychiatric assumption because it plays a primary role in delimiting the investigative scope for better understanding psychosis.

---

[11] An examination of Jaspers' views concerning the incomprehensibility of psychosis is undertaken in Chapter Four, Section 4.3.2.

The parameters of psychiatric practice are essentially defined by the presence of psychopathology, for it is a discipline concerned with diagnosing and remediating apparent pathological mental states and behaviours. This was clearly asserted ninety years ago by the German psychiatrist, Friedrich Moerchen, who held that "psychopathology asks but one question, normal or abnormal? Healthy or morbid?" (Moerchen in Bundy, 1922, p. xiii).[12] Similarly, Boisen (1936, p. 308) defined psychopathology as "the basic science upon which the practice of psychiatry is founded". More recently, Hamilton (1985, p. 2) notes that "psychiatry is concerned with pathological human psychology", and Andreasen (1997a, p. 592) explains that "psychiatry is the medical specialty that studies and treats a variety of disorders that affect the mind—mental illnesses". Verhagen et al. (2010, p. 209) make the generic assertion that "all psychiatrists would probably agree" that psychopathology is the "core business of psychiatry". Therefore, the perceived need for psychiatric intervention is evidently proportionate to the perceived degree of psychopathology.

Also, the jurisdiction of psychiatry terminates at the ostensible dividing line between psychopathology and normalcy. This is clearly suggested in the above neo-Kraepelinian tenets that 'there is a boundary between the normal and the sick' and that 'psychiatry treats people who are sick' with mental illnesses. Burang (1974, p. 107) sagely notes, however, that despite the pragmatic necessity of proposing provisional lines of differentiation between normal and abnormal, doing so can result in "a certain amount of arrogance" when done prescriptively. Furthermore, repeated attempts by psychiatrists to definitively identify and describe this boundary have been unsuccessful. Addressing this issue in his recent book, *Saving Normal*, psychiatrist Allen Frances (2013a, pp. 9, 82) holds that "many have tried and all have failed" to delineate mental health from mental illness, and that "the boundary between mental disorder and normality is so fuzzy that whenever we quickly expand the use of psychiatric labels to identify some few people who do need help, we misidentify many others who don't". Hence, establishing diagnostic lines of differentiation can be very fuzzy and problematic and this ambiguity is amplified when factoring in psychospiritual considerations. The problem of misidentification and the associated question as to what does, and does not, define psychopathology, is highly pertinent to diagnosing psychosis, especially in terms of differentiating it from non-pathological psychospiritual experiences.

While this psychopathology-seeking approach is evidently limiting, and the need for a more open-ended approach is called for, it is important to note that revealing the highly tenuous nature of the notion of psychopathology in psychiatric practice is *not* to suggest that psychic debilitation does not exist. It is apparent from the havoc and suffering often experienced by people in psychosis that something is distressingly awry. Therefore, the aim of my ensuing investigation is to show that pathways to better understanding psychosis can be opened when psychospiritual factors are seen as potentially informative, rather than routinely being ignored or pathologised. It is my contention that a heuristic approach enables such deepened and diversified

---

[12] Moerchen, F. (1908). *Die psychologie der heiligkeit: Eine religionswissenschaftliche studie.* C. Marhold.

understanding. Whereas the psychopathology-seeking approach used by psychiatry looks at psychosis through the predetermined belief that it is a 'mental disorder', the heuristic approach is comparatively neutral and, therefore, aims to let the phenomenon of psychosis reveal its meanings, rather than projecting preconceived meanings onto it. This enables open scope to see hidden potentialities and nuances of meaning that are invisible and, indeed, unthinkable, within the limited investigative scope of psychiatric medical materialism. Through this prism of heuristic investigation, it is shown that the notion of 'psychosis as intrinsically psychopathological' is not concrete, but rather, is highly mutable and open to interpretation. Indeed, it questions whether the notion of psychopathology hinders more than helps in understanding the nature of psychosis. The challenge and investigation throughout the ensuing focal settings of this book systematically demonstrate the potential and untapped value of drawing on psychospiritual considerations to better understand psychosis beyond the limited purview of psychiatric medical materialism and its axiomatic assumptions about psychopathology.

2.6 Conclusion

Having defined the term 'psychospiritual' and explicated the aim and scope of my challenge to medical psychiatry, the stage has been set for critically examining the psychosis-psychospiritual nexus within context of four focal settings. From this point forward, I systematically argue that the inclusion of psychospiritual considerations in psychiatric epistemology and research will enable a better understanding of psychosis than the traditional reductive materialist-based psychopathological approaches. Focal Setting One provides a historical and critical overview of psychiatric conceptualisations of psychosis which are nearly devoid of psychospiritual considerations. My attention to psychospiritual matters is then progressively developed throughout Focal Settings Two to Four.

FOCAL SETTING ONE

UNDERSTANDING PSYCHOSIS: THE PSYCHIATRIC VIEW

Focal Setting One provides a historical overview of evolving understandings of psychosis within the tradition of psychiatry, in which psychospiritual matters are generally not considered.

CHAPTER 3

Understanding psychosis: etymological and clinical origins

3.0 Introduction

This chapter formally begins my investigative process by examining three initial meanings attributed to the term 'psychosis': one, its psychospiritual etymological roots; two, its mid-nineteenth century clinical origins as a psychosomatic form of psychopathology; and three, the first vestiges of a biogenic depiction of psychosis during the latter nineteenth century. My aim here is to demonstrate the term's original conceptual plasticity and to identify the emergence of psychiatry's prescriptive and biogenic understanding of psychosis.

3.1 The etymology of psychosis

The word 'psychosis' derives from the root word 'psyche' and is, therefore, etymologically invested with an essential psychospiritual meaning. As Ayto (1994, p. 418) explains, the Greek *psūkhḗ*, which "started out meaning 'breath' and developed semantically to 'soul, spirit'", was later transcribed into the Latin *psȳchē*, and then adopted into English as *psyche*. Further to this, Barnhart (1988, p. 859) maintains that the term 'psychosis' is a combination of the Greek *psūkhḗ* (soul, mind) and the New Latin *–osis* (abnormal condition). Thus, from an etymological perspective, 'psychosis' essentially appears to denote an abnormal condition of the soul or mind. Andreasen (2005) accordingly notes that "literally, a psychiatrist is a healer of the spirit, not of the mind or brain". However, it appears mainstream psychiatry has eschewed its etymologically psychospiritual roots to adopt a biomedical understanding of psychosis.

As a pertinent aside, the Greek *psūkhḗ* is also directly connected to the word *psŷkhros* which represents the quality of coolness. As Onions (1966, p. 720) explains, a relationship exists between the Greek *psūkhḗ* (breath, soul, life), *psūkhein* (breathe, blow, cool), and *psŷkhros* (cool). It is, therefore, possible that the medical term 'psychosis' initially emerged in the 1830s as a derivative of *psŷkhros*.[13]

3.2 The clinical emergence of the word 'psychosis'

The term 'psychosis' first emerged from the crucible of mid-nineteenth century German Romantic medicine and psychiatry. Coining a new psychiatric word is a gesture that intimates the cause and meaning of a particular psychic anomaly, and works as a symbolic vehicle for breaking new ground in epistemological development. As Petitmengin & Bitbol (2009, p. 389) contend, the formation of new vocabulary "enables us to progressively refine our consciousness of this experience". What, then, did the original coining of the word 'psychosis' aim to communicate about the cause and meaning of mental disturbances?

3.2.1 Gottfried Eisenmann (1835)

As a medical term, the word 'psychosis' first appeared during the 1840s within the field of German medicine. However, just prior to this, a close approximation of it was used by the German physician Gottfried Eisenmann who, in his book *Die vegetativen Krankheiten und die entgiftende Heilmethode* (1835), coined the term 'psychrosen' to depict a specific form of neurosis. Emulating the system of scientific classification in botany, he proposed that, within the overall kingdom of diseases, 'psychrosen' was one of four orders of illness under the class 'neurosis'; namely, the order of "the mental diseases" (López Piñero, 1983, p. 40). Beer (1995a, p. 177) maintains that Eisenmann "used the word 'psychroses' in the same sense that psychoses was later to be used".[14] However, the word 'psychosis' has been used in many senses since it was first coined and Beer does not specify which of these he means. This aside, it appears that Eisenmann adopted the term 'psychrosen' from the etymological root word *psŷkhros*.

3.2.2 Carl Canstatt (1841)

The apparent first use of the word 'psychosis' was in 1841 by the German physician Carl Canstatt (Bürgy, 2008, p. 1200).[15] Six years after Eisenmann's coining of 'psychrosen', Canstatt used the words "psychosis" and "psychotic neurosis" interchangeably to

---

[13] The pertinence of this is clarified below in Section 3.2.1 in my examination of Eisenmann's clinical use of the term 'psychrose'.

[14] Beer cites the following article as his source regarding Eisenmann and psychrosis: Mechler A. (1965). Über den begriff der psychose. *Jahrbuch der Psychologie und Psychotherapie, XII*, 67–74. It is unclear why Beer uses the term 'psychroses' instead of Eisenmann's 'psychrosen'.

[15] Bürgy cites the text in which the term was used as: Canstatt, C. (1841). *Handbuch der medizinischen klinik.* Enke. I have been unable to source a copy of this book to ascertain the extent to which Canstatt used

designate "psychic manifestations of a disease of the brain", in contradistinction to other neurological disorders that were seen as "diseases of the nervous system" (Schultze-Lutter et al., 2008, p. 304). As Bürgy (2008, p. 1201) explains, for Canstatt "psychosis emphasized the psychic manifestation of an organically based neurosis". In other words, psychosis referred to a particular form of neurosis (i.e. a brain-centred neurosis) that expressed itself psychically rather than physiologically.

However, the nature and composition of the 'psychic' self remains unexplained by Canstatt. Indeed, he attests to its aetiological obscurity in acknowledging that "often causal indication lies beyond the scope of the doctor, and nothing else remains than direct combat of the psychosis" (Canstatt in Schultze-Lutter et al., 2008, p. 304).[16] According to Bürgy (2008, p. 1202), this inability to understand and empirically grasp the intangible nature of the human psyche led materialist psychiatrists to assert a physical aetiology of psychosis. From these roots stemmed the medical approach to understanding and treating psychosis that later prevailed throughout psychiatry's history.

3.2.3 Ernst von Feuchtersleben (1845)

The Austrian physician Ernst von Feuchtersleben is thought by many to have coined the word 'psychosis' in 1845,[17] though, as is evident above, it seems Canstatt, or even Eisenmann, did so before him. This aside, Feuchtersleben was the first person to use the term extensively and did so in his book *Lehrbuch der ärztlichen Seelenkunde* (1845), which was translated into English in 1847 as *The Principles of Medical Psychology*. Here, he used 'psychosis' synonymously with 'psychopathy', but offered no explanation or rationale for coining this new terminology (Beer, 1995a, p. 177). It is possible, however, that he borrowed it from Canstatt who is cited several times in his book.

Whereas the respective descriptions of psychosis by Canstatt and Eisenmann seem aetiologically obscure, Feuchtersleben was unambiguous in his view that the aetiology of psychosis was both psychic and physical. At the time, a longstanding dispute as to the cause of mental illness was still in progress between somatists and mentalists (Beer, 1995a, p. 178). In Feuchtersleben's (1847, p. 68) view, the former "assumes the operations of the mind to be an emanation from those of the body, and considers mental disorders to be merely bodily ailments", while the latter "assumes an independent operation of the mind, and considers its disorders as purely psychical derangements". Hence, somatists believed that mental illness was the result of a physical aberration, while mentalists believed that mental illness was the result of a psychical aberration. Although Feuchtersleben subscribed to the mentalist belief regarding the mind's independent nature, he also endorsed

---

the terms 'psychosis' or 'psychoses' ('psychose' and 'psychosen' in German), and Bürgy provides no examples.

[16] Canstatt, C. (1843). *Handbuch der medicinischen Klinik: Die specielle pathologie und therapie.* Ekne.

[17] For instance, see Middleton et al., 2008, p. 14; Berrios, 2008, p. 362; Laplanche & Pontalis, 1980, p. 372; Bowman & Rose, 1951, p.162.

a "mixed" view that "sees in its derangements a half psychical, half corporeal disease" (ibid.). This thinking was based on his observation that medical science had erroneously rejected the independent psychic reality of human nature in favour of an overly somatic fixation:

> If we consider the science of medicine in general, and especially its present state, there is perhaps nothing so essential to its advancement as psychology, carefully adapted to medical purposes ... In the study of medicine, the psychical element is almost obscured by the abundance and prominence of the somatic portion, and its claims to attention are more imperatively felt, when we come to the study of psychiatrics proper—the doctrine of the diseases of the mind (p. 7).

It is apparent here that Feuchtersleben viewed psychiatric research and practice as an ideally psychosomatic venture.

Within this framework of psychosomatic belief, Feuchtersleben engaged in a comprehensive analysis of what he called 'psychosis' (*Psychose*) or 'psychoses' (*Psychosen*). For example, he discussed psychosis/psychoses in terms of pathology, pathogeny, phrenology, phenomenology, co-morbidity, natural history, cause, course, duration, prognosis, forms, signs, symptoms, treatments, cures, and so on. As such, even though he may not have coined the term, it is evident that he was the first person to flesh it out thoroughly. Broadly speaking, he employed the word 'psychosis' (or psychopathy) to generically indicate "mental disorders" or "diseases of the personality":

> Psychopathies ... or diseases of the personality (insanity in the more comprehensive sense), is the name we give to those compound conditions, in which the psychophysical reciprocal relation is diseased in several directions, so that the empirical personality of the individual appears therefore to be disturbed—disordered (Feuchtersleben, 1847, p. 244).

It is evident from this description that, in Feuchtersleben's view, psychoses are the result of a "reciprocal etiology between body and mind" (ibid., p. 261) culminating in a series of imbalances within the 'psychophysical reciprocal relation'. His malleable approach of giving equal weight to both sides of the somatic and mentalist dispute, and investing the new notion of psychosis with a synthetic aetiological character, arguably enabled the prospective marriage of both psychological and physiological research. Subsequently, the scope for psychiatric investigation was extended from a singular to a threefold potential. That is, it was extended from a purely physiological focus, to the combination of:

1. a physiological focus;
2. a psychological focus; and
3. a dialectical focus that brings both worldviews together.

However, this opportunity for gleaning a broader psychosomatic understanding of psychosis was short-lived because it was soon superseded by the development of a materialist and biological model of psychiatry.

3.3 Feuchtersleben to Kraepelin: 1840s to 1890s

After Feuchtersleben's prolific use of the term 'psychosis' in his 1845 treatise, it was employed by few writers until adopted fourteen years later by the psychiatrist Carl Flemming, at a time when materialist thinking began to supersede the last vestiges of German Romantic psychiatry (Beer, 1995a, p. 182). Originally, in his book *The Pathology and Treatment of Psychoses* (1859), Flemming used the term "psychoses" analogously with "mental disorders" (Beer, 1996a, p. 275). According to Bürgy (2008, p. 1206), however, his use of the term specifically inferred "both mental disorders with identifiable organic findings and disorders of the soul which were assumed to have an organic cause". Hence, although maintaining its prior generic connotation, this constituted a transitional step into "the strong tide of organicity" (Beer, 1995b, p. 317) and away from Feuchtersleben's portrayal of a psychosomatically-based disease of the personality. Flemming's use of 'psychoses' as a term depicting somatically-based disorders was largely maintained by mainstream German psychiatry until the 1890s, when a further marked transition in the conceptualisation of psychoses occurred.

The 1890s was an era when psychosis became less a nebulous generic idiom and more a reference to discrete forms of psychiatric disorder within nosological classification systems. According to Beer (1996a, p. 275), it was during this decade that the term was "'hijacked' by materialistically minded psychiatrists". For example, in 1891 the German psychiatrist Julius Koch fashioned a "psychiatric-nosological system" that made a clear classificatory distinction between "psychopathic inferiorities" and psychoses, whereby the former consisted of "all abnormalities ... which influence a human's personal life, but which do not constitute ... mental illnesses" (Koch in Gutmann, 2008, p. 210),[18] while the latter referred to three forms of insanity, namely "idiopathic, constitutional, and organic psychoses" (ibid., p. 209). Similarly, the neurologist and psychiatrist Carl Wernicke proposed a multi-tiered classificatory system for psychoses in his lecture titled *On the Classification of Psychoses* (1899), whereby the three broad groups of somatopsychoses, autopsychoses, and allopsychoses could be further divided into twelve sub-categories of psychosis (Beer, 1995a, pp. 187–188). The nosological systems created by psychiatrists such as Koch and Wernicke established a new way of conceptualising psychosis, shifting from a generic to a reductionist use of the term.

Hence, throughout this fifty-year period, an epistemological transition transpired. First, Feuchtersleben's generic notion of *psychosomatic* psychoses was stripped of its psychological aetiology by Flemming to become a generic notion of *somatic* psychoses, and then transformed again by psychiatrists like Koch and Wernicke into discrete

---

[18] Koch, J. (1891). *Die psychopathischen minderwertigkeiten*. Maier, p. 1.

forms of somatically-based psychotic disorders. Arguably, this marked a gradual transition into a medical-based classificatory model that was further consolidated by the binary psychoses model proposed by the prominent psychiatrist Emile Kraepelin (see Chapter Four); a model which has prevailed in mainstream psychiatry ever since.

3.4 Conclusion

The term 'psychosis' has a psychospiritual etymology; however, this meaning was not reflected in any of its initial nineteenth-century psychiatry iterations (nor has it been since). While Feuchtersleben's 1845 construal of psychosis as a psychosomatic mental disorder enabled the conceptual flexibility to consider its psychological determinants, over the ensuing fifty years it was progressively perceived in biogenic terms. As evidenced in Chapter Four, this trajectory of biogenic understanding was further consolidated by key psychiatric commentators from 1890–1950.

CHAPTER 4

Understanding psychosis: key psychiatric influences: Kraepelin to Schneider

4.0 Introduction

This chapter describes and critically appraises the work of four key psychiatrists who have fundamentally influenced modern psychiatry's construal of psychosis. These are: Kraepelin's binary model of psychosis; Bleuler's coining of the term 'schizophrenia'; Jasper's phenomenological notion of the incomprehensibility of psychosis; and Schneider's identification of first-rank psychotic symptoms. Here, I illustrate the "persistent unclarity" (Janzarik, 2003, p. 3) of psychiatric depictions of psychosis and challenge the recurrent unsubstantiated assertion as to its biological aetiology.

4.1 The Kraepelinian binary model of psychoses

The German psychiatrist, Emil Kraepelin, established a clinical picture of psychosis that has essentially endured within the lexicon of medical psychiatry until the present day.[19] In the sixth edition of his consistently revised psychiatry textbook for students and physicians, Kraepelin (1899) proposed a model that reduced psychoses into two definitive types: i) deteriorating disorders clustered together as 'dementia praecox'; and ii) cyclic, non-deteriorating disorders clustered together as 'manic-depressive disorder' (Gach, 2008, p. 393; Jackson, 2008, p. 456). Hence, the transition from a

---

[19] Kraepelin has been identified by many commentators as the instigator of modern psychiatry due to his introduction of a descriptive classificatory diagnostic model to the field. According to Wu & Duan (2015, p. 106), the tradition of descriptive psychiatry was formally inaugurated with the publication of Kraepelin's (1921) paper titled "Psychological work experiments" which subsequently led to him being "regarded as the contemporary father of psychiatry".

psychosomatic to a biomedical picture of psychosis culminated in his formulation of a binary model of discrete psychoses. This instituted a significant crossroads in conceptualising psychosis because he depicted dementia praecox and manic-depressive disorder as distinct disease entities. The present-day psychotic disorders of schizophrenia and bipolar disorder are its direct descendants.

As with physical disorders, Kraepelin construed psychosis as a structured entity identifiable by key characteristic features and symptoms. In regard to dementia praecox he maintained that:

> the meaning of the term has been extended so as to include a larger group of cases appearing in earlier life, characterized by a progressively chronic course with certain fundamental symptoms, of which progressive mental deterioration is the most prominent. (Kraepelin, 1902, p. 152)

Hence, the three key features of dementia praecox were early onset, ongoing degeneration, and poor prognosis, while the 'fundamental symptoms' included "discrepancies between thought and emotion, negativism, stereotypical behaviours, hallucinations, delusions and disordered thoughts" (Middleton et al., 2008, p. 15). Assuming a biological aetiology, he saw "an organic defect as the basis of the illness, leading to the destruction of cortical neurons, possibly by a process of 'auto-intoxication'" (Hoff, 2003, p. 74). Kraepelin distinguished the thought disorders of dementia praecox from the affective states of manic-depressive disorder. He perceived the aetiology of manic-depressive illness as comparatively more obscure than dementia praecox and noted of the former that:

> thus far observation has failed to reveal any characteristic anatomical pathological changes. This fact, together with the recurrence of individual attacks, mostly independent of external causes, has led to the conclusion that the disease depends upon a neuropathic basis, which in the vast majority of cases is hereditary. (Kraepelin, 1902, p. 242)

He also observed that patients with manic-depressive illness had "a later onset and better outcome" (Bentall, 1993, p. 224). According to Owen et al. (2010, p. 70), Kraepelin's proposed psychoses taxonomy "introduced order in the previously chaotic field of nosology and laid down the foundation for the current classifications of psychotic disorders". However, upon closer investigation of literature relating to Kraepelin's work, it appears that his binary model of psychoses only established a stream of quasi-order within a continuing chaotic field of differing views.

Although Kraepelin's classification system marked a major turning point in psychiatric thinking, his hypotheses seemingly worked to complicate, rather than simplify, the task of understanding psychosis. For instance, contrary to his assertion that dementia praecox and manic-depressive disorder were distinct disease entities, a growing body of psychiatrists have observed that they are not discrete, but conjoint, for psychotic patients often exhibit many of the signs and symptoms common to both

(Bentall, 1993, p. 224). Additionally, Kraepelin's psychiatric textbook was a work in progress, therefore, his descriptions of psychosis consistently changed as he updated his views; a practice Read (2004, p. 23) rather cynically refers to as "creating the illusion of discovery where there is nothing more than yet another meaningless re-categorization". Yet another complicating factor was the often vague nature of Kraepelin's assertions and the confused interpretations stemming from these. For instance, in the 1899 edition of his psychiatric textbook Kraepelin (1902, p. 153) states:

> The nature of the disease process in dementia praecox is not known, but it seems probable, judging from the clinical course, and especially in those cases where there has been rapid deterioration, that there is a definite disease process in the brain.

This statement is clearly ambiguous and, indeed, self-contradictory. On the one hand, it acknowledges that the cause of dementia praecox is unknown, yet immediately proceeds to suggest the probability, and then the certainty, that dementia praecox stems from an anatomical flaw in the brain. This unresolved aetiological dilemma has continued to feature in psychiatric representations of psychosis since Kraepelin.

Furthermore, there are conflicting views in the literature regarding Kraepelin's later understanding of the aetiology of psychosis. For example, Gilman (2008, pp. 466–467) notes that although Kraepelin originally conceived of dementia praecox as a somatic disease, he later viewed it "as having a psychogenic rather than a somatic etiology". This is seemly corroborated by Jablensky (1987, p.167), who cites Kraepelin as stating, in a 1920 article,[20] that "the affective and schizophrenic forms of mental disorder do not represent the expression of particular pathological processes, but rather indicate the areas of our personality in which these processes unfold". In saying so, he appears to draw a conclusion similar to Feuchtersleben's original psychosomatic perception of psychosis. However, Jaspers (1997 v2, p. 853), a contemporary of Kraepelin,[21] unequivocally maintained that:

> Kraepelin's basic conceptual world remained a somatic one which in the company of the majority of doctors he held as the only important one for medicine, not only as a matter of preference but in an absolute sense. The psychological discussions in his Textbook are brilliant in parts and he succeeded with them as it were unwittingly. He himself regarded them as temporary stopgaps until experiment, microscope and test-tube permitted objective observation.

Regardless of whether or not Kraepelin's original, strictly anatomical understanding of psychosis later changed to an ambivalent or psychosomatic view, it is apparent that

---

[20] Kraepelin, E. (1920). Die erscheinungsformen des irreseins. *Zeitschrift der Gesamten Psychiatrie und Neurologie, 62*, 1–29.

[21] The text referred to here is from a 1997 edition of a book first published by Jaspers in 1913. Hence, the reference to its contemporaneity with Kraepilin is meant in the 1913 context.

mainstream psychiatry has inherited his initial and reductive physical disease theory, while overlooking, or ignoring, any later psychosomatic views he may have proffered as to the cause of psychosis.

4.2 Bleuler and the advent of schizophrenia

A further important development in the psychiatric epistemology of psychosis is the coining of the term 'schizophrenia' by the Swiss psychiatrist and psychologist Eugen Bleuler. Bleuler challenged Kraepelin's notion of dementia praecox and proposed the alternative term 'schizophrenia' in his book *Dementia Praecox oder die Gruppe der Schizophrenien* (1911). He proffered several reasons to support his view that this name change was necessary. Clinically, he believed Kraepelin's picture of dementia prae-cox was inaccurate in terms of prognosis and course. Whereas Kraepelin's prognosis for patients diagnosed with dementia praecox was pessimistic, Bleuler (1950, p. 8)[22] observed that the course of dementia praecox was not always degenerative, because many patients recovered:

> There is hardly a single psychiatrist who has not heard the argument that the whole concept of dementia praecox must be false because there are many catatonics and other types who, symptomatologically, should be included in Kraepelin's dementia praecox, and who do not go into complete deterioration.

Furthermore, he identified four pragmatic problems regarding both the term and concept of 'dementia praecox': i) "it seems too awkward"; ii) "it only designates the disease, not the diseased"; iii) "it is impossible to derive from it an adjective denoting the characteristics of this illness" (ibid., p. 7); and iv) a new name was "less apt to be misunderstood" (p. 8). The latter point was proffered in light of his assessment that British psychiatrists had generally misconstrued the essential meaning of Kraepelin's dementia praecox; that they "either have ignored or not understood the basic concept of this disease-entity" (ibid.). Acknowledging that psychiatry, by nature, was a work in progress, and that "it is really quite impossible to find a perfect name for a concept which is still developing and changing" (ibid.), Bleuler proposed that his provisional term 'schizophrenia' should supersede Kraepelin's dementia praecox.

Bleuler's schizophrenia embodied several clinical refinements pertaining to the nature of psychosis which, in his view, were not evident in Kraepelin's dementia praecox. First, in coining the term 'schizophrenia', he broadened Kraepelin's binary model of psychoses to denote a singular umbrella term with its constituent variet-ies of psychotic disorders, or schizophrenias (p. 8). For Bleuler, the defining charac-teristic common to schizophrenia (singular) and the schizophrenias (plural) was the "more or less clear-cut splitting of the psychic functions" (p. 9). Also, in contrast to Kraepelin's perceived course of steady degeneration in dementia praecox, Bleuler's

---

[22] Bleuler's 1911 book was translated into English in 1950.

schizophrenia depicted "a group of psychoses whose course is at times chronic, at times marked by intermittent attacks, and which can stop or retrograde at any stage, but does not permit a full *restitutio ad integrum*" (ibid.). He asserted that schizophrenia was diagnosable as a disease entity via the presence of certain primary and secondary symptoms, and that it was necessary to distinguish between the former ("the symptoms stemming directly from the disease process itself"), and the latter ("symptoms which only begin to operate when the sick psyche reacts to some internal or external processes") (p. 348). However, despite the differences between Kraepelin's dementia praecox and Bleuler's schizophrenia, they shared in common an ambiguous and biogenic depiction. For instance, like Kraepelin, Bleuler (p. 349) averred that "we do not as yet know with certainty the primary symptoms of the schizophrenic cerebral disease" (p. 349). Arguably, then, rather than illuminate the clinical picture of psychosis, the advent of schizophrenia simply established a different form of ambiguity, shifting from a disease entity defined by its course and prognosis, to a disease entity defined by an uncertain symptomatology set.

As with his predecessors and contemporaries, Bleuler also underscored the fundamental enigma of the process and aetiology of psychosis. For instance, he stated that "*we assume the presence of a process*" (p. 461) from which the primary symptoms stem, and more candidly that "*we do not know what the schizophrenic process actually is*" (p. 466). Similarly, due to the limits of psychiatric knowledge at the time, he was unable "to establish valid etiological groups of schizophrenia" (p. 242). Additionally, although he personally presumed an underlying somatic aetiology for the schizophrenic psychoses, he cautioned that "it is not absolutely necessary to assume the presence of a physical disease process. It is conceivable that the entire symptomatology may be psychically determined" (p. 461). Although medical psychiatry gradually accepted Bleuler's schizophrenia into its nosology, his caveat regarding the possible psychic aetiology of psychosis has been ignored. In addition, despite Bleuler's more positive prognosis for schizophrenia, psychiatry has generally invested the term with "Kraepelin's original pessimism" (Warner, 2004, p. 29). Hence, it appears that psychiatry has exercised a selective bias in choosing from evolving theories about the nature of psychosis. Arguably, this sort of epistemological cherry-picking has been guided by an underlying bias towards a biogenic understanding of psychosis.

Since its formulation by Bleuler, the term 'schizophrenia' has become analogous with psychosis and features prominently in the annals of psychiatry. However, despite Bleuler's clear distinction between schizophrenia and dementia praecox, psychiatrists often used the terms interchangeably until the former superseded the latter around the mid-twentieth century. As Edelston (1949, p. 960) wryly observed at the time, "even to-day the change from dementia praecox to schizophrenia is not much more than an alteration in nomenclature, with no corresponding change in understanding". Notwithstanding his intention to clarify the psychiatric conceptualisation of psychosis, Bleuler (1950, p. 277) also recognised that "our literature is replete with complaints about the chaotic state of the systematics of psychoses and every psychiatrist knows that it is impossible to come to any common understanding on the basis of the old diagnostic labels". His coining of the new diagnostic label 'schizophrenia', then, was ostensibly a step toward reconciling this clinical confusion. If so, it was a gesture in vain, for research conducted by Jansson & Parnas (2007, p. 1178) indicates that schizophrenia "remains an elusive entity, and the history of psychiatric research is replete with the attempts at formalizing its definition ... In fact, since the introduction of the concept, psychiatry has produced not less than 40 definitions". Regardless, the term has become ubiquitous within psychiatric nosology where it connotes a psychotic type of psychopathology of assumed biological aetiology.

4.3 Jaspers' phenomenological approach

The work of German psychiatrist Karl Jaspers played a fundamental role in shaping the nosological and diagnostic systems of global mainstream psychiatry, and significantly, though inadvertently, influenced the conceptualisation of psychosis as a disorder of somatic origin. Mishara & Fusar-Poli (2013, p. 278) maintain that Jaspers was "the first major psychiatrist to bring scientific foundation to psychopathology" and this foundation was principally established via his landmark book *General Psychopathology* (1963).[23] The impact of his work on the developing epistemology and practice of psychiatry has been substantial, a fact iterated by many commentators over the decades. For instance, Anderson (1959, p. v) referred to it as "epoch-making", while Fusar-Poli (2013, p. 268) describes it as "one of those major works that have become a classic in psychiatric literature". In terms of shaping psychiatric thinking and practice, Stanghellini (2004, p. 31) claims that "the Jasperian approach to the phenomenology of madness was practically the law for a whole century in psychopathology", while Mullen (2007, p. 113) contends that Jaspers' work was "to exert a profound influence on the development of psychiatry in general and psychiatric nosology in particular. The current *Diagnostic and Statistical Manual of Mental Disorders* and *International Classification of Diseases* both reflect, at least in part, that legacy". Hence, facets of Jaspers' work were incrementally adopted and adapted to set both the clinical parameters for comprehending anomalous mental experiences, and for categorising them into diagnosable psychotic disorders.

4.3.1 Key notions and principles of Jaspers' phenomenological approach

It is first apposite to outline the key ideas of Jaspers' work to provide a background context for later examining his influential views on psychosis. Jaspers' overarching vision in writing *Allgemeine Psychopathologie* was to harness phenomenology as a scientific medium for better understanding psychopathology and to incorporate

---

[23] This book was first published in 1913 under the title *Allgemeine Psychopathologie* (Jaspers, 1913). Jaspers made extensive revisions and additions over the next several decades, with seven updated editions published in total. The seventh edition (1959) was translated into English and published as *General Psychopathology*.

this into the body of psychiatry. This was his innovative response to an intractable nineteenth and early twentieth century debate called *Methodenstreit* (Methodological Controversy), in which opposing camps argued for and against adopting the methodology of the natural sciences into the human sciences (Beveridge, 2011, pp. 82–83; Thornton & Schaffner, 2011, p. 128). For Jaspers (1968 [1912], pp. 1315–1316), the key to settling this disagreement was implementing a phenomenological approach:

> The first step towards a scientific comprehension must be the sorting out, defining, differentiating and describing of specific psychic phenomena, which are thereby actualized and are regularly described in specific terms … [A]t this stage we must put aside altogether such considerations as the relationships between experiences, or their summation as a whole, and more especially must we avoid trying to supply any basic constructs or frames of reference. We should picture only what is really present in the patient's consciousness; anything that has not really presented itself to his consciousness is outside our consideration.[24]

In effect, then, Jaspers' project aimed to resolve this dispute by establishing a methodology for *"reconciling meanings and causes"* (Stanghellini et al., 2013, p. 288), whereby the concerns of both human and natural sciences, and subjective and objective lines of psychopathological inquiry, were considered.

Broadly speaking, Jaspers held that *meaning* and *cause* constituted the two primary and interrelated lenses for understanding mental disorders. His elucidation on this is comprehensive and complex, therefore, only those aspects related to the Jaspersian conceptualisations of psychosis adopted by mainstream psychiatry are outlined here. For Jaspers, *meaning* referred to "'understanding' or 'perception of meaning'—Verstehen", and *cause* to "'explanation' or 'perception of causal connection'—Erklären" (Jaspers, 1997 v1, p. 27). Moreover, he explained that the notion of *understanding* pertains to "the understanding of psychic events 'from within'" in contrast to the notion of *explanation* which denotes "the appreciation of causal connections, which … can only be seen 'from without'" (ibid., p. 28). Further to this, he differentiated between subjective and objective modalities—"*Objective* means everything that can be *perceived by the senses* … *Subjective* then means everything that can be comprehended by *empathy* into psychic events" (p. 26). Hence, his phenomenological approach aimed to first foster an understanding of a psychopathological event by employing empathy to fashion a picture of a person's subjective experience. The repetition of this procedure with many patients over time worked to "provide a theory-neutral set of descriptions from which the science of psychiatry could begin" (Owen & Harland, 2007, p. 105). Jaspers (1968 [1912], pp. 1313, 1314) referred to this process as the "systematic study of subjective experience" which enables a practitioner to draft a compilation of

---

[24] This text is quoted from a 1968 English translation of an article Jaspers published in 1912. The translated article appears in the *British Journal of Psychiatry* "on the initiative of Dr. J. N. Curran" (Jaspers, 1968 [1912], p. 1313).

subjective symptoms that "cannot be perceived by the sense-organs, but have to be grasped by transferring oneself, so to say, into the other individual's psyche; that is, by empathy". He understood that the proficient exercise of empathy essentially entailed an abandonment of absolute theories:

> We must set aside all outmoded theories, psychological constructs or materialist mythologies of cerebral processes; we must turn our attention only to that which we can understand as having real existence, and which we can differentiate and describe ... And so this phenomenological attitude is to be acquired only by ever-repeated effort and by the ever renewed overcoming of prejudice (ibid., p. 1316).

In fact, he underscored the necessity of an atheoretical stance by insisting that "phenomenology can gain nothing from theory: it can only lose" (p. 1322). The combined application of these notions and principles characterises the phenomenological approach. While this approach differentiates psychological understandings from causal explanations, it also posits the former as complementary to the latter. Together, these constitute a more holistic approach to psychiatric practice whereby both modalities of knowledge formation are deemed component parts of the science of psychopathology.

4.3.2 The incomprehensibility of psychosis

Jaspers' notion of the incomprehensibility of psychosis has been adopted by psychiatry as fundamentally delineating psychotic from non-psychotic experiences and has had significant sway on the development of psychiatric thinking. Indeed, Estroff (1989, p. 190) refers to incomprehensibility as "the hallmark of psychosis". Jaspers asserted that the application of his systematic phenomenological approach led to the identification of a particular defining feature of psychotic disorders, which he referred to as "incomprehensibility" or "ununderstandability" (Stanghellini, 2013, p. 168). Hence, in his view, the empathic approach generally leads to what he called "genetic understanding" whereby "psychic events 'emerge' out of each other in a way which we understand ... *our understanding is genetic*" (ibid., p. 302). In other words, the genesis of a presenting clinical problem (i.e. psychic event d) can be logically traced as the end product of a series of preceding causal psychic events ($a \rightarrow b \rightarrow c \rightarrow d$). In such instances, the emergence of a particular psychic event is genetically understandable.

In contrast to most psychological problems, however, which can be empathically understood in terms of their discernible genetic unfolding, Jaspers held that a psychotic disorder is marked by its "complete inaccessibility to any empathic understanding" (1968 [1912], p. 1318), for it seemingly "rises spontaneously ... and is unrelated to the patient's life-history and experiences" (1997 v1, pp. 384–385). Elsewhere he explained that such psychic occurrences "appear suddenly as something entirely new ... One psychic event follows another quite incomprehensibly; it seems to follow arbitrarily rather than emerge" (ibid., p. 27). For him, psychotic delusions exemplified the incomprehensible, as they "cannot be understood in terms of prior psychological origin or motivation. They seem to come from nowhere and cannot be derived from anything else" (Mishara & Fusar-Poli, 2013, p. 279). Jaspers subsequently concluded that "the most profound distinction in psychic life seems to be that between what is meaningful and *allows empathy* and what in its particular way is *ununderstandable*, 'mad' in the literal sense, schizophrenic psychic life" (Jaspers, 1997 v2, p. 577). Psychiatry has subsequently recognised incomprehensibility as a defining feature of psychosis.

4.3.3 Psychiatry's biogenic and reductive adaption of Jaspers' thinking

Psychiatry not only adopted but also adapted Jaspers' notion of incomprehensibility to buttress its views concerning the ostensible somatic aetiology of psychosis. On this point Stanghellini (2004, p. 27) maintains that "much of the contemporary medical model followed the spirit (if not the letter) of Jaspers' axiom of incomprehensibility or ununderstandability of schizophrenic experiences. It ... treated schizophrenia as merely an epiphenomenon of some biological dysfunction". Bentall (2004, p. 29) holds a similar view, purporting that "the irony" of Jaspers' enterprise was that "he tried to identify a role for psychological explanations in psychiatry. In the process, he gave madness to the biologists and inadvertently discouraged the psychological investigation of the psychoses". This is an odd development for he repeatedly expressed the need to be cautious of biological reductionism. Indeed, his *General Psychopathology* is replete with statements to this effect. For instance, he referred to the purported relationship between the brain and psychic events as "brain mythologies" that are "somatic constructions [with] no real basis" (Jaspers, 1997 v1, p. 18). Further to this, he warned that "we should be particularly wary of regarding known cerebral processes as such direct bases for particular psychic events" (Jaspers, 1997 v2, p. 460), and elsewhere asserted that:

> the assumption that what is physical and what is psychic coincide somewhere in the brain is pure fantasy, and must always remain an untestable hypothesis ... It is a vague, general truth that the psyche is tied to the body, but how and where this connection takes place fragments into a multitude of possibilities awaiting exploration. (Jaspers, 1997 v1, p. 225)

His views, therefore, seem to offer little leeway for supporting a biogenic psychiatric view. While he did state that "one must ... assume that many of these psychoses have a somatic base which one day will be known" (Jaspers, 1997 v2, p. 607), his method rejected the adoption and utilisation of any unsubstantiated theory, be it psychological or biological, as a presumed factual foundation for clinical research and practice.

Through empathic, methodical, and repeated observation, a phenomenological approach aimed to identify and systemise the veiled nuances of psychopathological experiences and in doing so, emulate the rigour of research development in the medical sciences. To further this undertaking, Jaspers (1997 v1, pp. 58–60) promoted the idea of focussing on the *form* rather than the *content* of patients' experiences and collating these into a provisional classification system for diagnostic and empirical research purposes (ibid., pp. 43–44; Jaspers, 1997 v2, pp. 604, 616). As Walker (1991, p. 94) explains, "Jaspers accepts that all experience or knowledge entails both an incoming sensation and an organising concept. The former is matter or content, the latter is form". In terms of psychotic symptomology, for example, a hallucination constitutes a *form* of psychotic experience that is the object of phenomenological investigation, whereas its subjective *content* is of no interest in strict observational terms (Jaspers, 1997 v1, p. 58). However, while this focus on form over content has been embedded into psychiatric research and classification systems worldwide, it has inclined towards a reductivism which Jaspers eschewed.

Jaspers did not intend his phenomenological views to be used prescriptively or reductively by psychiatry, but more as a heuristic tool for advancing understanding. Hence, his depiction of psychosis as being incomprehensible was not absolute, but provisional. Heinimaa (2008, p. 47) alludes to this in positing that "'incomprehensibility' is not a form of understanding at all, but marks the limits of understanding in human life". In other words, Jaspers was not inferring that psychotic experiences are absolutely and irrevocably incomprehensible, but that their comprehension is beyond the grasp of conventional modalities for understanding reality. In fact, he warned against limiting the scope of traditional psychiatric understanding via reductionism:

> The chaos of phenomena should not be blotted out with some diagnostic label but bring illumination through the way it is systematically ordered and related. Psychiatric diagnosis is too often a sterile running round in circles so that only a few phenomena are brought into the orbit of conscious knowledge. (Jaspers, 1997 v1, p. 20)

In other words, although psychosis seems to be incomprehensible, it is not to be dismissed as basically meaningless. It therefore seems Jaspers intended his approach to be used heuristically, and not reductively, for it allowed scope to incrementally understand that which is *seemingly* incomprehensible as phenomenological research was developed and refined. Indeed, as is argued throughout the ensuing Focal Settings Two to Four of this book, psychotic experiences and phenomena are considerably more comprehensible when viewed in light of psychospiritual and cross-cultural considerations.

Overall, it seems Jaspers' work both opened and closed potential pathways for better understanding psychosis. Regarding the former, his introduction of phenomenology into psychiatry called for an open-minded observation of psychotic experiences, which, free from the blinkers of preconceived theoretical constructs, enabled the practitioner to delve more deeply into the forms of psychosis and, hopefully, their latent meanings. It also required that a psychiatrist engage his or her patients in a caring manner, exchanging clinical distance for active listening, in order to "become a fellow-actor [who] participates in the patient's destiny and goes through his crisis with him" (Jaspers, 1997 v2, p. 676). Some commentators have subsequently referred to Jaspers as a humanist for advocating this approach (Jablensky, 2013; Ghaemi, 2008; Giorgi, 1997). In terms of hindering understanding, Jaspers' notion of the incomprehensibility of psychotic disorders has arguably and ironically been misconstrued by psychiatry. Consequently, his thinking has been used to serve reductive diagnostic practices and to bolster the biogenic belief that the ultimate answers to the enigma of psychosis lay hidden in the physical body, thus limiting the primary focus of psychiatric research to an anatomical scope.

4.4 Schneider and 'morbid' psychotic disorders of 'unknown etiology'

The final key contributor to the evolution of modern psychiatric thinking that I shall consider here is the German psychiatrist Kurt Schneider. As a student of Kraepelin, Schneider "consolidated and developed" his mentor's binary classification of psychoses (Beer, 1996b, p. 21), and played a significant role in refocussing the attention of psychiatric diagnostics to the Kraepelinian model during the 1930s (Beer, 1995b, p. 319). Hence, he acted as a clinical lynchpin between Kraepelinian thinking and the development of modern psychiatry. He also generated a set of first and second rank symptoms for diagnosing schizophrenia that strongly influenced the development of contemporary psychiatric diagnostics. Andreasen & Flaum (1991, p. 28) assert that DSM-III "placed great emphasis on Schneiderian first-rank symptoms", while Tsuang et al. (2000, p. 1042) maintain that these symptoms "formed the basis of DSM-III criteria for schizophrenia". As such, Schneider was another primary player in medical psychiatry's clinical trajectory towards construing psychosis as a particular type of biogenic and psychopathological disorder that can be diagnosed via the identification of specific symptoms.

4.4.1 Schneider's model for diagnosing schizophrenia

Schneider drew and built upon the work of Kraepelin, Bleuler, and Jaspers to inform his own understanding of psychosis. In devising his diagnostic model, he adopted the works of Kraepelin and Bleuler as a baseline for this project and redressed perceived limitations within both to invest them with a refined clinical capacity (Nordgaard et al., 2008, p.137). For instance, he divested Kraepelin's dementia praecox of its "positivist theories and inappropriate clinical characterizations" (Hoenig, 1983, p. 554), to propose a diagnostic formula that highlighted symptom specificity for identifying the two forms of psychosis (Tsuang et al., 2000, p. 1042). Additionally, counter to the Kraepelinian prognosis of degeneration in dementia praecox, Schneider believed that recovery was possible, though rare (Hoenig, 1983, p. 554). He also composed a modified and more succinct version of the Bleulerian primary symptoms, which he saw as overly vague in meaning (ibid.) and as "often continuous with normality" (Andreasen, 1997b, p. 108). It was his conviction that "somatically speaking there are no transitions with normality" in psychoses (Schneider in Beer, 1995b, p. 319),[25] hence, he endorsed the basic medical psychiatric view that insanity and sanity are discrete states of being. Jaspers' phenomenological approach also influenced Schneider's thinking (Huber, 2002, p. 52; Schneider, 1959, p. v), particularly his rationale regarding the imperviousness of psychotic disorders to empathic understanding (i.e., their apparent incomprehensibility) (Mundt, 1993, p. 1245). Conversely, Schneider played a significant role in helping Jaspers shape his fourth edition of *General Psychopathology* (Huber, 2002, p. 50), and was subsequently acknowledged in the book's preface.[26]

In 1946, when Schneider published the first edition of his book that was later titled *Klinische Psychopathologie* (*Clinical Psychopathology*),[27] many psychiatrists used the term 'psychosis' loosely in reference to various mental disorders, despite Kraepelin's proposal of a binary model of psychoses. Hence, a driving aspiration of his venture was to crystallise the application of psychiatric diagnostics by asserting a more precise clinical picture of psychosis (Beer, 1995a, p. 195). As Heinimaa (2008, p. 29) states:

> Schneider dismissed the use of the concept of psychosis in the broad sense: for him it was a narrowly defined scientific concept, referring specifically to an organic illness, and did not lie on the continuum between illness and healthy personality function ... He distinguished sharply between psychoses and 'understandable abnormal reactions'.

As such, he was a staunch advocate of "an empiric dualism of psyche and soma" (Schneider, 1959, p. 1), and his objective was to unambiguously delineate psychosis from the throng of other mental disorders by depicting it in psychopathological juxtaposition to health and normality, and by stamping it with the status of biological disease. This is evident in his assertion of the "fact" that "a psychic disturbance, no matter how severe, should never be termed a psychosis if no morbid condition has given rise to it" (ibid., p. 3). Schneider (p. 7) defined a morbid condition as follows: "When we speak of morbid psychic disturbances, we mean that they are conditioned by organic processes and their functional and local effects. Thus, our concept of psychiatric illness is based entirely on morbid bodily change". In other words, if a psychic disturbance is not caused by an underlying somatic malfunction, then it is not a psychosis.

---

[25] This is Beer's translation of a journal article published by Schneider (1933).
[26] In the preface to the fourth edition of *General Psychopathology*, Jaspers (1997 v1, p. xix) states: "I want to thank Professor Kurt Schneider of Munich. Not only has he stimulated me with penetrating criticism and valuable suggestions but he has greatly encouraged my work through his positive and exacting attitudes".
[27] Cutting et al. (2016, p. 339) explain that Schneider published a book in 1946 "entitled *Beiträge zur Psychiatrie* (Schneider, 1946) which then ran through nine editions. From the third edition, the title became *Klinische Psychopathologie*, and the fifth edition was translated into English as *Clinical Psychopathology* (Schneider, 1946/1959)".

In order to instrumentalise this view, Schneider categorised two modes of mental illness in *Clinical Psychopathology*. These were the non-somatic "Abnormal variations of psychic life", and the somatic "Effects of illness" (Beer, 1996c, p. 245). The latter included the two Kraepelinian forms of psychosis: namely, a "Condition of unknown etiology causing schizophrenia" and a "Condition of unknown etiology causing cyclothymia" (manic-depressive disorder) (ibid.). He subsequently established an unequivocal differentiation between psychological and somatic mental disorders, with schizophrenia and cyclothymia designated as belonging to the latter. In his own words, "psychosis is a matter of disease. In the end one could conclude that schizophrenia is an organic-constitutional, perhaps a primary cerebral disorder" (Schneider in Beer, 1995b, p. 319). It is pertinent to note here the incongruity between his classifying psychosis as being 'of unknown etiology' and his assertion that the cause of psychosis is almost certainly anatomical. This reflects the perennial practice throughout the history of medical psychiatry of professing a somatic core to psychosis, while simultaneously acknowledging its aetiology is yet to be scientifically substantiated.

Further to this, Schneider compiled a set of first and second rank symptoms to differentiate schizophrenia from cyclothymia and psychological disorders. He upheld the value of his suggested first rank symptoms "in helping us to determine the diagnosis schizophrenia … from cyclothymia", and further stated that they "have a decisive weight above all others in establishing a differential typology between schizophrenia and cyclothymia" (Schneider, 1959, pp. 133, 135). These symptoms were comprised of "abnormal experiences" in the form of "disturbances in perceptions, sensations, feelings, impulses and volition" (Pull, 2002, pp. 2–3), or what Carpenter et al. (2009, p. 2032) refer to as "reality distortion phenomena". According to Bruijnzeel & Tandon (2011, p. 292), Schneider endorsed Jaspers' view that psychosis was essentially defined by its incomprehensibility, and on this understanding he based the formulation of his ranked diagnostic symptoms. Schneider (1959, pp. 133–134) listed these symptoms as follows:

> audible thoughts, voices heard arguing, voices heard commenting on one's actions; the experience of influences playing on the body (somatic passivity experiences); thought-withdrawal and other interferences with thought; diffusion of thought; delusional perception and all feelings, impulses (drives), and volitional acts that are experienced by the patient as the work or influence of others.

He maintained that "the decisive clinical diagnosis of schizophrenia" can be made if any these signs or symptoms appear in the absence of a known somatic disease (ibid., p. 134). Hence, they were identified as being emblematic of schizophrenia. His proposed second rank schizophrenic symptoms consisted of supplementary experiences of diagnostic significance such as "other hallucinations, delusional notions, perplexity, depressed and elated mood, experiences of flattened feeling, and so on" (ibid.). Schneider's ranked symptom model had significant influence in the formation of the modern medical diagnostic system.

4.4.2 Appraising Schneider's model for diagnosing psychoses

When considering that Schneider's work on psychosis was fundamentally informed by the works of Kraepelin, Bleuler, and Jaspers, it is apposite to appraise its veracity. Although the respective works of Kraepelin, Bleuler, and Jaspers each represent a distinctive attempt to better clinically grasp the enigmatic nature of psychosis, in Schneider's work they are drawn together to mark the end of a particular era of psychiatric investigation into the phenomenon of psychosis. Therefore, if Schneider's construal of psychosis represents the incorporation, refinement, and culmination of nearly seventy years of psychiatric research into psychosis, does it hold veracity within the fabric of its own assertions and assumptions?

Although Schneider's work may appear to be authoritative and clinically sound at face value, it is actually fraught with ambiguity. In particular, this is the case with his ranked symptoms for diagnosing schizophrenia and also his contention regarding the likely biological aetiology of psychosis. To begin, the clinical validity of his first rank symptoms is debatable. For instance, psychiatrist Clive Mellor (1970, p. 15) claims that first rank symptoms possess pragmatic legitimacy because Schneider formulated them by drawing on his extensive clinical experience. However, Crichton (1996, p. 538) maintains that Schneider's clinical expertise in itself does not constitute medical validity, and consequently, psychiatrists "can really only guess how he determined which symptoms should be promoted to the first rank". He also claims "no scientific evidence was found in Schneider's writings to establish the special importance of FRS [First Rank Symptoms] for the diagnosis of schizophrenia. He presented no data to suggest that FRS are anything more than a chance cluster" (ibid., p. 539). If so, then Schneider's ranked symptoms are seemingly more supposition than scientific fact.

The ambiguity of his ranked symptoms is further evident in quantitative research conducted to test their veracity. When his first rank symptoms were initially utilised on a broad scale, they indeed seemed highly effective in identifying schizophrenia. For instance, their first widespread use was in 1966, when adopted for their perceived diagnostic efficacy by the World Health Organization (WHO) and incorporated into the International Pilot Study of Schizophrenia (IPSS), "a large-scale cross-cultural collaborative project carried out simultaneously in nine countries" (Sartorius et al., 1974, pp. 21, 29). The results of this study indicated that Schneider's first rank symptoms were highly indicative of schizophrenia, for "if they were present, the chance that the clinical diagnosis would be schizophrenia was at least 95 percent" (ibid., p. 30). Hence, at first, Schneider's first rank symptoms appeared to offer psychiatry a breakthrough instrument for understanding and diagnosing schizophrenia. Recent research, however, seems to counter this view. For example, Škodlar et al. (2008) conducted a study to ascertain the incidence of changing symptomatology in psychiatric diagnostics in Slovenia from 1881–2000, paying particular attention to change rates after the introduction of Schneiderian first rank symptoms. They found that "Schneiderian first-rank symptoms were reported dramatically more frequently after Schneider's ideas became known", and tentatively concluded, "we presume that it was the attention of clinicians and not actual change in the first-rank symptoms that contributed to the increase ascertained in their percentages" (ibid., pp. 104, 108). In other words, it is likely that through exposure to Schneider's symptoms set, clinicians subjectively found what they expected to find.[28]

Schneider's contradictory reference to 'morbid' psychotic disorders of 'unknown etiology' also casts doubt on the validity of his postulations. The fact that he saw psychosis as biogenic is evident in his claim that "we are firmly postulating that cyclothymia and schizophrenia are psychopathologic symptoms of some unknown illness" and that "there is no question at this point whether some morbid condition does in fact underlie these psychopathologic forms" (Schneider, 1959, p. 5). Additionally, he stressed that "our definition of illness in psychiatry is strictly a medical one … our concept of psychiatric illness is based entirely on morbid bodily change" (ibid., p. 7). Yet, despite this show of biomedical certitude he also concedes that the somatic theory "is undoubtedly a confession of faith and it can be contested" (p. 10). Elsewhere, he mixes concession with assertion in stating that "it is true we have no precise knowledge of the basic morbid processes leading to cyclothymia and schizophrenia but that they are in fact at the root of these disorders is an extremely well-supported postulate, a well-founded hypothesis" (p. 8). In a similar vein, he concludes:

> What then is to be the nature of these psychoses that lack any known somatic base? We are totally averse to identifying them as developments arising from psychic reaction to experience … We are quite adamant about this, though we cannot give conclusive grounds … We stand by our hypothesis, therefore, as a heuristic principle. (pp. 9–10)

This dubious practice of asserting an unsubstantiated biological aetiology of psychosis has been a common feature, and point of contention, within the discipline of medical psychiatry since its inauguration. It also represents the prime obstacle to opening exploration into possible psychological and psychospiritual causes of psychosis. Intriguingly, Schneider acknowledged the vexing fact that "if we were to keep strictly to what is actually known … our concept of psychosis, with its accent on basic illness, could no longer hold" (p. 9). It appears, then, that Schneider's biomedical-based assertions regarding the nature and diagnosis of psychosis have dubious veracity, as does the general medical model of psychiatry with its propensity towards reductive diagnostics based on unproven biogenic theories.

---

[28] The questionable validity of psychiatry's use of core symptoms in defining and diagnosing psychotic disorders, and the corollary assumption that sanity and insanity are discrete states of being, is critiqued in further detail throughout Focal Settings Three and Four of this book.

4.5 Conclusion

Despite six decades (1890–1950) of rigorous psychiatric theorising and research into the ostensible biogenic nature of psychosis, it remained enigmatic and 'incomprehensible'. Arguably, this was due to psychiatry's general adherence to an unsubstantiated, materialist-based, biogenic view of psychosis, coupled with a reductive categorisation approach, which eclipsed the consideration of possible psychosocial and psychospiritual determinants in psychosis and stripped its symptomatic manifestations of any intrinsic meaning. As is shown in Chapter Five, the advent of a psychoanalytic model of psychiatry in America (1952–1980) temporarily stemmed this biogenic trajectory. However, it was firmly reinstated in 1980 and has prevailed to the present date.

CHAPTER 5

Understanding psychosis: historical developments via the Diagnostic and Statistical Manuals

5.0 Introduction

This chapter provides a historical overview of conceptualisations of psychosis throughout respective editions of the *Diagnostic and Statistical Manual of Mental Disorders* (DSM). My concomitant critical review identifies key factors that have influenced the shift from a psychoanalytic model of psychiatry in DSM-I and DSM-II, to a medical model in DSM-III, and a prevailing biomedical model in DSM-IV and DSM-5.

5.1 Background to the Diagnostic and Statistical Manual of Mental Disorders

The *Diagnostic and Statistical Manual of Mental Disorders* (DSM) was devised by the American Psychiatric Association (APA) as a diagnostic guidebook for clinicians and researchers. In terms of this book's core objective of investigating the notion of better understanding psychosis, the DSM manual is of especial interest due to the dynamic nature of conceptual developments throughout its history.[29] The first edition (DSM-I) was published in 1952 and the current edition (DSM-5) was published in 2013.

---

[29] My rationale for examining only the DSM, and not also the World Health Organisation's *International Classification of Diseases* (ICD), is as follows. Although the ICD contains a section on mental disorders, it has not seen the same degree of dynamic change throughout its development as has the DSM. While the ICD iterations have generally reflected a medical understanding of psychopathology, the DSM iterations reflect both psychodynamic and medical approaches. Hence, a historical and critical investigation of DSM developments proffers insights into various factors and forces not evident with ICD that can shape, and have shaped, how mainstream psychiatry has understood psychopathology and psychosis.

According to Kraemer (2008, p. 8), "the process of DSM development is analogous to a spiral ... Each successive iteration is expected to move closer to the true disorder". Overall, then, the DSM series has been provisional in nature, with each edition aiming to gradually advance the clinical and aetiological understanding of mental disorders by psychiatry.

Since its inception, there have been three key developmental phases within the DSM series. The first phase, in DSM-I and DSM-II, reflected a psychodynamic model of understanding, while the second phase, in DSM-III, saw a revival of the medical model of understanding. Finally, throughout the third phase, in DSM-IV and DSM-5, this medical view has been reinforced. For each of these phases and associated manuals, this chapter provides: i) an elucidation of key process developments and the resultant construal of psychosis; and ii) a critical appraisal of related conceptual issues. The aim of doing so is to present an unfolding picture of the variant ways in which psychosis has been understood and to highlight the degree to which social, political, and economic factors have worked to shape the present and prevailing biomedical view.[30]

5.2 DSM-I and DSM-II: the psychoanalytic model

Since the 1800s, when psychiatry first emerged as a discipline, it has predominantly been governed by a biomedical model of understanding. However, the DSM-I and DSM-II manuals reflect a twenty-eight-year American epoch wherein a psychoanalytic model of psychiatry prevailed. The publication of DSM-I by the APA in 1952 represented a significant development in American and international psychiatry. It fulfilled the need to establish a generic classification and nosological system of mental disorders for consensus diagnostic purposes, and to correspondingly create names for newly identified post-war disorders (APA, 1968, p. ix). DSM-I also marked the advent of an era of psychoanalytic understanding of mental illness in American psychiatry. Its success is evident in the fact that it was reprinted twenty times (ibid.) before being replaced by the DSM-II update in 1968. While DSM-II remained a psychoanalytic-based manual there were ostensible signs throughout its review process that indicated an emergent ideological shift back toward a biomedical model. These dynamics, and how they shaped the understanding of psychosis, are examined below.

5.2.1 DSM-I process

A salient feature of the DSM-I manual was that it superseded psychiatry's long-standing biogenic view with a psychogenic theory of mental illness. In contrast to the traditional medical view, DSM-I highlighted a dialectical interplay between psyche and soma which was akin to Feuchtersleben's original depiction of mental illness

---

[30] This chapter completes the investigative process for Focal Setting One, beyond which the prevailing materialist view of psychosis is challenged and further explored in the context of psychospiritual considerations throughout Focal Settings Two to Four.

and psychosis. Although informed by Freudian psychoanalytic theory (Barton, 1987, p. 134), the manual was fundamentally shaped by the psychobiological theory of the Swiss-born American psychiatrist Adolf Meyer, whose work shows the capacity for psychiatrists to understand psychopathology as a phenomenon caused by a mix of biological and psychic determinants.

Meyer's complex and comprehensive psychobiological theory and practice had a significant influence on American psychiatry during the early-to-mid twentieth century (Menninger et al., 1977, p. 467; Lidz, 1966) and worked to fundamentally change the nature of American psychiatric practice via DSM-I. He rejected the Kraepelinian notion of discrete disease entities of purely organic aetiology (Lidz, 1966, p. 328), and the biomedical model of psychiatry in general. For instance, he spoke of the "fruitless debates" and conceptual cul-de-sacs stemming from "the desire to understand the peculiar reaction of mind as signs of irritation or other lesions of its organ, and the effort to use in a dogmatic way the medical formula of specific diseases" (Meyer, 1908, p. 250). From this psychobiological perspective, mental illnesses were viewed as "reactions of the personality to psychological, social, and biological factors" (APA, 1980, p. 1). In order to reconcile the classic psyche-soma divide, Meyer proposed that "we must expect of the psychiatrist sound medical training along all the specifically medicinal lines, but with just as much of a sound grasp on the 'person and setting', situational and personal, psycho-biological, physiological and sociological and biographic" (Meyer, 1940, p. 275). He maintained that "a 'science of life' without full respect for life where it lives and as it lives is not true science" (Meyer, 1941, p. 156). This view was at odds with mainstream psychiatric theory as to the primacy of biological causes in mental disorders.

Meyer understood mental illnesses to be stress-induced psychological reactions (Gaines, 1992, p. 8) and DSM-I highlighted the pivotal role of stress in activating mental illnesses and psychoses:

> While it is recognized that multicausal factors operate, the apparent or obvious external stress precipitating the condition is to be evaluated as to type, degree, and duration. The stress will generally refer to the immediate emotional, economic, environmental, or cultural situation which is directly related to the reaction manifest in the patient. (APA, 1952, p. 47)

In adopting key tenets of psychobiological thinking, DSM-I was published as a compendium of "Diseases of the Psychobiologic Unit"[31] in which "Psychotic Disorders" were listed under a section titled "Disorders of Psychogenic Origin or Without Clearly Defined Physical Cause or Structural Change in the Brain" (APA, 1952, pp. 1, 6).

---

[31] According to Stevenson (1937, p. 742):

> the psychobiologic unit is the feeling-acting-thinking person, the living man as contrasted ... with the cadaver ... In brief, the psychobiologic unit is the person as he is busied with his work, his pleasure, his rest, his growth and creativeness, his safety or whatever else may occupy him.

These were further subdivided into four types of psychotic reaction; namely, "Affective reactions", "Schizophrenic reactions", "Paranoid reactions", and "Psychotic reaction without clearly defined structural change, other than above" (ibid., pp. 5–6). The term "psychotic reaction" was defined as "one in which the personality, in its struggle for adjustment to internal and external stresses, utilizes severe affective disturbance, profound autism and withdrawal from reality, and/or formation of delusions or hallucinations" (p. 12). The advent of this model represented a marked breakaway from psychiatry's history of promoting an anatomical conceptualisation of psychoses.

5.2.2 DSM-I construal of psychosis

In DSM-I, psychosis was understood to be a meaningful reaction to environmental stressors. However, the manual not only abandoned the premise of a biological aetiology for psychoses, but also rejected the identification of psychoses as discrete diseases. For instance, the majority of American psychiatrists throughout the 1950s believed mental illnesses existed "along a continuum of severity—from neurosis to borderline conditions to psychosis", and that "the boundary between the mentally well and the mentally ill is fluid because normal persons can become ill if exposed to severe enough trauma" (Wilson, 1993, p. 400). This view ushered a unitary conceptualisation of psychosis into mainstream psychiatry. In contrast to the discrete disorder model endorsed by Kraepelin and adopted by mainstream psychiatry prior to the advent of DSM-I, the unitary model conceived of a single form of psychosis which manifested variously (Berrios & Beer, 1994). Aetiologically, the unitary model saw the various manifestations of psychosis as major stress-related adaptive failures (Wilson, 1993, p. 400). In DSM-I, then, the "tradition-determined" view of psychoses (Meyer, 1957, p. 128) was replaced by a mental illness model whereby psychotic reactions were understood to be the product of multiple interacting and coalescing forces; psychosocial, psychodynamic, cultural, and biological. Although as theoretical as the traditional biogenic model it replaced, it arguably opened several new research avenues for psychiatry to better understand psychosis.

5.2.3 DSM-II process

After sixteen years in print, DSM-I was revised and replaced by DSM-II. Broadly speaking, the DSM-II revision process represented an attempt to reconcile the DSM and ICD frameworks; hence, it was a preliminary step towards establishing a multilateral and uniform classification system of mental illnesses. A collaborative process transpired between WHO and APA representatives culminating in the publication of the revised ICD-8 and DSM-II in 1968 (APA, 1968, pp. xii–xv). Although the revised DSM-II was based on the ICD-8 classification of mental disorders (APA, 1980, p. 1), the final product represented a compromise between adapted ICD-8 categories and existing DSM-I categories (APA, 1968, p. xv). Its publication constituted a historical watershed in advancing parity between different international psychiatric classification systems. The upgraded DSM-II manual has been described as "similar to DSM-I" (APA, 2000, p. 3), however, it appears that the review process resulted in significant changes to the construal of mental disorders, including psychosis.

5.2.4 DSM-II construal of psychosis

The most significant change in DSM-II was the Review Committee's decision to remove the term 'reaction' from many disorders, including most of the psychoses. The official explanation for this exclusion was that it "tried to avoid terms which carry with them implications regarding either the nature of a disorder or its causes", however, the authors assured that this "has not changed the nature of the disorder" (APA, 1968, pp. viii–ix). Spitzer & Wilson (1969, p. 358) mirrored the official view in assuring that "some individuals may interpret this change as a return to a Kraepelinian way of thinking, which views mental disorders as fixed disease entities … [but] this was not the intent of the APA Committee". Many clinicians, however, were concerned that this omission reflected a significant conceptual or ideological change. Indeed, when considering that the aetiological term 'reactive' was integral to the unitary understanding of mental disorders, it is reasonable to conclude that removing the former equates to abandoning the latter. This change was particularly evident in the DSM-II psychotic disorders section. For instance, whereas the 'struggle for adjustment to internal and external stresses' was core to the DSM-I definition for reactive psychoses, in DSM-II, the terms 'reactive' and 'stress' were expunged from the psychosis definition (APA, 1968, p. 23). This raises the pointed questions: if schizophrenic, affective and paranoid illnesses are not *reactive* psychoses, then what type of psychoses are they? And what substantiates the claim that their essential psychogenic nature remains unchanged? Arguably, removing the term 'reactive' represented a fundamental change to the understanding of the nature of psychosis. Hence, it is apposite to suggest that this terminological change in DSM-II signified an attempt to precipitate an ideological shift away from ideas of the psychobiological aetiology of psychosis, and presumably back towards the biogenic model traditionally endorsed by medical psychiatry. The following critical appraisal of conceptual dynamics throughout the DSM-II process supports this suggestion.

5.2.5 Conceptual issues

While the formulation of mental disorder categories within the DSM manual was guided by psychiatric research, it was also significantly influenced by administrative and ideological factors. Hence, to a considerable degree, the construal of psychosis reflected a compromise between clinical observation, administrative expediency, and personal opinion. In terms of administration, the manual was created for both diagnostic and *statistical* purposes, with a strong emphasis on expediting the latter. For instance, in DSM-I, the descriptive material on mental disorders was about half that dedicated to elucidating statistical matters. On this matter, the authors explained that:

the construction of a practical scheme of classification of disease and injury for general statistical use involves various compromises ... to meet the varied require-ments of vital statistics offices, hospitals of different types, medical services of the armed forces, social insurance organizations, sickness surveys, and numerous other agencies. (APA, 1952, p. 88)

This attention to statistical needs was replicated in DSM-II, wherein the reader was informed that the "preservation of statistical continuity has been considered at every stage in the development of this Manual" (APA, 1968, p. x). Although establishing enhanced statistical precision was a laudable goal, this entailed compromising epis-temological integrity to administrative necessity, and had the effect of construing mental disorders as units of measure. Accordingly, Menninger (1969, p. 415) critically described the DSM-II review process as serving "the interest of pigeonholing for sta-tistical purposes". While such 'pigeonholing' enabled easier and effective counting, it had the reductive effect of rendering DSM mental illness categories, including the psychoses, into ontologically clipped units of measure. Hence, the understanding of mental disorders was not based purely on the clinical observation of their respective characteristics, but reflected, to a considerable degree, a diagnostic construct shaped by the empirical requirements of statisticians. Analogously speaking, this was tan-tamount to proclaiming that water is box-shaped because technicians measure the volume of swimming pools in cubic litres.

The revised DSM-II manual was also the product of ideological influences in that apparent rudimentary steps were taken to reinvest it with a biomedical character. Despite assurances that DSM-II changes did not signify a move back to a medical model, there were indicators that suggested otherwise. For instance, several years prior to the commencement of the revision process, Cole & Gerard (1959, p. 10) observed that, in American psychiatry, "the pendulum is again swinging back a bit toward the importance of material biological factors". Furthermore, Henry Brill, the DSM-II Review Committee Chairman from 1960–1965, was described as hav-ing "had considerable impact on the form and content of the final classification" in DSM-II (APA, 1968, p. xv). According to Whitaker (2002, p. 156), Brill was a staunch biomedical advocate who played a critical role during the late 1950s in influencing "the final stamp of science" on the pharmacological treatment of psychiatric disor-ders. Indeed, two years after his nomination as Chairman, Brill (1962, pp. 489–490) published an article in which he concluded that "it would seem that the clinical foun-dation for research in schizophrenia remains firm. Modified by experience and by technical advances, the broad outlines of a true entity appear to emerge more clearly than before". This evidently eschews the DSM-I unitary understanding of psychosis in favour of a Kraepelinian 'disease entity' view. He also asserted that "failure to get laboratory confirmation is not conclusive disproof; it is only failure to find proof ... Final laboratory correlates of the concept of clinical schizophrenia will soon be estab-lished" (ibid., p. 490). It is, therefore, feasible to assume that the decision to remove the term 'reaction' from DSM-II was influenced by Brill and his biomedical view of psychopathology.

Another occurrence of putative ideological bias was that the draft DSM-II manual was sent to only 120 American psychiatrists for evaluation (APA, 1968, p. ix). This led Jackson (1969, p. 388) to comment that "one is left wondering how these psychiatrists were chosen and what biases may have influenced their choice", and to wryly assert that "as far as its Kraepelinian status is concerned, *DSM-II* in many respects is a progressive step in a backward direction". Additionally, despite a formal declaration that the DSM-II review process "included representatives of many views" (APA, 1968, p. ix), proponents of the psychobiological term 'reactive' were not included in the Review Committee (Gruenberg, 1969, p. 371). Therefore, contrary to assurances that DSM-II remained essentially the same as DSM-I, it appears that preliminary steps toward an ideological shift were afoot. Indeed, the DSM-II revision process was viewed by many as a step toward reviving a medical model of psychiatry in DSM-III. For example, Skodal (2000, p. 432) purports that expunging the word 'reaction' from DSM-II "was seen by many as the first sign of a return of a Kraepelinian conceptualization", while Rogler (1997, p. 10) holds that the manual's architects "anticipated the paradigm shift in the DSM-III". Combined, these factors suggest the likelihood of a nascent ideological shift of a biomedical nature having occurred with the publication of DSM-II. Overall, while the degree to which biomedical ideology influenced the shaping of DSM-II is debatable, it had unequivocal sway throughout the ensuing DSM-III review process.

5.3 DSM-III and DSM-III-R: the medical model revived

The 1980 publication of DSM-III represented a tectonic shift in modern psychiatric thinking and practice. In America, it saw an explicit change from a psychodynamic model of psychiatry back to a model based on the tenets of medical science. If the quest to reassert a medical model of psychiatry was veiled and ambiguous in DSM-II, then this was not the case with the publication of DSM-III, which was unambiguously identified as a manual based on the tenets of medical materialism. This change, which was precipitated and orchestrated by a complex mix of converging forces, correspondingly saw a significant alteration in how psychosis was understood.[32]

5.3.1 DSM-III process

The restitution of an American medical model of psychiatry with DSM-III was a momentous event which ended nearly thirty years of a psychodynamic understanding of psychosis and other forms of psychopathology. The magnitude of this

---

[32] See Appendix Two for a comprehensive critical appraisal of various factors and forces that influenced the DSM-III review process. Although many authors have examined the history of DSM-III's formulation, none have drawn together an exposition that maps the variety of socio-political forces, and other determining factors, that collectively influenced its production. Therefore, my extensive research into and critical appraisal of this historical transition provides a unique explication of the socio-political and economic influences that shaped the reinstitution of a medical model of psychiatry in DSM-III. In terms of better understanding the nature of psychosis, it also illuminates the generally invisible dynamics that have operated to maintain a restrictive clinical view of this enigmatic phenomenon.

change is reflected in descriptors used by various authors. For instance, DSM-III has been referred to as: "a major turning point" (Klerman, 1984, p. 539); a revolutionary occurrence (Rogler, 1997, p. 10; Decker, 2007, p. 350); a "sea change" (Tsuang et al., 2000, p. 1042); a "dramatic shift in orientation" (Gruenberg et al., 2005, p. 3); and a "major paradigm change" (Heinimaa, 2008, p. 50). This change was engineered by a minority faction of medically oriented American psychiatrists who saw the psychodynamic nature of DSM-I and DSM-II as overly theoretical. They subsequently worked to supersede this in DSM-III with an ostensible "atheoretical" model that eschewed assumptions of aetiology in preference for identifying specific diagnostic criteria (Spitzer, 1985, p. 522). In their view, this process re-established the professional legitimacy of psychiatry which, in its psychodynamic form, was censured by some as being redundant because it was essentially indiscernible from psychology (Mayes & Horwitz, 2005, p. 257; Hackett, 1977, p. 434). Klerman (1978, p. 106) described this transformation as "a Kraepelinian revival", which seemingly justifies Jackson's aforementioned view that the DSM-II revision represented a 'step in a backward direction' toward Kraepelinian thinking.

The review process began in 1974 (APA, 1980, p. 2). Although there was little initial indication of impending ideological changes (Kirk & Kutchins, 1992), these became increasingly overt during the ensuing years, culminating in what Healy (2002a, p. 304) referred to as "a successful palace coup" by medical psychiatrists with the 1980 publication of DSM-III. While the task force hailed the new manual for its scientific value, and Klerman (1984, p. 541) optimistically described it as "science in the service of healing", others were less approving. For example, Faust & Miner (1986, p. 962, 966) referred to it as an empirical "throwback" and "quick fix", Schacht (1985, p. 515) as a "*political* document", and Vaillant (1984, p. 545) as the product of "a bold series of choices based on guess, taste, prejudice and hope". The formulation of DSM-III, then, was marked by much controversy and conflict of opinion.

The review process saw the instigation of three key developments which reflected its ideological shift back to a biomedical model of psychiatry.[33] First, a generic definition for 'mental disorder' was formulated in an attempt to consolidate the discipline's scope of clinical focus (APA, 1980, p. 363). According to Spitzer & Endicott (1978, p. 15), this was a landmark endeavour which had not previously occurred in DSM, ICD, or other "standard textbooks of medicine and psychiatry". A second novel development was the formulation of a framework of operational diagnostic categories and criteria, which have since been incorporated into global psychiatry (Mayes & Horwitz, 2005, p. 250).[34] A final innovation was the development of a multiaxial evaluation system

---

[33] For a more detailed account of these developments, see Appendix Two, Section A2.3.

[34] In psychiatric terms, a mental disorder is invested with an operational definition as follows:

> Instead of stating that the typical features of a disease are features, A, B, C, D and E, etc., an unambiguous statement is presented in the operational definition defining precisely how much of A, B, C, D and E must be present (or about) to fulfil the definition, e.g. a disorder X may be diagnosed if the patient has one of the symptoms listed under A, two of the symptoms under B, one of the symptoms under C, etc. Thus proceeding operationally facilitates precise, reliable, unambiguous features of disorder to be defined. (Farmer, 1997, p. 56)

by which "every case be assessed on each of several 'axes', each of which refers to a different class of information" (APA, 1980, p. 23). This consisted of five axes of evaluation, which formed a complete clinical picture when combined.[35] Overall, these new DSM-III developments established a medical model of psychiatry with ostensibly increased diagnostic reliability, which Allardyce et al. (2010, p. 1) define as "diagnostic agreement ... among practitioners". This also resulted in a very reductive depiction of psychosis.

5.3.2 DSM-III construal of psychosis

The DSM-III project instigated a significant shift in American psychiatric conceptualisations of psychosis. Three decades of psychodynamic understanding was superseded by a medical model that compressed psychotic symptomatology into an operationalised system whereby boxes were progressively ticked to arrive at a diagnostic label. This saw the understanding of psychosis narrowed to the simple identification of symptoms, with potential psychological determinants being eclipsed, or given peripheral clinical value (Blashfield, 1984, p. 123). Frances & Cooper (1981, p. 1199) noted that while this method provided an effective structure for collating symptom sets, it was phenomenologically superficial because it "generally selects material on the psychological surface". This change resulted in the reification of psychotic disorders. For example, the construal of schizophrenia as a homogenous psychopathological entity was established through a system of operationalised selection criteria that represented "a modification of the criteria used in the Research Diagnostic Criteria",[36] combined with a selection of Schneider's first rank symptoms (Spitzer, Andreasen & Endicott, 1978, pp. 490, 492). In contrast, then, to the unitary depiction of schizophrenia in DSM-I and DSM-II, schizophrenia in DSM-III was invested with relatively distinct boundaries via operationalised diagnostic criteria.

Despite the DSM-III authors understanding that the manual's diagnostic categories and criteria were provisional, they had the general effect of investing mental disorders with an artificial solidity. As Andreasen (1997b, p. 108) explained, the DSM-III diagnostic criteria were "intended only as a 'provisional consensus agreement'" for ongoing scientific research and diagnostic refinement, but became "reified and given power that they were originally never intended". In her view, this was a development that

---

[35] See Appendix Two, Section A2.3.4.
[36] The Research Diagnostic Criteria (RDC) is a diagnostic tool fashioned by Spitzer et al. (1975). It is an adapted version of Feighner et al.'s (1972) operational diagnostic criteria for fourteen psychiatric illnesses, which, in turn, were modelled on a method developed by Robins & Guze (1970, p. 983) for "achieving diagnostic validity ... in five phases: clinical description, laboratory study, exclusion of other disorders, follow-up study, and family study". According to Spitzer, Robins & Endicott (1978, p. 1):

> The Research Diagnostic Criteria (RDC) were formally developed to enable research investigators to apply a consistent set of criteria for the description or selection of samples of subjects with functional psychiatric illness ... The purpose of this approach to psychiatric diagnosis is to obtain relatively homogenous groups of subjects who meet specified diagnostic criteria.

worked to "discourage creative or innovative thinking about the psychological and neural mechanisms of schizophrenia" (ibid.). Overall, then, despite DSM-III medical model developments, an understanding of the nature of psychosis remained obscure. Arguably, this was largely due to the empirical reification of the diagnostic picture of psychosis in DSM-III, which has consequently seen the potential psychological determinants of psychosis increasingly eclipsed from the psychiatric picture.

5.3.3 DSM-III-R process

In 1987, an upgraded manual was published in the form of DSM-III-R. Although some minor changes were made, the manual basically followed the same DSM-III formula of a categorised descriptive system with operationalised diagnostic criteria. The review process began in 1983 when updated research revealed diagnostic shortcomings in the recently released DSM-III. As explained by the task force, the manual "needed to be reviewed for consistency, clarity, and conceptual accuracy, and revised when necessary" (APA, 1987, p. xvii). Accordingly, Mayes & Horwitz (2005, p. 264) observed that DSM-III-R "reaffirmed and solidified the transformation of psychiatry and mental health that the DSM-III began in 1980". Hence, the upgraded manual aimed to further validate and consolidate the legitimacy of psychiatry as a medical profession. The transition from DSM-III to DSM-III-R saw no major clinical changes in conceptualisations of psychosis. Indeed, the DSM-III-R definition for 'psychotic' remained essentially the same as in DSM-III. The only difference was that, while DSM-III defined 'psychotic' as "gross impairment in reality testing" (APA, 1980, p. 367), DSM-III-R redefined it as "gross impairment in reality testing and the creation of a new reality" (APA, 1987, p. 404). No explanation was provided as to why the extra criterion of 'creating a new reality' was added or how or if this reflected a new development in understanding psychosis.

5.3.4 DSM-III-R construal of psychosis

Although DSM-III-R saw no major medical changes in relation to psychosis, significant changes did occur within a cultural context. While cultural matters had been addressed in earlier DSM issues as marginal considerations (APA, 1980, p. 188; 1968, pp. 21–22; 1952, p. 47), in DSM-III-R they became more central to diagnostic practice, especially in consideration of psychotic disorders. In regards to schizophrenic-like symptoms, for example, the manual stipulated that "when an experience or behavior is entirely normative for a particular culture … it should not be regarded as pathological" and that "the experience of hallucinating the voice of the deceased" is an example of a symptom that may be considered culturally normal (APA, 1987, p. xxvi). Additionally, whereas DSM-III defined bizarre delusions as a state whereby "content is patently absurd and has *no* possible basis in fact" (APA, 1980, p. 188), DSM-III-R redefined them as "involving a phenomenon that the person's culture would regard as totally implausible", such as "being controlled by a dead person" (APA, 1987, p. 194). In justifying this cultural addition Kendler et al. (1989, p. 954) explained that: "a culture-free definition of bizarreness is difficult to defend, since what would not be bizarre in one culture (e.g., spirit possession) could be bizarre in another". Although the introduction of a cultural context was laudable it was also diagnostically and conceptually problematic. For instance, from a purely medical perspective, the presence of bizarre delusions alone can warrant a diagnosis of schizophrenia because they are deemed intrinsically psychopathological (Pull, 2002, p. 3). However, from the perspective of cultural relativity it appears that the *social context* of a bizarre belief, rather than the belief per se, is the essential marker of psychopathology. Hence, incorporating cultural relativity into medical psychiatry paradoxically established a situation whereby a defining diagnostic psychotic marker may also be construed as not implicitly psychotic.[37]

5.3.5 Conceptual issues

The ideological swing from a psychodynamic to a medical model in DSM-III was shaped by a complex mix of scientific, social, economic, and political forces that converged to mould an understanding of psychosis that has been passed onto subsequent DSM editions. First, as a social force, medical-minded advocates refashioned psychotic disorders into reified diagnostic entities, thus establishing the appearance of improved medical certitude. This group, which became known as "the neo-Kraepelinians", championed key tenets of Kraepelinian thinking as "part of a general movement of psychiatry towards greater integration with medicine", particularly the categorisation of mental disorders (Klerman, 1978, pp. 104–106).[38] Second, forces of economic expediency coalesced with this development to influence the diagnostic parameters of DSM-III disorders. The foremost influence was from health insurance companies that pressured psychiatry to provide medically legitimate diagnoses so as to differentiate psychiatric illnesses from non-medical psychological problems (Decker, 2007, p. 345). Consequently, Schacht (1985, p. 514) concluded that DSM-III had become "an official document that participates in the organization and distribution of social and economic power".[39] Third, psychiatry's political imperative of establishing scientific legitimacy and jurisdiction resulted in psychotic disorders being forged in a medical mould. As Schacht (ibid., p. 516) explained, the belief that science and politics should be separate is erroneous because "political forces are an integral part of the rational-scientific knowledge-producing process". He subsequently asserted that "DSM-III is a *political* document" (p. 515); a view mirrored by DSM-III and DSM-III-R task force Chair, Robert Spitzer (1985, p. 523), who observed midway through the divisive DSM-III-R review process that the "ultimate outcome will be determined by a political process involving rhetoric and negotiation among groups with different goals and

---

[37] This conundrum is further examined in Chapter Twelve within a psychospiritual context, because it proffers potential new pathways for better understanding psychosis.
[38] See Appendix Two, Section A2.4.1 for further detailed discussion of this issue.
[39] See Appendix Two, Section A2.4.2 for further detailed discussion of this issue.

perspectives, as was the case with DSM-III".[40] Overall, then, it appears that ideological and socio-economic-political forces considerably influenced the depiction of psychotic disorders in DSM-III and DSM-III-R.

The problems in DSM-III of defining 'mental disorder' and the parameters of psychiatric practice also featured in DSM-III-R. This is evident in Gaines' (1992, p. 15) critique of the ambiguity of definition in DSM-III-R:

> In looking at the disorders classified by DSM-III-R, one finds a variety of diseases but not an explicit common feature, aside from their inclusion … One might well ask, What do all the various disorders listed have in common? This very question appears in the Introductions of both DSM-III and III-R. Yet, no common element or elements could be offered uniting all the pathological conditions, behaviors, emotions, beliefs, states and processes.

The inability to define 'mental disorder' is a vexing problem for psychiatry because its professional legitimacy and jurisdictional scope are dependent on doing so. Without this, the designated body of mental disorders have no unifying core that, collectively and individually, identifies them as belonging to the psychiatric domain. This important issue was not redressed in DSM-III-R. Indeed, it appears that despite assurances about the veracity of DSM disorders, their essential nature remains elusive. It also seems that a combination of social, economic, and political influences, more than scientific evidence, has been the foremost decider about which mental disorders are included in each revised manual. Furthermore, these socio-economic and political forces have seemingly played a significant role in establishing a reductive construal of psychosis in DSM-III and DSM-III-R.

5.4 DSM-IV, DSM-IV-TR and DSM-5: the medical model reinforced

While DSM-III and DSM-III-R saw the reinstitution and consolidation of a medical model of psychiatry in America, the manuals since then, (i.e. DSM-IV (1994), DSM-IV-TR (2000), and DSM-5 (2013))[41] have reinforced this model. All three manuals have maintained the same basic structure established in DSM-III of descriptive categories and operationalised diagnostic criteria, though the multiaxial system became optional in DSM-IV and was abandoned in DSM-5. A significant development throughout this era, however, was the close relationship formed between psychiatry and pharmaceutical companies. This has arguably operated as a socioeconomic force to entrench and preserve a medical understanding of psychopathology and psychosis. Also, instructions for diagnostic cultural considerations have been substantially advanced.

---

[40] See Appendix Two, Section A2.4.3 for further detailed discussion of this issue.
[41] The shift from Roman to Arabic numerals, that is, from DSM-V to DSM-5, occurred in December 2009 as an attempt by the task force to distance itself, and the manual, from the considerable controversy and criticisms surrounding the initial DSM-V review process (Decker, 2010, online).

While this is a progressive development it has also amplified the aforementioned diagnostic conundrum regarding the seeming discord between cultural relativity and clinical positivism.[42]

5.4.1 DSM-IV process

The diagnostic reign of DSM-III-R was short-lived. In May 1988, only four months after its publication, the APA appointed a task force to review the manual in preparation for DSM-IV (Kirk & Kutchins, 1992, p. 207). Allen Frances was nominated as the new task force Chair, and Spitzer was relegated to an advisory role. A chief aim of the DSM-IV review process was to achieve improved empirical legitimacy. As explained by Francis et al. (1991, p. 171),[43] "the major difference between the preparation of DSM-IV and that of DSM-III and III-R is its emphasis on explicit review and documentation of the available data". This task was undertaken via: "1) comprehensive and systematic reviews of the published literature, 2) reanalyses of already-collected data sets, and 3) extensive issue-focussed field trials" (APA, 1994, p. xviii). Although the increased attention to empirical rigour in DSM-IV represented a proactive diagnostic development, this change arguably implied that the empirical processes employed in formulating DSM-III and DSM-III-R were perceived as somehow lacking. Indeed, it seems the instigation of the DSM-IV review process, so soon after the publication of DSM-III-R, was an attempt by the APA to distance the discipline from criticisms about the empirical veracity of the DSM-III manuals. For instance, Kirk & Kutchins (1992, p. 209) maintained that DSM-III-R was empirically dubious because, in their view, its diagnostic categories were arbitrary constructs born chiefly of political decision-making processes. Skodal (2000, p. 447) later observed that "DSM-III and DSM-III-R were both the results of expert group consensus … In contrast, each DSM-IV work group was responsible for conducting comprehensive literature reviews to explicitly document evidence supporting the fourth edition's text and criteria". It therefore appears that the DSM-IV empirical upgrade was deemed necessary in order to redress criticisms regarding the subjective and political influences inherent to formulating the DSM-III manuals.

5.4.2 DSM-IV construal of psychosis

Although the categories of psychotic disorders in DSM-IV generally remained the same as in DSM-III-R, the DSM-IV definition for 'psychotic' was markedly different. Whereas DSM-III-R provided a descriptive snapshot of various symptomatic manifestations of the generic psychotic state of "gross impairment in reality testing" (APA, 1987, pp. 404–405), DSM-IV portrayed the psychotic state as manifold, explaining that "different disorders in DSM-IV emphasize different aspects of the

---

[42] See my closing sentence in Section 5.3.4 above.
[43] In this article Allen Frances' surname is misspelt as 'Francis'. I have adopted the incorrect spelling of 'Francis' for citation purposes.

various definitions of *psychotic*" (APA, 1994, p. 770). Put simply, DSM-III-R proffered one essential definition for 'psychotic' as the common denominator for all psychotic disorders, while DSM-IV provided several nuanced definitions that respectively reflected different contexts of psychotic experience. Additionally, while DSM-III-R clearly depicted impaired reality testing as the constitutive marker of psychotic experience, DSM-IV was ambiguous about this. For instance, although it stated that "the term [psychotic] has been defined conceptually as ... a gross impairment in reality testing", this is proffered as one among several definitions, "none of which has achieved universal acceptance" (ibid.). Consequently, the definition of 'psychotic' in DSM-IV seems more ambiguous than in DSM-III-R. In terms of psychotic symptomatology, some minor fine-tuning of psychotic diagnostic criteria occurred (Tsuang et al., 2000, p. 1042), resulting in minimal changes. For instance, the duration of active symptoms for schizophrenia was increased from a week to a month, and a couple of negative symptoms were added (e.g., alogia and avolition) (APA, 1994, p. 779). Also, the DSM-III Brief Reactive Psychosis was renamed Brief Psychotic Disorder and updated so a diagnosis could be made without the presence of a precipitating stressor (ibid.). Arguably, this alteration represented a further incremental development in the neo-Kraepelinian effort to distance psychiatry from psychodynamic principles and terminology.

In DSM-IV, the DSM-III-R cross-cultural instruction was significantly upgraded. This included four innovations to help cultivate cultural sensitivity:

1. An "Outline for Cultural Formulation" that provided a "systematic review of the individual's cultural background, the role of the cultural context in the expression and evaluation of symptoms and dysfunction, and the effect that cultural differences may have on the relationship between the individual and the clinician" (APA, 1994, pp. 843–844).
2. A "Glossary of Culture-Bound Syndromes" that listed "the best-studied culture-bound syndromes and idioms of distress that may be encountered in clinical practice ... and ... includes relevant DSM-IV categories when data suggest that they should be considered in a diagnostic formulation" (ibid., pp. 844–849).
3. Discussions and descriptions throughout the manual about "specific cultural factors relating to many of the axis I and axis II disorders" (Turner et al., 1995, p. 442).
4. A new V-Code (62.89) titled "Religious or spiritual problem" (APA, 1994, p. 685).[44]

Prior to publication, the DSM-IV Cultural Committee proposed that cultural considerations about schizophrenia be given diagnostic primacy (Jenkins, 1998, p. 361), however, the task force did not accept this proposition and relegated cultural concerns to the multiaxial system of optional diagnostic considerations (APA, 1994, p. 843).

---

[44] The transpersonal origins of the 'Religious or spiritual problem' category, and dynamics pertaining to its eventual inclusion in DSM-IV, are examined in Chapter Seven, Section 7.1.

This presumably designated cultural considerations as an optional adjunct in psychosis diagnostics. Additionally, the manual proffered the perplexing instruction that "determining whether a behavior is normative or pathological" is dependent on "cultural elements of the relationship between the individual and the clinician" (ibid., p. 844). How this translates to discerning between psychotic and culturally normative situations is very vague. What exactly is inferred by the notion of 'cultural elements of the relationship'? Does this speak of the level of proficiency in intercultural communication between patient and clinician? If so, is the incidence of the diagnosis of psychosis proportionate to achieved levels of intercultural proficiency (i.e., more proficient intercultural communication between clinician and patient results in less misdiagnoses of psychosis)? And why may a given behaviour be deemed essentially psychotic in a Western cultural context but not in a non-Western cultural context? Again, it appears the introduction of cultural relativity to a medical framework of psychiatry has raised many vexing questions and conundrums in relation to diagnosing psychotic disorders.

Finally, it is pertinent to note that psychiatry forged deeper ties with drug companies after the publication of DSM-IV, resulting in the advancement of a biomedical understanding of psychosis and the promotion of physical (i.e. pharmaceutical) treatments. Indeed, all six members of the DSM-IV Schizophrenia and Other Psychotic Disorders Work Group had financial ties to drug companies (Cosgrove et al., 2006, p. 154),[45] which ostensibly influenced how psychosis was construed in the manual. Yet, despite this biogenic trend, DSM-IV acknowledged that "no laboratory findings have been identified that are diagnostic of Schizophrenia" (APA, 1994, p. 280). Biogenic assertions by psychiatrists and drug companies have increasingly shaped the construal of psychosis beyond DSM-IV, despite the lack of substantiating biological evidence.

5.4.3 DSM-IV-TR process

The DSM-IV-TR review process was, again, headed by Allen Frances, with the upgraded manual being published in 2000. This process began in 1997 (APA, 2000, p. xxix) with the updated text and structure remaining much the same as in DSM-IV. As stated by the authors, "no substantive changes in the criteria sets were considered, nor were any proposals entertained for new disorders, new subtypes, or changes in the status of the DSM-IV appendix categories" (ibid.). However, some moderations were made. Whereas the DSM-IV task force chiefly aimed to invest the manual with a sounder empirical research foundation, the DSM-IV-TR task force worked to update and fine-tune the original content. Overall, this entailed a detailed revision of DSM-IV content and related literature in order to update the descriptive

---

[45] Cosgrove et al. (2006, pp. 154, 158) interviewed 170 DSM-IV panel members regarding their financial links with the pharmaceutical industry, of which 95 (56%) indicated having such ties.

text. The authors described this as a process of "reviewing the text carefully to identify errors or omissions and then conducting a systematic, comprehensive literature review that focused on relevant material that has been published since 1992"
(p. xxx). DSM-IV-TR also operated as a bridging document between DSM-IV and
DSM-5 (p. xxix). The content of the final published product remained much the same
as its predecessor.

5.4.4 DSM-IV-TR construal of psychosis

The bulk of DSM-IV-TR text regarding psychotic disorders replicated that in DSM-
IV. There were few changes to the psychotic disorders section of the updated
manual and no changes to the cross-cultural section. However, two updates in the
DSM-IV-TR 'Schizophrenia and Other Disorders' section ostensibly reflect efforts
to consolidate a medical and biogenic understanding of psychosis. First, the DSM-
IV term psychotic "disturbance" (APA, 1994, p. 274) was changed to read as psychotic "disorder" in DSM-IV-TR (APA, 2000, p. 298). No explanation is given for this
change. At face value this may appear to be inconsequential, however, it possibly
represents an intentional attempt to invest the term 'psychotic' with a more medically concrete meaning (i.e., whereas the term 'disturbance' is ambiguous and has
a psychological connotation, the term 'disorder' is more medical in connotation).
A second notable change was evident in the DSM-IV-TR Schizophrenia 'Associated
laboratory findings' text. This section reported on neurophysiological research that
found apparent anatomical aberrations in schizophrenic patients that did not occur
in control groups. The DSM-IV-TR version was about triple the length of that in
DSM-IV and also included a bio-aetiological emphasis that was absent in DSM-
IV (APA, 2000, pp. 305–306; 1994, p. 280). For instance, the DSM-IV-TR version
suggested that this neurophysiological finding "may have important pathophysiological implications, because it is suggestive of an early (i.e. prenatal) midline
developmental brain abnormality" (APA, 2000, p. 305). This identification of causality as 'prenatal' represents a distinct leaning towards a biogenic and genetic construal of schizophrenia for it proscribes possible psychosocial or environmental
determinants.

5.4.5 DSM-5 process

DSM-5 was published in 2013 and is the seventh and latest manual in the DSM series.
Compared to other medical model DSM updates the DSM-5 review process was a
somewhat protracted affair. The first phase began in 1999 with an appraisal of the
DSM conceptualisation of mental disorders, and culminated with the 2002 publication of a conference proceedings monograph (Kupfer et al., 2002) titled *A Research
Agenda for DSM-V* (APA, 2013, p. 6). The next five-year phase, from 2003 to 2008,
consisted of: "13 international DSM-5 research planning conferences, involving 400
participants from 39 countries, to review the world literature in specific diagnostic

areas to prepare for revisions in developing … DSM-5"; the selection of David Kupfer as task force Chair in 2006; and the inauguration of the task force in 2007 (ibid., pp. 6–7). Finally, the ensuing years, until the manual's publication in 2013, involved an intensive process of:

> conducting literature reviews and secondary analyses, publishing research reports in scientific journals, developing draft diagnostic criteria, posting preliminary drafts on the DSM-5 Web site for public comment, presenting preliminary findings at professional meetings, performing field trials, and revising criteria and text. (p. 7)

Since then, a new work group has formed to consider possible changes for the next planned update in the form of DSM-5.1 (APA, 2021; Appelbaum, 2017). Hence, the DSM series remains a provisional work in progress.

Despite this rigorous process of extensive research and multiple reviews, the DSM-5 project was plagued by controversy and marked by criticism from many quarters, far beyond that which occurred with its predecessors. Overall, key points of concern were that:

- the review process lacked adequate transparency;
- proposed new diagnostic parameters threatened to include normal human behaviours and experiences within the threshold of psychopathology; and
- many task force members had a conflict of interest due to close ties and investments with pharmaceutical companies.[46]

This controversy was exacerbated by the fact that two prior DSM task force Chairs, Robert Spitzer and Allen Frances, were among the most vocal of critics (Greenberg, 2010). In light of the controversy surrounding DSM-5, Katschnig (2010, p. 21) rhetorically questioned whether or not psychiatrists were becoming "an endangered species" due to the dubious "validity of psychiatry's diagnostic definitions and classification systems". Indeed, soon after the publication of DSM-5, Funnell (2014) reported that "psychiatry is currently experiencing a global schism" and that psychiatrists were "split on whether to ditch DSM" due to inherent problems with its observational and symptoms-based categorical approach. Additionally, due to the manual's many issues, there were calls on numerous fronts to boycott it when published, which Frances (2013b) described as "completely understandable [because] there is lots in DSM 5 to be angry at or frightened about". Yet, despite such robust criticism from prominent psychiatrists, the manual has been published and now

---

[46] For more details on these and other related issues see: Funnell, 2014; Frances, 2013a; American Psychological Association, 2011; British Psychological Society, 2011; Chapman, 2011; Pilecki et al., 2011; Citizens Commission on Human Rights, 2010; Decker, 2010; Frances, 2010; Greenberg, 2010; Horwitz, 2010; Katschnig, 2010; Citizens Commission on Human Rights, 2009; Frances, 2009.

represents the latest iteration of expert opinion on psychosis and other forms of psychopathology.

The DSM-5 review process also entailed updates to cultural considerations and the ongoing attempt to define mental illness. Several cultural-related changes and additions were made: the Outline for Cultural Formulation, which first appeared in DSM-IV, was updated; a "Glossary of Cultural Concepts of Distress" was composed; and a new comprehensive "Cultural Formulation Interview" was included (APA, 2013, pp. 749–757, 833–837). However, the updated DSM-5 definition of 'mental disorder' remained essentially the same as definitions proffered in the DSM-III and DSM-IV manuals. This ongoing quest to formulate a basic definition for 'mental disorder' is understandable because it delineates the parameters of clinical focus for the discipline of psychiatry. Without such a definition, psychiatry's operational field is rendered vague, as are related factors such as diagnostic reliability, treatment approaches, clinical research data, and medical rebate coverage for patients. However, a dilemma for psychiatry is that this ultimately appears to be an impossible task.

Finally, a significant new development in DSM-5 was the suggestion that a dimensional model should supersede the traditional categorical model due to apparent deficits in the latter (ibid., p. 5). For example, the task force maintained that:

- "a too-rigid categorical system does not capture clinical experience or important scientific observations" (ibid.);
- a transition to a dimensional model was a way to reduce "the inevitable reification that occurs with diagnostic conceptual approaches" (ibid., p. 9);
- "identifying homogeneous populations for treatment and research resulted in narrow diagnostic categories that did not capture clinical reality" (ibid., p. 12);
- and "the historical aspiration of achieving diagnostic homogeneity by progressive subtyping within disorder categories no longer is sensible; like most common human ills, mental disorders are heterogeneous at many levels" (ibid.).

However, the task force decided that, despite these factors, DSM-5 would maintain the traditional categorical model (ibid., p.13). It therefore appears that a future transition to a dimensional diagnostic model is imminent.

5.4.6 DSM-5 construal of psychosis

In general, the construal of psychosis in DSM-5 has remained much the same as in the DSM-IV series. For instance, the manual's section titled "Highlights of Changes from DSM-IV to DSM-5" has only a brief paragraph explicating some minor modifications to diagnostic criteria for several types of psychotic disorder (APA, 2013, p. 810), including two alterations to the diagnostic criteria for schizophrenia (see Table 2).

Table 2. Comparative DSM-IV-TR and DSM-5 Criterion A diagnostic criteria for schizophrenia.

Criterion A diagnostic criteria for schizophrenia

DSM-IV-TR	*DSM-5*
A. *Characteristic symptoms:* Two (or more) of the following, each present for a significant portion of time during a 1-month period (or less if successfully treated).	A. Two (or more) of the following, each present for a significant portion of time during a 1-month period (or less if successfully treated). At least one of these must be (1), (2), or (3):
1. delusions.	1. Delusions.
2. hallucinations.	2. Hallucinations.
3. disorganized speech (e.g., frequent derailment or incoherence).	3. Disorganized speech (e.g., frequent derailment or incoherence).
4. grossly disorganized or catatonic behavior.	4. Grossly disorganized or catatonic behavior.
5. negative symptoms i.e., affective flattening, alogia, or avolition.	5. Negative symptoms (i.e., diminished emotional expression or avolition).
Note: Only one Criterion A symptom is required if delusions are bizarre or hallucinations consist of a voice keeping up a running commentary on the person's behaviour or thoughts, or two or more voices conversing with each other.	(APA, 2013, p. 99)
(APA, 2000, p. 312)	

The most obvious change here is that the DSM-IV-TR note pertaining to Criterion A symptoms (i.e. bizarre delusions and particular manifestations of auditory hallucinations) has been removed from the DSM-5 diagnostic criteria specifications. Additionally, while DSM-IV-TR allowed a diagnosis of schizophrenia to be made in the absence of delusions, hallucinations, or disorganised speech (e.g., if negative symptoms combined with grossly disorganized or catatonic behaviour occurred), this is no longer possible in DSM-5 because primary diagnosis has been restricted to the first three Criterion A symptoms. The DSM-5 authors have proffered no explanation for these diagnostic changes.

A final point of note is the apparent increased emphasis on advancing an empiric and biogenic understanding of psychosis in DSM-5. This is not so much evident in text pertaining to the main diagnostic categories, but in forward-looking statements regarding future psychiatric research and practice. For instance, the new provisional dimensional assessment measure provided in DSM-5 is hailed for its promise to aid in the identification of "neurobiological deficits" and "pathophysiological mechanisms" (APA, 2013, p. 89). Furthermore, although psychological determinants are discussed, they are couched in bio-empirical language. For example, the assertion that "clinical neuropsychological assessment can help diagnosis and treatment" (ibid., p. 90) seemingly anchors psychological determinants into a neurobiological frame. Indeed, this heightened trend towards developing a mechanistic and scientific view of psychosis, in both physiological and psychological terms, is evidenced in the DSM-5 review process book titled *Deconstructing Psychosis: Refining the Research Agenda for DSM-V* (Tamminga et al., 2010). In this text, which guides present psychosis research by mainstream psychiatry, Regier (2010, pp. xvii–xix) asserts that "we will incorporate into our current understanding of psychosis new information gleaned from research now under way", which includes a particular focus on "somatic, or somatoform, features of mental illness" and a general focus on "multiple areas, ranging from molecular genetics to brain imaging to social, behavioural, and anthropological science". This view clearly places primacy upon scientific biological research. Indeed, Gur et al. (2010, p. 111) maintain that using brain imaging methods in psychosis research will "enable integration of genetic and neuroimaging paradigms in our efforts to elucidate neurobiological mechanisms that *underlie* these disorders" (italics added) To reiterate, this emphasis on biological research approach to better understanding psychosis is highly restrictive, for it fails to give due consideration to the possibility that psychosocial and psychospiritual factors may be fundamental in effecting psychotic or psychotic-like human experiences.

5.4.7 Conceptual issues

A prominent and controversial issue in the DSM-5 review process was the relationship between psychiatry and the pharmaceutical industry. This has been particularly so in regards to pharmaceutical companies seemingly shaping psychiatric diagnostics. Indeed, some commentators have alleged that political and fiscal interests, rather than good science, are increasingly shaping psychiatric diagnostics. For instance, Pilecki et al. (2011, pp. 197, 199) propose that:

> at the very least such a high degree of financial connectedness constituted a powerful influence on the decision making process that produced the DSM-IV … At worst, these relationships may indicate that psychology and psychiatry are increasingly shaped and influenced by profit-seeking corporations who are exerting their economic powers in self-serving ways.

Furthermore, Robbins et al. (2011, p. 33) have concluded that "current psychiatric research and practice have become so biased by economic interests that the public health of patients served by psychiatry may hang in the balance". This issue, which began with DSM-IV, has continued in DSM-5. For example, the task force Chair, David Kupfer, was listed as having close ties with multiple drug companies (Citizens Commission on Human Rights, 2009) while about a third of the authors who contributed to the DSM-5 psychosis research text titled *Deconstructing Psychosis: Refining the Research Agenda for DSM-V*, had declared financial or professional ties with pharmaceutical industries (Tamminga et al., 2010, pp. xii-xiii). In fact, Frances (2009) viewed the DSM-5 project as a move by medical psychiatry to fulfil "their ambition to achieve a paradigm shift when there is no scientific basis for one", and scathingly predicted the consequent

> wholesale imperial medicalization of normality that will trivialize mental disorder and lead to a deluge of unneeded medication treatments—a bonanza for the pharmaceutical industry but at a huge cost to the new false-positive patients caught in the excessively wide *DSM-V* net.

It therefore appears that the pharmaceutical industry aims to maintain a medical model of psychiatry so as to boost its profits via the sale of psychiatric medications, and that the perception and formation of psychiatric diagnostic categories are being influenced accordingly.

A related and significant issue is the ongoing quest by psychiatry to scientifically identify the putative biological cause of psychosis, an endeavour that has intensified with the DSM-5 review process. The DSM-5 manual's prominent biogenic focus is limiting in that, while it offers one pathway for attempting to better understand the enigma of psychosis, it is problematic when posed as the *ultimate* investigative method, for this effectively eclipses other investigative pathways, such as psychosocial and psychospiritual approaches. Indeed, there is no substantive evidence to support the biogenic theory of psychopathology and psychosis. As Frances (2009) observed when contesting the validity of updated and newly formulated DSM-5 mental disorder categories, "not even 1 biological test is ready for inclusion in the criteria sets for DSM-V". In this light, Andreasen (2005) contends that:

> We tend to over-biologise, we oversimplify the mechanisms of mental illness: in a reductionist framework, depression is a serotonin disease, schizophrenia a dopamine disease. But if we look only at brains, we fail to recognise the important role that personal life experiences may play in losing our minds.

Here, she clearly warns against adopting an overly stringent biomedical approach and, correspondingly, advocates the value and clinical importance of considering psychosocial determinants in the quest to better understand psychosis. Arguably, then, the present and prevailing biogenic view enables only limited scope for better understanding the enigmatic complexities of psychotic experience, while the forces and factors that hold this view in place largely proscribe an investigation by psychiatry into possible psychospiritual determents in psychosis.

5.5 Conclusion

This chapter's critical examination of DSM depictions of psychosis culminates my Focal Setting One exposition. While psychiatry has viewed psychosis variously throughout its history, including psychosomatic and psychoanalytic understandings, a prevailing biogenic trend is evident. However, socioeconomic and political factors have apparently shaped these conceptual iterations more than robust science has. The consideration of possible psychospiritual determinants has generally been absent throughout this history of understanding psychosis, which seemingly suggests such investigation is antithetical to psychiatric research. The ensuing Focal Setting Two examination of marginal yet significant occurrences of psychospiritual research within mainstream psychiatry, challenges this idea.

FOCAL SETTING TWO

UNDERSTANDING PSYCHOSIS: PSYCHIATRY AND PSYCHOSPIRITUAL CONSIDERATIONS

Focal Setting Two aims to demonstrate that while psychiatry has traditionally eschewed psychospiritual considerations, such investigation is possible. This sets the conceptual stage for my deeper investigation of the psychosis-psychospiritual nexus throughout Focal Settings Three and Four.

CHAPTER 6

A historical overview of psychospiritual considerations by psychiatry: part one: pre-1980

6.0 Introduction

This chapter aims to challenge the view that psychospiritual considerations are essentially extraneous to psychiatric practice and discourse by examining three significant pre-1980 occurrences within mainstream psychiatry that counter this perception. These are: assertions by APA presidents as to the psychiatric relevance of psychospiritual matters; Dean's notions of metapsychiatry and ultraconsciousness; and the Group for the Advancement of Psychiatry's (GAP) investigative report on mysticism.

6.1 Psychospiritual assertions by APA presidents

Since the late 1800s, at least three APA presidents have championed the importance of psychospiritual considerations in psychiatry.[47] Although their views do not reflect those of the psychiatric majority, they do demonstrate that mainstream psychiatry is not devoid of psychospiritual standpoints.

6.1.1 Richard M. Bucke

Richard Bucke, the 1890 president of the then American Medico-Psychological Association (now the APA), exemplified the merging of metaphysical and psychiatric concerns. Integral to his work was the notion of 'Cosmic Consciousness', a phrase he

---

[47] These are the only three instances I am aware of. It is possible, however, that other APA presidents have also endorsed the value of psychospiritual considerations in psychiatric practice.

coined after a brief experience of mystical illumination in 1872, at the age of thirty-six (Bucke, 1901, pp. 9–10). He presented a paper on Cosmic Consciousness at the Association's 1894 annual meeting in Philadelphia where he proposed that the human mind was verging on a further phase of evolutionary development:

> Cosmic Consciousness is not simply an expansion or extension of the self conscious mind with which we are all familiar, but the superaddition of a function as distinct from any possessed by the average man as self consciousness is distinct from any function possessed by one of the higher animals. (1894, p. 7)

Hence, he understood Cosmic Consciousness as representing a transformative paradigm shift in the evolutionary development of humanity. He described this as "a consciousness of the Cosmos … a consciousness of the life and order of the universe; not … a knowledge of this, but a consciousness of it" (ibid., p. 10) and also referred to it variously as a state of "intellectual illumination" (ibid.), "instantaneous illumination" (p. 12), and an "unusual spirituality" (p. 14). In his view, this state of consciousness represented the pinnacle of human evolution.

Bucke's treatise on Cosmic Consciousness ostensibly represents the first, if not only, instance within mainstream psychiatry whereby a psychospiritual aetiology of psychosis is proposed. While others have noted correlations between psychopathological and psychospiritual experiences, Bucke is unique in depicting the former as having its causal roots in the latter. He hypothesised that, in human evolution, newly emergent faculties initially appear and develop within relatively few people of a particular race, and that these faculties are often tenuous and unstable (Bucke, 1897, p. 645). Cosmic Consciousness, in his view, characterised such an embryonic faculty. Furthermore, in keeping with the social Darwinist belief of the time, he maintained that, due to its advanced mental status, the Aryan race was at the vanguard of an evolutionary transition from self consciousness into Cosmic Consciousness, and that cases of insanity signified unstable instances of this faculty emerging (ibid.). Accordingly, he concluded that the high incidence of insanity in America and Europe was the result of "the rapid evolution in late millenniums of the mind of the Aryan people", while, conversely, for other races of supposedly less mental advancement "there exists comparatively little insanity" (Bucke, 1901, p. 60). Objectionable racial elitism aside, this view largely depicts madness as being an inevitable part of an unfolding metaphysical evolutionary process, and as disruptive and harrowing as it might seem, it actually heralds the emergence of an eventual apotheosis of human evolution via the achievement of Cosmic Consciousness. Hence, Bucke's notion of Cosmic Consciousness depicts the aetiology of mental disorders as fundamentally psychospiritual.

Bucke's work also represents the apparent first attempt within mainstream psychiatry to differentiate psychopathological from metaphysical experiences. For instance, he explained that:

> in every, or nearly every, man who enters into cosmic consciousness apprehension is at first more or less excited, the person doubting whether the new sense may

not be a symptom or form of insanity. The first thing each person asks himself upon experiencing the new sense is: Does what I see and feel represent reality or am I suffering from a delusion? … How, then, shall we know that this is a new sense, revealing fact, and not a form of insanity, plunging its subject into delusion? (Bucke, 1901, pp. 69–70)

His response to this conundrum was to identify four differentiation criteria for discerning psychopathological from psychospiritual experiences. In short, these were that:

1. the predispositions of those experiencing psychopathology are "distinctly amoral or even immoral", while those experiencing Cosmic Consciousness "are moral in a very high degree";
2. "self-restraint" or "inhibition" is diminished in the former and enhanced in the latter;
3. "if … cosmic consciousness is a form of insanity, we are confronted by the terrible fact … that our civilization, including all our highest religions, rests on delusion"; and
4. there exists a high degree of epistemological and experiential concord between those who have experienced Cosmic Consciousness throughout history (ibid., pp. 71–72).

Arguably, the latter two points are more an attempt at validating the experience of Cosmic Consciousness, for they seem to stray from the objective of differentiating insanity from valid mystical experience. This issue aside, Bucke's proposal demonstrates that psychospiritual dynamics can be, and have been, considered within the corpus of mainstream psychiatry's quest to better understand psychotic or psychotic-like experiences.[48]

6.1.2 Francis J. Braceland

Francis Braceland's 1957 presidential address to the APA convention in Chicago represents another instance of an APA president advocating the importance of including psychospiritual considerations in psychiatric epistemology and practice. Braceland (1957, pp. 3–4) held that psychiatry was but one discipline in the composite "science of man" and that psychiatrists should ideally "achieve wisdom" of the

---

[48] Despite Bucke's presidential status, it appears the psychiatric community did not take him seriously. For instance, subsequent issues of *The American Journal of Insanity* featured no articles, or commentaries, in response to his theory. The only rejoinder (that I was able to find) was the sardonic comment in an 1896 *British Journal of Psychiatry* review that "we fear that if and when his prediction comes true, it will be time for the sane to build themselves asylums" (The Editor, 1896, p. 177). Nonetheless, it appears Bucke was a man ahead of his time, for his recognition of the phenomenological parallels between psychospiritual and psychotic experiences has since been reiterated by many psychiatrists, clinicians, and scholars. This issue is further examined and critically appraised throughout Focal Setting Three.

"encompassing and well ordered knowledge" of being human. He endorsed an integrative, holistic, and scientific approach, asserting that clinical psychiatry and neurophysiology had demonstrated that "the various aspects of human existence and nature interpenetrate each other" (ibid., p. 7). Further to this, he maintained that "the net result of the evidence we have underscores the need to approach psychological problems from the humanistic point of view which affirms man's spiritual nature" (ibid.). In terms of zeitgeist, or "the general cultural atmosphere in which a person grows up and lives", he observed that "psychiatry is finding it rewarding to give consideration to these cultural—in the widest sense, spiritual—conditions, as much as to the factors constituting the social situation of the individual" (p. 8). In sum, while Braceland failed to define what 'man's spiritual nature' is, or articulate how clinicians might consider this in therapeutic practice, he clearly stressed the importance for psychiatry to take psychospiritual considerations seriously. Indeed, he ostensibly depicts them as being integral aspects of the global 'science of man'. Overall, then, he demonstrates the capacity for psychiatry to extend its epistemological parameters beyond the strictures of materialism to include metaphysical realities as part of scientific investigation.

6.1.3 Jules H. Masserman

Jules Masserman's 1979 Chicago presidential address represents another instance of an APA president attesting to the value of incorporating psychospiritual matters into psychiatric thinking and practice. In his speech, Masserman (1979, p. 1014) delivered an appraisal of psychiatry's ideal role in fostering mental health and identified three key areas of human need that "may serve as a template into which we may partially fit the past, present, and future of APA". These were physical needs, social needs, and "a system of values and mystic beliefs to provide metapsychological serenity" (ibid.). Strongly influenced by his internship under Adolf Meyer and his subsequent exposure to the Meyerian model of "integrative psychobiology", Masserman averred that "traditional classifications of personality types and mental diseases thus appeared to me to be nosologically, prognostically, and therapeutically inadequate" (p. 1013). He also claimed that "our current manuals almost never fulfill the essential purposes of a truly adequate *dia-gnosis* (Greek, thorough knowledge)" (p. 1016) and proposed that a more effective model of psychiatry would employ a comprehensive and integrated knowledge of the manifold domains of human needs and nature in its diagnostic practices (p. 1015). Although he did not use the word 'spiritual' throughout his address, his references to 'mystic' and 'metapsychological' needs in human mental health apparently connote this.

Masserman's address was titled "The future of psychiatry as a scientific and humanitarian discipline in a changing world", which suggests he understood metapsychological considerations to be part and parcel of the astute scientific practice of medical psychiatry. This is exemplified in his concluding comments on interdisciplinary "scientific sessions" (p. 1018):

The scientist has scaled the mountains of ignorance; he is about to conquer the highest peak; as he pulls himself over the final rock, he is greeted by a band of theologians who have been sitting there for centuries. (Jastrow[49] in Masserman, ibid.)

Here he obviously infers that spiritual adepts are ahead of their scientific counterparts in the quest to understand the nature of reality and, presumably, insanity. Arguably, he also suggests that both materialist and metaphysical investigative approaches are valid pathways to the mountain peak of knowledge formation, an idea that was absent from the updated DSM-III medical model manual, published the year after his address.

6.2 Stanley Dean: ultraconsciousness and metapsychiatry

The emergence of the notion of 'metapsychiatry' in American psychiatry during the 1970s exemplifies the capacity for the discipline to centrally include psychospiritual matters within its investigative remit. The instigator and champion of metapsychiatry was Stanley Dean who was "one of the leading psychiatrists in North America" (Canadian Press, 1976, p. 11). As a noted Clinical Professor of Psychiatry (Dean, 1975a, p. 43) and a self-professed "conservative medical man" (Harakas, 1985, p. 1) he was an unlikely candidate to urge the exploration of psychospiritual matters by psychiatry. His proposed remit for metapsychiatry as a branch of psychiatric interest was to investigate ultraconscious phenomena (Dean, 1971, p. 662).[50] Whereas the metaphysical views of the aforementioned APA presidents found little support from fellow psychiatrists, Dean's proposal to establish a branch of metapsychiatry within mainstream psychiatry attracted considerable support and interest. Indeed, his endeavour resulted in metaphysical and psi research[51] being incorporated, albeit briefly, into the lexicon and language of mainstream American psychiatry.

6.2.1 Ultraconsciousness

Before examining the advent and development of metapsychiatry, it is prudent to first investigate its origins in Dean's initial notion of 'ultraconsciousness'. His interest in this field of knowledge was triggered by four separate, yet related, events during the early 1960s:

1. his exposure to Zen Buddhist meditative and healing practices (Dean, 1970a, p. 33);
2. his discovery that "great numbers of sensible, rational people from all walks of life, lay and professional, believed in the ultraconscious" (American Press, 1984, p. 16);

---

[49] Jastrow, R. (1978). *God and the astronomers*. W.W. Norton, p.116.
[50] The terms 'ultraconsciousness' and 'metapsychaitry' are defined and examined below in Sections 6.2.1 and 6.2.2.
[51] According to Varvoglis (c2009), *psi* is "the term parapsychologists use to generically refer to all kinds of psychic phenomena, experiences, or events that seem to be related to the psyche, or mind, and which cannot be explained by established physical principles".

3. his perception that many of these people "heard voices, saw visions, communicated with spirits ... Yet I found in them no other indication of psychosis" (Harakas, 1985, p. 1); and

4. his experience in clinical practice of "observing paranormal phenomena of schizophrenics" (Rothman, 1982, p. 20).

Later, in 1972, his "observations of psychic healings in Bali" further fuelled his interests (Dean, 1975b, p. 4). In his first published mention of ultraconsciousness in a Letter to the Editor of *The American Journal of Psychiatry*, Dean (1965, p. 471) maintained that despite psychiatry's "amazing advances in recent years ... the secret of mental health still remains a secret". This set the stage for his subsequent introduction of the notion of 'ultraconsciousness' as a proposed key to the elusive secret of mental health. Indeed, he stated that the aim of his letter was "to argue for the systematic investigation of the ultraconscious and its integration into current psychiatric and psychotherapeutic usage ... because of its extraordinary ability to bring about freedom from mental and physical suffering" (ibid.). As such, Dean's primary focus was to promote the potential of ultraconsciousness for fostering mental health, a stance he maintained throughout his ensuing two-decade endeavour to establish a rapprochement between ultraconsciousness and psychiatry.

Dean coined the term 'ultraconsciousness' to reflect the spiritual knowledge and experience espoused within many religious, cultural, and mystical traditions over millennia. For instance, he defined it as "a supra-sensory, supra-rational state of mentation whose existence has been known since antiquity ... [and] has been called many names: *nirvana, satori, samedhi, shema, kairos,* cosmic-consciousness, *unio-mystica,* Godliness, etc." (ibid.). However, he also saw the term as being congruent with modern psychiatric language and explained that "for the purposes of standardization I have proposed the term 'ultraconsciousness' to provide a semantic tie to current psychiatric terminology" (Dean, 1973, p. 1036). He originally referred to this as "the summit of the ultraconscious mind" (Dean, 1965, p. 471), then "the summit of the Ultraconscious" (1970a, p. 36), and finally as "the ultraconscious summit" (Dean, 1973, p. 1037), all of which designate a peak psychospiritual state of consciousness. Dean also used the term 'ultraconsciousness' in relation to other metaphysical occurrences. For instance, he referred to it in context of psi phenomena, which he described as "flashes and *formes frustes* ... probably latent in all of us" (Dean, 1965, p. 471).[52] He later stated that "though total ultraconsciousness is rare, a great variety of lesser manifestations is extremely common" (Dean, 1975a, p. 46). Thus, he posited two meanings for the term: one inferring an ultimate state of mystical illumination, and the other inferring forms of paranormal human experience or capacity. Both of these metaphysical realities, however, are generally regarded as illusory by medical science and as potentially indicative of psychotic delusional ideation by mainstream psychiatry.

---

[52] Dean did not articulate what these *formes frustes* or psi phenomena were until six years later when he introduced the notion of 'metapsychiatry' in 1971. These are listed below in Section 6.2.2.

Hence, Dean faced the formidable challenge of establishing the validity of his ultra-consciousness theory.

In order to support his notion of ultraconsciousness, Dean drew attention to similar views expressed by APA presidents, Braceland and Bucke. For example, he frequently cited Braceland's appeal for psychiatry to heed "Man's spiritual nature" (Dean, 1970a, p. 33; 1970b; p. 58; 1974a, p. 18; 1975b, p. 6). His incorporation of Bucke's work, however, was far more significant. For example, he asserted that Bucke's proposed signs of Cosmic Consciousness reflected "the ultimate peak of ultraconsciousness" and listed these as follows:

1) Awareness of intense light.
2) Emotions of supreme rapture and transcendental love.
3) Intellectual illumination and uncovering of latent genius.
4) Identification with creativity, infinity and immortality.
5) Absence of all physical and mental suffering.
6) De-emphasis of material wealth.
7) Enhancement of physical vigour and activity.
8) A sense of mission.
9) A charismatic change in personality. (Dean, 1970b, p. 61)

Intriguingly, Dean gave the impression that this was Bucke's original list and did not explain it was his own adaptation.[53] It is possible that this adaptation of Bucke's work was an attempt by Dean to make these points reflect his personal vision and to invest them with significance and utility that would be meaningful and acceptable to conventional psychiatry of the time. For instance, Dean's (1970b, p. 60) explication on point 5 directly reflects his core belief in the potential utility of ultraconscious knowledge for psychiatry: "This property alone should be of particular interest to ... the psychiatrist ... and should give us an incentive to understand and use it in the treatment of the ... mentally ill". Also, the notion of a reduction in materialist interests (Dean's point 6) was more likely to pass the test of conventionality than Bucke's notion of a 'loss of a sense of sin', which many psychiatrists would likely have rejected as outdated religious dogma. Although it is unclear why Dean did not explain his adaptation of Bucke's original points, he subsequently instituted them as being fundamental to his idea of metapsychiatry.

A few years later, Dean added a tenth point to this list of indicators. He explained that "from the welter of literature and liturgy, ancient and modern, I have summarised

---

[53] Bucke (1901, p. 79) originally posited eleven signs or "marks of the Cosmic Sense":

> a) The subjective light; b) The moral elevation; c) The intellectual illumination; d) The sense of immortality; e) The loss of fear of death; f) The loss of sense of sin; g) The suddenness, instantaneousness of the awakening; h) The previous character of the man—intellectual, moral, physical; i) The age of illumination; j) The added charm to the personality so that men and women are always (?) [sic] strongly attracted to the person; k) The transfiguration of the subject of the change as seen by others when the cosmic sense is actually present.

ten distinguishing characteristics of the ultraconscious summit" (Dean, 1973, p. 1037). His tenth point stated that:

> There is a sudden or gradual development of extraordinary perception, telepathy, precognition, or healing. Though generally regarded as occult, such phenomena may have a more rational explanation; they may be due to an awakening of the transhuman powers of perception latent in all of us. (ibid.)

Here Dean eschewed the general view maintained by psychiatry that belief in occult phenomena is irrational and potentially psychopathological. In his view, such phenomena were natural, conceivably beneficial, and within the scope of rational understanding. Hence, he saw psychospiritual matters as being a legitimate concern for psychiatric research, thinking, and practice. From such thinking emerged his notion of 'metapsychiatry'. Whereas ultraconsciousness was principally a theoretical notion, the term 'metapsychiatry' represented the transposition of theory into a modality of psychiatric practice.

6.2.2 Metapsychiatry

In 1971, after six years promoting ultraconsciousness and its potential therapeutic benefits for psychiatry, Dean coined the term 'metapsychiatry' as the name for a prospective branch of psychiatry that engaged in the scientific study of metaphysical experiences, phenomena, and reality. This marked a shift from simply advocating an idea, to creating a vessel to officially actualise it. When first introducing the term, Dean (1971, p. 662) stated that metapsychiatry aims to "delimit the psychiatric ramifications of the subject", and further explained that:

> The special province of metapsychiatry would be the cogitative and scientific investigation of such diverse 'psi' categories as mental telepathy, ESP, clairvoyance, prophecy, precognition, premonitions, intuition, *déjà vu*, sixth sense, premonitory dreams, miracles, spiritualism, trances, hallucinations, hypnosis, charisma, faith healing, personal magnetism, psychedelic states, auras, psychokinesis (PK), catalepsy, graphoanalysis, tactile sight, radiesthesia, bioluminescence, cosmobiology, etc. (ibid.)

This heralded a marked transition, whereby his prior tentative and nebulous approach to discussing psi phenomena was superseded by an explicit spelling out of the *formes frustes* of ultraconsciousness that metapsychiatry might investigate.

As Dean developed his idea of metapsychiatry he increasingly began to conceptualise it in the context of mysticism. For instance, in 1973 he described metapsychiatry as the "important interface between psychiatry and mysticism" (Dean, 1973, p. 1036), and reiterated a year later that it constituted the "confluence of psychiatry and mysticism" (Dean, 1974b, p. 3). At this juncture he adopted the *American Heritage Dictionary* (Morris, 1969) definition of mysticism as the "belief in the existence of realities beyond perceptual or intellectual apprehension, but central to being and accessible to consciousness" (Dean, 1974b, p. 3). However, in his subsequent and influential edited book *Psychiatry and Mysticism*, he proffered a personal definition of mysticism, stating that "it simply means that very exceptional kinds of knowledge and awareness may reach consciousness through channels other than those known to us at present" (Dean, 1975c, p. 1). He also predicted that "it is only a matter of time before those channels are identified—a matter of time before the mysticism of yesterday ... becomes the science of today" (ibid., p. 2). As such, he posited metapsychiatry as a prospective bridge to span the perceived gulf between mystical and scientific worldviews.[54]

Dean's conviction about the scientific study of psychospiritual realities opening new frontiers to psychiatry was reinforced by his formulation of twelve psychic aphorisms. These aphorisms distilled and encapsulated his understanding of ultra-consciousness, and provided a guiding conceptual framework for the practice of metapsychiatry.

1. Faith is not fantasy; it is a form of precognition that has divined for countless years what science is just beginning to understand.
2. Science and mysticism are fraternal twins, long separated, but now on the verge of reunion.
3. Psychogeny recapitulates cosmogony—i.e. the developing mind includes an innate awareness of the origin and meaning of the universe.
4. Evolution is not homogeneous, but proceeds in two divergent streams; mental and physical. Mental evolution is far ahead of the physical.
5. The ultraconscious state bridges the evolutionary gap and produces cosmic awareness.
6. Psi power is latent in all, and an experiential reality to many.
7. Thought is a form of energy; it has universal 'field' properties which, like gravitational and magnetic fields, are amenable to scientific research.
8. Thought fields, like the theoretical 'tachyon', can interact, traverse space, and penetrate matter more or less instantaneously.
9. Thought fields survive death and are analogous to soul and spirit.
10. Thought fields are eternal; hence, past existence (reincarnation) is as valid a concept as future immortality.
11. Psychic research is on a par with other important courses of study; it should be included in academic curricula and lead to degrees and doctorates.
12. A new age is dawning—the Psychic Age—on the heels of the Atomic Age and Space Age. (Dean, 1974b, p. 9)

---

[54] As mentioned in Chapter Two, Section 2.1, the literature on mysticism is vast and proffers manifold meanings regarding the nature of mystic reality. While I generally use the terms 'mystical' and 'psychospiritual' synonymously, here, in the instance of Dean's work where mysticism per se is the subject of focus, it is apposite to expound upon its key meanings. Therefore, Appendix Three provides an overview of the term's meaning according to two prominent scholars in the field, and also from the perspective of the mystic Franklin Merrell-Wolff. This elucidates the nature and qualities of mystic experience and introduces some related ramifications for better understanding psychosis.

Overall, his aphorisms reflected his self-perception as an "eclectically-oriented psychiatrist", and scoped metapsychiatry as a central medium for the scientific exploration of various epistemological fields, including religion, mysticism, parapsychology, Bucke's spiritual evolutionary theory, and quantum physics (Dean, 1970a, p. 33). Indeed, Dean (1975c, p. 1) described metapsychiatry as "strongly interdisciplinary, having synergistic relationships with parapsychology, philosophy, religion, and empirical logic", and elsewhere as "the base of a pyramid whose other sides are psychiatry, religion, parapsychology and mysticism" (Dean, 1976, p. 115). Hence, his vision for metapsychiatry widened the remit of conventional psychiatry beyond the bounds of scientific materialism to an attitude that "strikes a harmonious chord with *metaphysics* ... and seeks to explain the nature of being or reality and the origin and structure of the universe" (Dean, 1975c, p. 1). Metapsychiatry, it seems, aimed to establish a branch of psychiatry that extended beyond simply contending with mental illness, to fulfilling a catholic and almost 'religious' role in engaging with ultimate questions pertaining to mental health, life, and supreme reality.

6.2.2.1 The promise of metapsychiatry

It might be expected that, due to its metaphysical nature, Dean's concept of metapsychiatry was spurned by the majority of psychiatrists. Conversely, it met with considerable success. Indeed, the article in which he first introduced the term 'metapsychiatry' was also published in the *Congressional Record* (1971), lending it immediate credibility.[55] Next, spurred by Dean's work, the APA hosted a symposium at its 1972 annual meeting titled "Science and psi: Transcultural trends" (Panati, 1975, p. 27). Two subsequent symposia on "psychic phenomena" were also presented at the 1973 and 1974 APA general meetings, with the latter being attended by "an audience of 650 lay and professional people—the largest panel attendance in APA history" (Dean, 1975d, p. xx). Papers presented at these three symposia were compiled and published in Dean's *Psychiatry and Mysticism*. At this point, the term 'metapsychiatry' was also included in the 1975 edition of *A Psychiatric Glossary: The Meaning of Terms Frequently Used in Psychiatry*, in which it was defined as:

> The interface between *psychiatry* and such psychic phenomena as *parapsychology*, mysticism, transcendental meditation, *biofeedback*, and other suprasensory, suprarational, esoteric manifestations of consciousness that are in any way relevant to the theory and practice of psychiatry. (APA et al., 1975, p. 101)

Subsequent to being accepted as an official and 'frequently used' psychiatric term, 'metapsychiatry' was also included in the 1977 edition of the prestigious *International Encyclopedia of Psychiatry, Psychology, Psychoanalysis and Neurology*

---

[55] The *Congressional Record* is the official record of the proceedings and debates of the United States Congress. It is published daily when Congress is in session.

(Dean, 1977). Furthermore, in his 1979 APA presidential speech, Jules Masserman (1979, p. 1015) averred that "there is a growing interest among us in what we call metapsychiatry, reflecting parallel preoccupations among the general public with esoteric faiths and transcendental seekings for the ultimate". He cited Dean's *Psychiatry and Mysticism* as an exemplar. It is evident from these occurrences that psychospiritual considerations have not only been conceptually entertained by mainstream psychiatrists but have also been taken seriously enough to merit entry into key psychiatric texts.

Taking these developments a step further, Dean also attempted to found the American Metapsychiatric Association (AMPA). He first mooted the idea in 1971, inviting inquiries regarding the formation of the AMPA (Dean, 1971, p. 662), which attracted some supportive comments in subsequent editions of *The American Journal of Psychiatry* (Magier, 1972; Ehrenwald, 1973). For Dean (1975a, p. 47) the AMPA objectives were "to give special emphasis to the relationship between psychiatry and psychic phenomena" and to "replace strangeness, sensationalism, and fraud with logic, common sense, and professional responsibility" (Dean, 1975b, p. 14). His reference to 'fraud' here inferred that the AMPA may act as a supervisory body to detect, regulate, and counter the charlatanism and cultish behaviour that abounds in the paranormal field (ibid., pp. 13–14). By 1975, about two thousand correspondents, including more than two hundred psychiatrists and physicians, had expressed an interest in becoming AMPA members (Dean, 1975d, p. xx). In 1976, Dean (1976, p. 115) reported that efforts were still under way to formally establish this body, but he did not mention the AMPA again in subsequent articles.[56] Nevertheless, these various occurrences indicate that many psychiatrists at the time believed it was feasible, if not necessary, to consider the ramifications of metaphysical phenomena in clinical practice.

Dean's final enterprise was to advocate for the inclusion of metapsychiatric knowledge in mainstream psychiatric training. At the 1975 APA general meeting, in a speech titled "A quest for purpose in psychic research", he discussed the theory and potential application of metapsychiatric research, and highlighted the perceived need, by himself and others, "to include psychic subjects in mental health education" (Dean, 1976, p. 115). Indeed, he saw metapsychiatric research as being "a sorely needed objective standard for psychiatric research and therapy" (Sandweiss quoting Dean, 2011, p. 318).[57] Several years later, Dean et al. (1980) published the results of research they conducted on medical professional opinions about the inclusion of psychic studies in psychiatric education. Questionnaires were sent to "293 deans of medical schools, 109 heads of departments of psychiatry, 261 professors of psychiatry, 419 residents in psychiatry, and 68 other medical faculty", and of the 228 respondents, "fifty-eight percent … believed that an understanding of psychic

---

[56] I have been unable to ascertain whether or not efforts to formally establish the AMPA were successful.
[57] The source of this quote, of which I am unable to find a copy, is: Dean, S. (1978). Metapsychiatry and psychosocial futurology. *MD*, December, 11–13.

phenomena is important to future graduates of psychiatry, and 44% believed that psychic factors are important in the healing process" (ibid., p. 1247). From these results the authors concluded that "including psychic studies in psychiatric education would attract more medical students to psychiatry" (ibid.). The implications of these findings are surprising. They indicate that, despite the shift back to a medical model of psychiatry with the 1980 publication of DSM-III, and the attendant materialist spurning of 'non-scientific' metaphysical matters in psychiatric practice, there was a significant, if not majority, support within late 1970s mainstream American psychiatry for including psychospiritual considerations in clinical training programs.

Over the following year, eight 'Letters to the Editor' responding to this research were published in *The American Journal of Psychiatry*; four disapproving and five approving. Excerpts from each are listed in Table 3 below.

Table 3. 'Letters to the Editor' in response to Dean et al. (1980).

Comments of disapproval
The history of metapsychiatry is that of poorly controlled studies, outright fraud, dependence on anecdotal reporting, and repeated failures at replication ... Therefore, it might be more appropriate to study those who accept such parapsychological phenomena. (Berman, 1981, p. 395)
I was disturbed by Dr. Dean and associates' recommendation to include psychic studies in residency curricula ... I would caution against inclusion of such scientifically unfounded ideas ... until they have been much more thoroughly studied. (Casher, 1981, p. 395)
I was surprised by Dr. Dean and associates' peculiar article ... Time and again psychiatry has been embarrassed by psychiatrists going strange ... It is time that our profession learned to deal with these difficult and controversial topics rather than indulge in idle speculation that feeds the popular need to believe in the bizarre. (McDonald, 1981, p. 396)
I strongly disagree with the recommendation of Dr. Dean and associates that psychic studies be included in the curriculum of medical education. The subjects of ESP, telepathy, precognition, and the like are all interesting matters to chat about but lack a scientific basis ... I object to such material being offered as medical knowledge. (Sturges, 1981, p. 396)

Comments of approval
It is gratifying to see that the *Journal* gives recognition to the field of metapsychiatry ... Practicing psychiatrists, as well as those in training, should be made aware of and have the opportunity to express interest in the investigation of psychic factors in the healing process. (Bowen, 1981, p. 540)

(Continued)

Table 3. (Continued)

The inclusion of metapsychiatry within resident's training is appealing ... Psychic studies may provoke the resident by demanding an openness to various theories and modalities ... Metapsychiatry could be offered as an elective during the fourth postgraduate year. (Granet, 1981, p. 703)

Metapsychiatry can provide excellent training in complex research design and disciplined conceptualization, besides having the potential to add new facts to our relatively inaccurate and inadequate knowledge of human psychology. (Twemlow, 1981, p. 1397)

It takes courage to publicly solicit support for unconventional concepts in education. I strongly urge that we support Dr. Dean and others who strive to extend our curricula by including psychic studies on our residency training programs. (Steele, 1981, p. 1398)

I think it is important to teach psychiatric residents about issues relating to psychic phenomena ... including these kinds of themes in the postgraduate psychiatric curriculum would have great value in attracting some medical students into the field. (Ruiz, 1981, p. 1515)

In response to the four critics, Dean (1981, p. 396) argued the legitimacy of his "interest in nonpsychotic paranormal (psychic) phenomena" by calling attention to some of his more renowned publications on the subject, highlighting the occurrence of APA panels on metapsychiatry, and noting an endorsement of his work by Swiss psychiatrist Manfred Bleuler,[58] who observed that "there are strong trends towards similar teachings as the ones of Professor Dean in Europe". It is evident from Bleuler's comment that the readiness to accept psychospiritual considerations into the body of psychiatric knowledge and research was not simply an American idiosyncrasy, but was also supported within European mainstream psychiatry. Dean seemingly published no further articles on metapsychiatry beyond this point. However, news articles indicate that he continued his campaign about psychic education for several more years (Rothman, 1982, p. 20; American Press, 1984, p. 16; Harakas, 1985, p. 1). Despite strong seeming support for including psychic studies in psychiatric training, Dean's efforts to this effect were unsuccessful, and the term metapsychiatry disappeared from psychiatric literature during the early 1980s.

6.2.2.2 Metapsychiatry, psychosis and healing

A key driving rationale behind Dean's endeavour to establish a confluence between psychiatry and ultraconscious phenomena, via the vessel of metapsychiatry, was that of advancing healing. Although he made few allusions to psychotic illnesses per se throughout his considerable literature on ultraconsciousness and metapsychiatry,

---

[58] Manfred Bleuler was the son of Eugen Bleuler, the psychiatrist who coined the term 'schizophrenia'.

there is some evidence he believed that psychiatrists educated in metaphysical realities would be better able to diagnostically differentiate between psychotic and mystical occurrences. For instance, Dean (1973, p. 1037) asserted that, "we psychiatrists are conditioned to equate hallucinations with schizophrenia and other psychoses, but a great many non-psychotic individuals also hear voices, see visions, and have supernatural experiences". Elsewhere he noted resemblances between "psychogenic culture-bound reactive syndromes … usually associated with primitive societies" and "our psychiatric concepts of acute schizophrenic episodes" (Dean & Thong, 1975, pp. 271–272). Indeed, as a clinical "first step", he advocated the idea that psychiatrists ask all patients about their potential metaphysical experiences, and that the resulting data be collated in order to advance the field's understanding of ultraconscious phenomena (Dean, 1970a, p. 36; 1970b, p. 61; 1973, p. 1038; 1975a, p. 46). Hence, he highlighted the potential for developing psychiatric practices steeped in ultraconscious (or metapsychiatric) understanding, whereby a knowledge base could be established for making differential diagnoses, and for informing therapeutic approaches.

The central thrust of Dean's thinking in terms of metapsychiatry was that of the implicit healing power of ultraconscious faculties. In regards to forms of psychopathology, he maintained that "a common denominator underlies them all", which he identified as a composite of two ultraconscious faculties, namely "the charisma of the therapist and the faith of the patient, both of which apparently involve a suprasensory, suprarational level of mentation" (Dean & Thong, 1972, p. 91). He further posited that these faculties could be harnessed for advancing therapeutic practices along a spectrum of diverse cultural settings, "from the native witch doctor at one extreme to the academically trained psychiatry at the other" (ibid.). Dean (1976, p. 119) later identified five common denominators in ultraconscious healing capacity:

> (1) Nature's remarkable self-reparative mechanisms. (2) The awesome power of suggestion. (3) The reputation and therapeutic personality (charisma) of the therapist. (4) The expectant faith of the patient. (5) The growing belief in a mysterious transfer of energy between healer and patient.

He saw the healing efficacy of medical interventions as secondary to these facilities (Rothman, 1982, p. 20). Hence, from this perspective, the metapsychiatrist, through his or her understanding of ultraconscious phenomena and personal development of ultraconscious capacities, would ostensibly be better equipped than conventional psychiatrists to diagnose and remediate mental illnesses.

This outlook exemplifies the type of psychiatric thinking that is possible when stepping beyond the strictures of materialist thinking, for it conceptually enables a rapprochement between metaphysical and scientific worldviews. Furthermore, such an approach bridges the putative gap between traditional shamanism and modern psychiatry, for each is seen as a different, but equally valid, cultural manifestation along a therapeutic continuum. Ideally, the metapsychiatrist would become adept at moving fluidly between these therapeutic paradigms and bring the best of both medical and psychospiritual considerations into clinical settings.

In sum, the above overview of Dean's metapsychiatric project demonstrates that psychospiritual considerations are not utterly foreign to mainstream psychiatric thinking and terminology. Indeed, the existence of metapsychiatry within the historical stream of conventional psychiatry is of import, for it represents an unprecedented step towards the potential incorporation of psychospiritual knowledge into psychiatric thinking and practice. Additionally, it heralded the prospective emergence of a new chapter in psychiatric treatment approaches through harnessing the alleged healing potential of ultraconscious knowledge and capacities. Although metapsychiatry was ultimately not incorporated into psychiatric teaching and practice, it did engender considerable interest in, and support from, many psychiatrists, thus indicating that psychospiritual and biological approaches are not antithetical.[59] Be this as it may, the rising tide of post DSM-III medical psychiatry appears to have eclipsed metapsychiatry and its psychospiritual viewpoint. However, this does not mean such a viewpoint has been invalidated. My examination in Focal Settings Three and Four of psychosis and related psychospiritual factors, both within and beyond psychiatric thinking, demonstrates that a holistic investigative approach may likely result in better understanding psychosis and other related anomalous and enigmatic states of consciousness.

6.3 The 1976 GAP report on mysticism

This section provides an explication and critical appraisal of the Group for the Advancement of Psychiatry's (GAP) report on mysticism. The GAP investigation and report constitutes a significant milestone in the consideration of psychospiritual matters by mainstream psychiatry, for it represents the only official attempt within global psychiatric research to comprehensively appraise the nature of mysticism, and how

---

[59] See Appendix Four for an overview of the American mystic Franklin Merrell-Wolff's critical appraisal of Dean's work on metapsychiatry. Although Dean promoted metapsychiatry as a rapprochement between psychiatry and mysticism, and unflaggingly attempted to institute metapsychiatry as a professional body, he never personally experienced psi phenomena or any other mystical occurrences (Dean, 1965, p. 471). Unlike Bucke, whose work was born of direct mystical experience, Dean's view was more a theoretical construct born of secondary observation and literature study. In this sense, his construct of metapsychiatry, despite its merits, was a treatise *about* mysticism and lacked input from the standpoint of somebody who had direct mystical experience. As a mystic, Merrell-Wolff's appraisal offers an insider's perspective on both the merits and shortcomings of Dean's work in light of metaphysical experience and knowledge. He also highlights the importance of incorporating mystic considerations into psychiatric epistemology and identifies some problems that are implicit to this venture. Although Merrell-Wolff's critical appraisal is tangential to the core focus here in Focal Setting Two, it provides an introductory foray into matters pertaining to better understanding the differences and commonalties between psychospiritual and psychotic experiences, which are further explored in Focal Setting Three.

it might relate to clinical practice and thinking.[60] Also, the GAP authors attempted to formulate a typology for differentiating psychotic from mystical experiences. This constitutes a significant breakthrough in psychiatric thinking, because doing so intrinsically validates the existence of psychospiritual realities. However, a critical appraisal of this typology indicates that it embodied flaws that are reflective of axiomatic psychiatric assumptions. Regardless, the GAP report process of attempting to understand mysticism from a psychiatric perspective indicates that such an enterprise is possible.

6.3.1 The GAP report: rationale and objectives

In 1976, a year after Stanley Dean published his book *Psychiatry and Mysticism*, the Committee on Psychiatry and Religion, a branch of GAP, published a report titled *Mysticism: Spiritual Quest or Psychic Disorder?* (GAP, 1976). The committee was comprised of six "psychoanalytically oriented psychiatrists" (Frank, 1977, p. 1057), hence, the report's findings generally reflected interpretations from a psychoanalytic perspective. Input was also invited from several past members, consultants, and committee guests (GAP, 1976, p. 711). As such, this venture represented an eclectic appraisal of views from various epistemological standpoints. As the secondary title of the report suggests, the committee's primary objective was to "contribute to an understanding of *the psychology of mysticism*" because of "the fact that mysticism has become a significant force in our time" (ibid., p. 713). Here, the term 'significant force' refers to a social trend of the time whereby a growing number of American "young people" were being attracted to "mystical movements" (pp. 811–812). Surprisingly, apart from a passing reference to the fact that the subject of mysticism drew "the largest audience ever to attend a meeting of the American Psychiatric Association" (p. 815), the report makes no mention of Dean's work or the formal adoption of his term 'metapsychiatry' into psychiatric vocabulary. However, whereas Dean's theories regarding metapsychiatry and ultraconsciousness had very little to say about psychotic states, the GAP report attempted to redress the problem of differentiating between psychotic and psychospiritual experiences.

6.3.2 Critical appraisal of the GAP report

Did the GAP report fulfil its stated objective of providing an informed appraisal of the psychology of mysticism and subsequently enhance psychiatry's understanding of the phenomenon? The answer to this question is a matter of opinion. Therefore, the opinions of two noteworthy commentators will be used to scope and structure a response, namely, a book review by Professor Jerome Frank, and a critical review

---

[60] A search of *The American Journal of Psychiatry*, *The British Journal of Psychiatry*, *European Psychiatry*, and the World Psychiatric Association's journal *World Psychiatry* reveals that no other investigations akin to the one conducted on mysticism by the GAP team have since been undertaken.

by Professor Arthur Deikman.[61] These commentators are noteworthy because their reviews apparently constitute the only published responses to the GAP report at the time. Also, Frank gave the report a glowing commendation, while Deikman was mostly condemnatory; hence, a closer examination of these conflicting views provides a balanced evaluation of the GAP report and its contribution to better understanding mystic and psychotic experience.

Frank proffered a brief, one-column review of the GAP report in *The American Journal of Psychiatry*. Much of this consisted of a synopsis of the report's structure and conceptual focus, though his closing comments were very commendatory. For instance, as a clinical empiricist, he praised the authors for prudently confining their investigation to the "consideration of features that can be empirically studied" and observed that the document "offers much fascinating information, objectively presented and thoughtfully discussed" (Frank, 1977, pp. 1057–1058). Overall, he concluded that the report "can be highly recommended as an introduction to the psychology of mysticism" (ibid., p. 1058). Intriguingly, Frank's (p. 1057) justification for praising the report's empirical felicity was his understanding that "when all is said and done, essential features of the mystical experience remain inexplicable in terms of Western cosmology". Hence, incongruously, his reasoning was that because mysticism is ultimately ineffable the GAP authors wisely chose to reduce their scope of research to that which could be clinically observed.

While Frank considered the GAP report to be an informative boon to clinical psychiatry, Deikman was less glowing in his four-page critical review in the *Association for Humanistic Psychology Newsletter*. Although he concurred with Frank in observing that "certain of the sections, especially those on Christian and Hindu mysticism, show an objectivity and scholarship that are quite commendable" (Deikman, 1978, p. 16), beyond this, he was very critical. Indeed, in stark contrast to Frank's view that the report is 'highly recommended as an introduction to the psychology of mysticism', Deikman (ibid.) concluded that "as a whole ... the report displays extreme parochialism, a lack of discrimination, and naive arrogance in its approach to the subject". It is apposite to examine more closely why Deikman drew this conclusion, because his critical appraisal of the report highlights some key issues pertaining to introducing psychospiritual matters into psychiatry.

Deikman's chief criticism of the GAP report was the authors' failure to discriminate between mystical experience proper and its attendant metaphysical phenomena. He remonstrated that they "have selectively ignored the central issues of mysticism and have made traditional interpretations of the secondary phenomena" and that the report "emphasizes lurid, visionary phenomena which lend themselves readily to standard psychiatric interpretations" (pp. 18, 16). To clarify, he further argued that the essence

---

[61] Jerome Frank was an American "clinician scholar" and hailed in his obituary as "a giant in the field of psychotherapy research" (The JHU Gazette, 2005). Arthur Deikman (2012) is a Professor of Psychiatry and "a pioneer in the scientific investigation of meditation, the mystical experience, and consciousness". He was one of the aforementioned GAP committee guests.

of mysticism was to transcend the indirect sensate and cognitive modes of construing reality and to ultimately achieve a spiritual state of consciousness whereby there
is an "immediate knowledge of reality" (p. 17). In neglecting to establish this critical
distinction as a cornerstone for examining mysticism, the GAP report, in Deikman's
view, failed to fulfil its objective of educating psychiatry about this phenomenon.

> To confuse lower level sensory-emotional experiences with the transcendent
> 'Knowledge' that is the goal of mysticism seriously limits the usefulness of the
> report and tends to perpetuate in the reader the ignorant parochial position that
> was standard in most psychiatric writings before the GAP publication and now,
> unfortunately, is likely to be reinforced. (p. 17)

This is a legitimate criticism, for the mystical literature abounds with quotes from
mystics underscoring this distinction. Hence, Frank's acclaim of the report's empirical
utility arguably demonstrated a poor understanding of the essential nature of mysticism, because the mystic domain is ultimately beyond empirical measure.

However, while Deikman was ultimately correct in criticising the GAP authors for
their biased, narrow focus, he appears not to have considered that mysticism can also
be viewed in terms of a journey. For instance, the GAP authors' understanding of
mysticism was partly based on Underhill's notion of "the mystic way" (GAP, 1976,
pp. 720–722), a term that infers the key developmental stages that mystic adherents
pass through during their unfolding passage towards spiritual illumination (Underhill, 1912, p. 96). From this perspective both the path and the goal are composite parts
of the mystic process. Hence, the mystic way is a journey of incremental spiritual
development that features both the experience of spiritual illumination and the antecedent passage to achieving it. This journey can often include experiences of psychic
phenomena (e.g., voices and visions) that are analogous to psychiatric symptoms of
psychosis (e.g., auditory and visual hallucinations, ibid., p. 319). In this context, the
GAP authors' focus on 'visionary phenomena which lend themselves readily to standard psychiatric interpretations' was justified.

Deikman's other main bone of contention with the GAP report was its strong psychoanalytic bias. Indeed, the GAP authors acknowledged that their interpretations
were informed by a "psychoanalytic orientation" (GAP, 1976, p. 816). However, what
they clearly saw as a legitimate methodological approach, Deikman (1978, p. 18) saw
as ideological parochialism that he disparagingly referred to as "monotonous clouds
of reductionism". He subsequently concluded that "our profession, when it comes to
mysticism, does not feel the need to ask serious questions about its own assumptions,
nor to take the devil's advocate's position toward its too-easy conclusions" (ibid.). It
appears this admonition has merit, because there was a definitive trend in the report
towards psychoanalytic reductionism. For instance, the GAP authors (1976, p. 731)
maintained that mystics who "show good object relations" in their attempt to escape
a problematic world "show *less psychopathology* than those who do not maintain them"
(italics added). Arguably, this depicts mysticism as a form of morbid escapism and

infers that *all* mystics exhibit some degree of psychopathology, but less so if good object relations are upheld. In a similar reductive and biased vein, they concluded that:

> at some point … the mystical defence breaks down. Then troublesome symptoms may appear, or possibly frank depression or psychosis … The psychiatrist will find mystical phenomena of interest because they can demonstrate forms of behaviour intermediate between normality and frank psychosis; a form of ego regression in the service of defense against internal or external stress; and a paradox of the return of repressed regression in unconventional expressions of love. (Ibid.)

This not only portrays mysticism as an unconscious psychological defence mechanism and form of escapism, but also identifies it as a phase of quasi-psychopathology that some people may pass through in their decline from normalcy to madness.

The GAP authors' appraisal of mysticism beyond this point was replete with comments and conclusions of a similarly psychoanalytic ilk, particularly in the context of psychotic symptoms, as understood by psychoanalytic psychiatry. For instance, they described mystic trance states as "hallucinatory experiences" (p. 776) and further deduced that:

- Mystic and schizophrenic experience share in common a sense that "the external world has been removed from the individual's awareness and therefore seems destroyed" (p. 778).
- In such experiences "the sense of reality is usually transferred from the outside inward with the permission of an indulgent ego" (ibid.).
- This can be understood as problem-solving displacement, whereby the "fantasy represents a reunion of some kind" with an alienated other, usually the person's parents (ibid.).
- Whereas "schizophrenic detachment … is usually precipitated by some disappointment in relations with other individuals", mystical detachment can also be "a way of escaping" unsettling and oppressive "community demands" (p. 779).
- Trance, for both the schizophrenic and the mystic: i) represents "the psychic functioning of an infant"; ii) is a means for "hallucinating the fulfilment of his needs"; and iii) is therefore a form of "primary narcissism" that can establish a predisposition to mental illness (pp. 779–780).

Having unpacked this line of reasoning, the GAP authors (p. 784) concluded by defining "the mystical way of life" as:

> first, a minimizing of one's sensitivity to external reality and a complementary maximizing of sensitivity to inner 'reality' by partial regression to primary narcissism; second, the deployment of one or more of the manoeuvres commonly used to ward off depression.

It is evident here that the GAP authors have presented a reductive and biased interpretation of mysticism that reflects psychoanalytic theory.

Overall, then, the GAP authors' distorted depiction of mystic experience as essentially psychopathological arguably shows a near absence of the objectivity for which Frank applauded the report. Hence, it appears Deikman's criticism was accurate and justified. Indeed, such reductive distortion is common to both psychoanalytic and medical psychiatry, and creates a formidable barrier to enabling psychiatry to be truly objective in considering psychospiritual matters in the context of better understanding psychosis.

6.3.3 GAP typology for differentiating psychotic from psychospiritual experiences

Despite the GAP report's apparent flaws, the authors' effort to compose a typology of indicators for differentiating psychotic from psychospiritual experiences was arguably a new and significant contribution to psychiatry. Whereas the works of Bucke and Dean on mysticism were primarily independent ventures, the GAP review was formally sanctioned by American mainstream psychiatry's governing body, the APA. Indeed, according to Grof (2000, p. 216), the GAP report represents "the kindest judgement about mysticism that has so far come from official academic circles". Albeit rudimentary, and reflective of the aforementioned psychoanalytic bias, this still constituted a progressive step, for no such formally sanctioned differential diagnosis had previously been attempted within mainstream psychiatry. The GAP authors (p. 784) maintained that while schizophrenic and mystic experience seems to include similar forms of regressive escapism, they differ in three significant ways:

> First, [the mystic's] retreat is facultative rather than obligatory; second, it is particular rather than complete ... third, he finds it possible, frequently desirable, to associate with others who share his view of the world—that is, he participates in mystical fraternities, while the schizophrenic rarely is able to form or maintain similar affectionate ties with others.

Although these points of discernment are seemingly sound, upon closer examination it is evident they are not absolute differential diagnosis markers.

The first point proposes that a 'retreat', or regressive trance state, is intentionally attained by the mystic, but involuntarily arrived at by the schizophrenic. Further to this the authors maintained that "when regression becomes obligatory to the extent that the subject cannot by an act of will prevent or reverse it, we consider him psychotic" (p. 780). Thus, they contend that the presence of regressive autonomy discerns the mystic from the psychotic state. Although this proposition may appear cogent within the fabric of its own psychoanalytic reasoning, its veracity as a fixed point for diagnostic differentiation can be disputed. Counter to the authors' claim, a rudimentary examination of the literature pertaining to mysticism shows that mystic trance states are often involuntary. Indeed, a chief resource used by the authors to inform their description of mysticism (i.e., Underhill's *Mysticism*) explains that mystics experience both "voluntary and involuntary trances" (Underhill, 1912, p. 428), while, more recently, Lukoff, Lu & Turner (1998, p. 34) suggest that one of the defining features of the mystical experience is "the sense of lacking control over the event". Similarly, the nineteenth-century Indian mystic Sri Ramakrishna, whom the GAP authors (1976, p. 748) identify as "one of the greatest mystics of all time", experienced frequent, sudden, and involuntary numinous trance states (Swami Budhananda, 1971). Hence, mystic and psychotic experience evidently cannot be differentiated according to whether the 'retreat is facultative rather than obligatory'.

The veracity of the second differentiation point is also questionable. According to the GAP authors, the atypical phenomenon of mystic trance represents a regressive 'retreat'. This line of thinking is unsubstantiated and speculative, as is the related suggestion that the mystic and psychotic can be differentiated according to whether the trance, retreat, or regression is 'particular rather than complete'. It assumes that regression represents a gradual trajectory of deepening psychopathology, and hence divests mystic experience (regression) of any transcendental or healing attributes. Yet, psychological models exist that see regression as playing a salutary role in a larger psychodynamic developmental process, a process that Washburn (1988) refers to as "regression in the service of transcendence".[62] Similarly, Prince & Savage (1966, p. 70) hypothesise that "mystical states are examples of regressions in the service of the ego". When considered in this light, the notion of differentiating between 'particular' and 'complete' regression is rendered unsound.

Of the three points of differentiation proffered by the authors, the third point is the least credible. To reiterate, they proposed that the mystic, who 'participates in mystical fraternities', can be differentiated from the person diagnosed as schizophrenic, who 'rarely is able to form or maintain similar affectionate ties with others'. Although history shows that spiritual followings, religious denominations, and entire religions have stemmed from the numinous experiences of a mystic (Cunningham, 2011a, p. 9; Merrell-Wolff, 1994, p. 173), these are generally the result of people being drawn to the mystic, and/or the mystic sharing his or her revelations with others. Therefore, it is not a case of 'escapism', as the GAP authors (1976, p. 786) claim, whereby the mystic "reinforces his retreat and overcomes the loneliness which it would create by joining with others to form an elite, democratic, and abstemious mystical fraternity". Additionally, the validity of this proposed point of differentiation is also undermined by the fact that many mystics have chosen a hermitic lifestyle of contemplative solitude over social interaction. For instance, the Christian mystic text titled *The Cloud of*

---

[62] 'Regression in the service of transcendence' is a transpersonal notion that refers to the apparently regressive nature of psychosis as actually being, in many instances, a psychic movement towards some form of psychological or psychospiritual healing or transcendence. This notion is discussed in more detail in Chapter Ten, Section 10.6.

Unknowing holds that there are four "degrees" of living that progressively take the adherent closer to union with God (Underhill, 1970, p. 59). The penultimate of these is "the third degree and manner of living, the which is called Singular ... [the] solitary form and manner of living, thou mayest learn to lift up the foot of thy love; and step towards that state and degree of living that is perfect, and the last state of all" (ibid., p. 60). Here the 'Singular' or solitary spiritual path is advocated as an advanced stage of mystic maturity. In light of these critical points of evaluation, it appears the GAP authors' third proposed differentiator is also untenable.

As already mentioned, a detailed consideration of problematic issues pertaining to the idea of differentiating between psychotic and psychospiritual experiences is undertaken in Chapter Nine. The above appraisal of the GAP authors' proposed typology is a prelude to this and demonstrates that such an enterprise is fraught with ambiguous tensions. Although it is clear that psychiatry can acknowledge the existence of psychospiritual realities, the challenging implications of this for clinical thinking and practice are not easy to resolve. Indeed, they call to question the fundamental assumptions and diagnostic practices upon which psychiatry is based. Arguably, the solution to this conundrum is not for psychiatry to disregard psychospiritual considerations or attempt to force-fit them into a limited modality of psychiatric thinking, but to interrogate its axiomatic assumptions in order to accommodate psychospiritual knowledge.

6.4 Conclusion

While the discipline of psychiatry has traditionally eschewed the consideration of psychospiritual determinants in psychosis research, it is evident from the instances examined above that such avoidance is a matter of choice rather than empirical necessity. The work of Bucke and Dean especially demonstrates that psychiatry can include metaphysical research within its epistemological ambit. This view is supported by Chapter Seven's further investigation of this matter, from 1980 to the present date.

CHAPTER 7

A historical overview of psychospiritual considerations by psychiatry: part two: post-1980

7.0 Introduction

Here, the challenge instigated in Chapter Six is continued by identifying post-1980 instances of psychiatry's understanding of psychopathology being significantly influenced by psychospiritual factors. This entails an examination of:

1. The psychospiritual roots of DSM-IV's 'religious and spiritual problem' category.
2. Contemporary neuropsychiatric research into human psychospiritual experiences.
3. 'Spiritual' psychiatric special interest groups.
4. Contemporary mainstream psychiatrists who endorse the inclusion of psychospiritual considerations in psychiatric research.

7.1 DSM-IV V-Code 62.89: religious or spiritual problem

The renaissance of medical psychiatry in America did not result in the complete occlusion of psychospiritual considerations from the discipline's research agenda. After Dean's promotion of metapsychiatry and the GAP report on mysticism in the 1970s, the next significant event of this nature occurred with the 1994 inclusion in DSM-IV of a new diagnostic category titled 'Religious or spiritual problem' (V62.89). However, the genesis of this idea began about ten years earlier with clinician David Lukoff's work on mysticism and psychosis. The ensuing historical and critical overview of this category's developmental trajectory, from its transpersonal roots to its adaption and final inclusion in DSM-IV and subsequent re-adaptation in DSM-5, provides further evidence of psychiatry's engagement with psychospiritual issues. It also elucidates some inherent problematic issues in psychiatry's endeavour to reconcile psychospiritual realities within its clinical framework, particularly in terms of diagnostically differentiating psychotic disorders from normative cultural-religious-spiritual experiences.

7.1.1 What is V-Code 62.89?

The DSM-IV V62.89 category of 'Religious or spiritual problem' was included in the manual to enable clinicians to account for factors that related to, but were not part of, a mental disorder. It applied to "other conditions or problems that may be a focus of clinical attention", such as:

1) The problem is the focus of diagnosis or treatment and the individual has no mental disorder;
2) The individual has a mental disorder but it is unrelated to the problem;
3) The individual has a mental disorder but it is related to the problem, but the problem is sufficiently severe to warrant independent clinical attention (APA, 1994, p. 675).

The inclusion of this category in DSM-IV represented a rudimentary but important step by psychiatry towards acknowledging the value of psychospiritual considerations to clinical practice. The new V62.89 V-Code was part of an innovative suite of developments whereby clinicians were encouraged to exercise "cultural sensitivity" in diagnostic practices (Turner et al., 1995, pp. 441–442). Indeed, Harold Pincus, the Vice Chairman of the DSM-IV task force asserted that the introduction of V62.89 was "a sign of the profession's growing sensitivity not only to religion but to cultural diversity generally" (McIntyre, 1994, p. 3). Hence, V62.89 entered DSM-IV as one of several measures developed to enhance the clinician's awareness of cultural considerations when diagnosing and treating patients.

The advent of V62.89 in DSM-IV has been hailed by many commentators as an important event in psychiatric diagnostics. For instance, it has been variously referred to as "a significant breakthrough" (Turner et al., 1995, p. 443), "a major innovation" (Lu et al., 1997a, p. 76) and "a significant first step towards explicit delineation of spiritual clinical foci" (Scott et al., 2003, p. 163). Furthermore, Scotton (2011, p. 199) described it as the product of a "groundbreaking effort in the period preceding the release of DSM-IV" to contend with the "embarrassing situation" in psychiatric diagnostics "of having to label normative spiritual and religious experiences ... as being grossly pathological if not outright psychotic". This latter comment by Scotton calls attention to a fundamental precipitating factor in the formulation of V62.89. While the DSM-IV authors depicted V62.89 as a culturally sensitive diagnostic category, they failed to explain that the initial impetus for its creation came from a group of transpersonal-oriented clinicians. This group aimed to redress: first, the problem of non-psychopathological symptoms relating to spiritual practices and crises being misdiagnosed as mental disorders; and second, the "iatrogenic harm" that can result from such misdiagnoses (Lukoff, Lu & Turner, 1992, p. 673). My ensuing examination of the development and eventual inclusion of V62.89 as a DSM-IV diagnostic category further elucidates the existent tensions between the worldviews of medical psychiatry and metaphysics, and how these may enhance or limit conceptualisations of psychosis.

7.1.2 From Lukoff's MEPF to V62.89: a chronology of key developments

The notion of "Mystical Experiences with Psychotic Features" (MEPF), formulated by American clinical psychologist David Lukoff (1985), was the transpersonal seed-idea from which V62.89 ultimately emerged as a formal diagnostic category in medical psychiatry. Brown (2005, p. 7) explains that "when transpersonal psychology developed, it acknowledged and sought to understand spiritual and transcendent experiences in actualizing the highest human developmental potential". It was from this transpersonal context that the idea for formulating V62.89 arose. Lukoff was one of many transpersonal-oriented clinicians affiliated with the Spiritual Emergence Network (SEN),[63] which provided therapeutic support for people experiencing "spiritual emergencies", a term designating "forms of distress associated with spiritual practices and experiences" (Lukoff, Lu & Turner, 1998, p. 22). His involvement with SEN subsequently inspired the formulation of MEPF as a proposed diagnostic category that delineated "the overlap between mystical experiences and psychotic states" (Lukoff, 1985, p. 156). Lukoff developed a simple model consisting of two overlapping circles, one symbolising 'Mystical Experiences', the other 'Psychotic Episodes', with the common overlapping region representing two diagnostic categories: 'Mystical Experiences with Psychotic Features' (MEPF) and 'Psychotic Disorders with Mystical Features' (PDMF) (see Figure 1).

For Lukoff, both of these proposed categories were applicable to situations in which a clinician might exercise diagnostic discernment regarding the possible psychospiritual dimensions of a seeming case of psychosis. His main focus at this point, however, was structuring MEPF as a clinically robust diagnostic category. Adopting the DSM-III "empirical descriptive approach" as a guiding model (ibid., p. 161), he composed a flowchart of operational diagnostic criteria[64] that "are intended to allow cases of positively-transforming psychotic episodes to be recognised with a high degree of accuracy" (p. 160). Overall, Lukoff's original proposal was concerned with

---

[63] The Spiritual Emergence Network was originally established in 1980 as the Spiritual Emergency Network. SEN was founded by the American clinicians Christina Grof, a psychotherapist, and Stanislav Grof, a psychiatrist (Grof & Grof, 1989, p. xiv). The association was formed "in response to the lack of understanding and respect for psychospiritual growth in the mental health profession" (Spiritual Emergence Network, n.d.). The Grofs' notion of 'spiritual emergency' is examined in Chapter Eight, Section 8.2.

[64] A copy of this flowchart is included in Chapter Eight, Section 8.3 (see Figure 2), which further examines Lukoff's work in context of the issue of discerning psychotic from psychospiritual experiences.

preventing misdiagnosis and iatrogenic harm by training clinicians to differentiate healthy or distressing psychospiritual experiences from psychotic episodes, and/or to identify situations of possible overlap between them. At this juncture there was no consideration of the cultural and religious factors that later took precedence in the DSM-IV V62.89 category.

Figure 1 – Lukoff's model of the relationship between mystical experiences and psychotic episodes

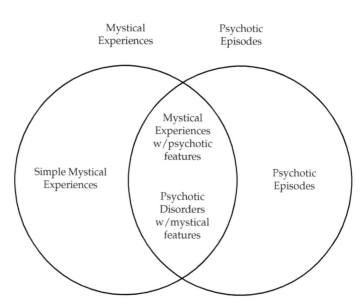

(Source – Lukoff, 1985, p. 156)

Figure 1. Lukoff's model of the relationship between mystical experiences and psychotic episodes.

Between 1985 and 1994, several further developments transpired before culminating in the DSM task force's acceptance of the proposed new V-Code. Having formulated MEPF as a diagnostic category, Lukoff (1988, p. 135) next likened it to the DSM-III-R V-Code titled "Uncomplicated Bereavement", which enabled clinicians to diagnose depression related to major losses in life (e.g. the death of a loved one) as "a normal reaction" (APA, 1987, p. 361). In light of the intrinsic resemblance between MEPF and Uncomplicated Bereavement, Lukoff (1988, p. 135) concluded that:

> individuals in the midst of a tumultuous spiritual emergence may appear to have a mental disorder if viewed out of their context, but are actually undergoing a transformative process. Delineating both the areas of overlap and nonoverlap between specific diagnostic categories and discrete transpersonal states of consciousness could yield some guidelines for clinicians faced with the task of differentiating mental disorders from spiritual emergencies.

In order to further bolster the efficacy of MEPF as a diagnostic category, Lukoff (1988, pp. 114–128; 1985, pp. 171–176) presented case studies of two patients he had worked with from a transpersonal perspective. Both had been diagnosed as having a psychotic disorder, yet an appraisal of descriptions of their respective experiences, and the meanings they attributed to these experiences, demonstrated that they were candidates for a being diagnosed with MEPF, because their beliefs, though apparently psychotic, were generally of a transpersonal or mystical nature (ibid.). Finally, using the DSM-III-R bereavement V-Code as a precedent, (Lukoff, Lu & Turner, 1998, p. 26) notified the DSM-IV task force in 1991 to say they were submitting a V-Code category titled "Psychospiritual Conflict" for prospective inclusion in DSM-IV as a "nonpathological category for a distressing and disruptive experience". Even at this advanced stage, the proposed diagnostic context was scoped to the psychospiritual-psychotic nexus, with seemingly no allusion to religious or cultural considerations.

Religious considerations were apparently not incorporated into their proposal until after the DSM task force had been notified of the impending submission of a psychospiritual V-Code. In order to "obtain greater support", Lukoff, Lu & Turner (ibid.) subsequently decided to add "psychoreligious problems" to their proposal and over the ensuing months they conducted two extensive literature reviews on psychoreligious and psychospiritual research (Lukoff, Turner & Lu, 1993; Lukoff, Turner & Lu, 1992). In the first of these reviews they explained that, in 1985, "Lukoff proposed a diagnostic category, Mystical Experience with Psychotic Features (MEPF), to identify intense *religious* experiences that present as psychotic-like episodes" (Lukoff, Turner & Lu, 1992, p. 43, italics added). However, in his 1985 proposal, Lukoff originally spoke of mystical rather than religious experiences, hence the sudden emphasis on a 'religious' context was seemingly part of their endeavour to sway the DSM authors to accept their V-Code category proposal.

A further step in formulating the V-Code was to associate it with the notion of cultural sensitivity. An article published at the time by key task force members stressed that "the DSM-IV must not be culture specific but instead be applicable cross culturally" (Frances et al., 1991, p. 409). Hence, Lukoff and company proceeded to anchor their proposal within a cultural context, undoubtedly as a measure to further enhance the likelihood of securing the task force's approval. After May 1991, Lukoff, Turner & Lu (1992, p. 44) began to investigate and consider the "cultural sensitivity implications" for both psychoreligious and psychospiritual problems. The end result of this process was the publication of an article aptly titled "Toward a more culturally sensitive DSM-IV: Psychoreligious and psychospiritual problems" (Lukoff, Lu & Turner, 1992), thus deftly linking their particular V-Code focus with the emergent cultural considerations for DSM-IV. In this article they argued that:

> in theory, research, and practice, mental health professionals have tended to ignore or pathologize the religious and spiritual dimensions of life. This represents a type of cultural insensitivity toward individuals who have religious and spiritual experiences in both Western and non-Western cultures. (ibid., p. 673)

This statement, situated psychoreligious and psychospiritual problems squarely within the realm of cultural sensitivity, as did their assertion that "the religious and spiritual dimensions of culture are among the most important factors that structure human experience, beliefs, values, behaviour, and illness patterns" (ibid.). Here, they also included *Western* religious and spiritual dimensions under the generic umbrella of 'culture' (ibid.), presumably to emphasise that Western people who experience distressing transpersonal events or spiritual emergencies also warrant clinical cultural sensitivity when being assessed. Regardless, strongly linking the proposed V-Code to cultural sensitivity appears to have played a vital role in its eventual acceptance, for as stated above, it was later adopted by the task force as one of four innovations to help foster cultural sensitivity in DSM-IV.

A formal V-Code proposal was finally submitted to the DSM-IV task force in December 1991, with definitions for psychoreligious and psychospiritual problems. The word 'conflict' had been substituted with 'problem' to complement DSM-III-R V-Code terminology, and the authors "stressed the need for this new diagnosis to improve the cultural sensitivity of the DSM-IV" (Lukoff, Lu & Turner, 1998, pp. 26–27). The working definitions in the submitted proposal were:

> *Psychoreligious problems* are experiences that a person finds troubling or distressing and that involve the beliefs and practices of an organized church or religious institution. Examples include loss or questioning of a firmly held faith, change in denominational membership, conversion to a new faith, and intensification of adherence to religious practices and orthodoxy.
>
> *Psychospiritual problems* are experiences that a person finds troubling or distressing and that involve that person's relationship with a transcendent being or force. These problems are not necessarily related to the beliefs and practices of an organized church or religious institution. Examples include near-death experience and mystical experience. This category can be used when the focus of treatment or diagnosis is a psychoreligious or psychospiritual problem that is not attributable to a mental disorder. (ibid., p. 27)

The second definition provided much latitude for the clinical consideration of a broad range of ostensible transpersonal experiences and incorporated the original notion of MEPF via the use of 'mystical experience' as a specific example of a psychospiritual problem. Like Dean's metapsychiatry proposal,[65] this clearly aimed to expand the parameters of psychiatric thinking for it encouraged clinicians to consider mystical, parapsychological, and psychospiritual experiences as innately human, rather than as probable signs of psychopathology.

---

[65] Surprisingly, despite the similarity between Lukoff's and Dean's respective visions for validating mysticism within psychiatric epistemology, Dean is not cited in any of the numerous articles published by Lukoff and company.

The DSM task force's response to this initial V-code draft appears to have either missed, or dismissed, the *raison d'être* of the proposed category, particularly its psychospiritual aspect. After reviewing the proposal, the task force maintained that psychoreligious and psychospiritual problems might best be subsumed under an existing DSM-III-R axis I category (e.g. adjustment disorder) or a V-Code category (e.g. identity problem) (Turner et al., 1995, pp. 436–437). Hence, in reductively situating these experiences under the umbrella of minor psychiatric categories, the task force seemingly failed to appreciate the essential idea from which the proposed V-Code stemmed; that is, the significance, legitimacy, and value of transpersonal, religious and psychospiritual domains of human experience, and their related problems. Lukoff and associates counterargued by:

1. pointing out that subsuming the V-Code would subvert its basic aim to "anchor the nonpathological end of the differential diagnostic spectrum regarding religious or spiritual problems" (ibid., p. 437); and
2. contending that the existent DSM-III-R categories did not provide the clinician with apposite information regarding the nature and treatment of religious and spiritual problems.

Hence, they reaffirmed that a fundamental aim of the proposed V-Code was to address situations of human distress, in the form psychoreligious and psychospiritual problems, which were not recognised within DSM diagnostics. The above counterarguments also subtly reasserted that religion and spirituality are not subsidiary to the likes of adjustment disorders or identity problems, but exist as primary realms of reality in their own right.

Despite the task force's initial reservations about accepting the new V-Code category, Lukoff and company gained support from the APA Committee on Religion and Psychiatry as well as the National Institute for Mental Health (NIMH) Workgroup on Culture and Diagnosis (Lukoff, Lu & Turner, 1998, p. 27). The latter group played a key formative role in instituting the DSM-IV cultural innovations (Mezzich et al., 1999, p. 457), and likely influenced the task force's final decision to adopt a revised version of the V-Code. The task force formally announced its acceptance of the proposed V-Code in January 1993, though the title was changed from "psychoreligious or psychospiritual problem" to the simplified "religious or spiritual problem", so as to maintain congruence with other V-Code titles (Turner et al., 1995, p. 436). The revised definition proposed that:

> This category can be used when the focus of clinical attention is a religious or spiritual problem. Examples include distressing experiences that involve loss or questioning of faith, problems associated with conversion to a new faith, or questioning of other spiritual values which may not necessarily be related to an organized church or religious institution. (Lukoff, Lu & Turner, 1995, p. 469; Task Force on DSM-IV, 1993, p. U:8)

Due to the significant changes to their original submission, Lukoff and company challenged this revised definition, but were unsuccessful (Turner et al., 1995, p. 436). The above definition was subsequently introduced into DSM-IV in 1994 as V62.89 "Religious or spiritual problem" (APA, 1994, p. 685), then, in 2000, replicated in DSM-IV-TR (APA, 2000, p. 741). This event constituted both a progressive step and a failing for American psychiatry. To have included the word 'spiritual' at all in a category heading was a novel development. However, divesting the category of its original transpersonal meaning and purpose seemingly reflected an unwillingness, or inability, to fully accept the reality of psychospiritual experiences.

Issues of semantics aside, the task force's approval of the V62.89 'Religious or spiritual problem' category precipitated a wave of interest in the subject. As Lukoff, Turner & Lu (1993, p. 12) noted at the time:

> an increasing number of presentations addressing religious or spiritual issues in clinical practice are being made at the American Psychiatric Association Annual Meetings. In 1993, there were at least a dozen workshops, courses and symposia in the scientific program. Topics included: 'Religious Issues in Residency Training', 'Transpersonal Psychiatry', 'Existential and Spiritual Issues in PTSD Treatment', and a 'Practicum on Spiritual Issues in Treatment'.

This mirrored the similar upsurge of clinical interest in metaphysical matters that occurred during the 1970s with Dean's introduction of the notions of metapsychiatry and ultraconsciousness, and further demonstrates the capacity for mainstream psychiatry to consider the ramifications of such matters in clinical practice.

7.1.3 V62.89 and the 'spiritual' problem

Although the inclusion of V62.89 'Religious or spiritual problem' in DSM-IV marked a breakthrough and a triumph in terms of establishing a clinical platform for considering religious or spiritual problems in psychiatric diagnostics, the revised definition seemingly stripped Lukoff and company's V-Code proposal of both its intended use as a differential diagnosis category, and its essential transpersonal meaning. For instance, whereas the original proposal centred on enabling the clinician to make a differential diagnosis between psychospiritual and psychopathological experiences, V62.89 was ostensibly limited to considering the clinical implications of dilemmas and difficulties relating to a person's religious and spiritual beliefs and practices. Additionally, apart from the word 'spiritual', all metaphysical language and meaning was expunged from the V62.89 definition. Yet the original definition depicted psychospiritual problems as 'experiences that a person finds troubling or distressing and that involve that person's relationship with a transcendent being or force', with mystical experiences proffered as an example. For this reason, Lu et al. (1997b, p. 1012) conclude that "the name change to 'religious or spiritual problem' might result in the loss of conceptual clarity that could aid the differential diagnosis and referral process". Teodorescu (c2008) also critically remarked that "the DSM revision committee changed the name of the diagnosis as well as excluded spiritual emergencies as proposed by Lukoff, Lu and Turner, turning it into a more general and less specific diagnosis". It therefore appears that the V62.89 definition portrays a spiritual problem as pertaining only to everyday spirituality and does not include experiences relating to mysticism, transcendent beings or forces, and psychotic-like spiritual emergencies.

It is unclear whether the task force intended the term 'spiritual values' to incorporate metaphysical considerations, but the fact that they purposefully removed any related terminology suggests not. Regardless, after the publication of DSM-IV, Lukoff and company continued to maintain that V62.89 was applicable as a 'spiritual problem' category that enabled a psychiatrist to consider whether or not a person's distress was associated with transpersonal experiences or crises.[66] Yet, despite these repeated assertions, Turner acknowledged in a 2005 interview that while the task force authors "allowed the word spiritual to be used" despite their discomfort in doing so, they also stripped the V-Code of its essential intended meaning "by dropping the words Mystical and NDEs" (Herrick, 2008, p. 82). Arguably, then, the modified DSM-IV version of 'spiritual' appears to be a psychologised and shallow clinical idiom, with a scope of meaning limited to everyday religious issues or spiritual anxieties, and devoid of deeper mystical connotations and application. If so, the DSM-IV 'Religious or spiritual problem' category did not have the clinical scope for diagnostically differentiating psychospiritual from psychotic experiences. The essential transpersonal vision and meaning of Lukoff and company's 'psychospiritual problems' definition was lost when modified by the DSM-IV task force. Furthermore, their aim to encourage psychiatry to recognise the veracity of mystic realities was also seemingly thwarted, for the task force reluctantly allowed the word 'spiritual' into the manual only after having divested it of its essential mystical associations.

7.1.4 DSM-5 and the 'Religious or spiritual problem'

With the advent of the DSM-5 review process, Lukoff and associates again attempted to have the 'Religious or spiritual problem' category invested with its original transpersonal scope and depth of meaning. In 2006, a symposium was held in which many "well-known clinicians and researchers" gathered to consider "the spiritual and religious aspects of major diagnostic categories including psychotic disorders", and

---

[66] For example see: Lukoff et al., 2010; Lukoff, 2009, p. 138; Lukoff, 2007, p. 637; Lukoff, 2001, p. 1; Yang et al., 2006, p. 169; Lukoff & Lu, 1999, p. 470; Lukoff et al., 1999, p. 68; Lukoff, Lu & Turner, 1998, pp. 32–39; Lu et al., 1997a, p. 76; Lukoff, Lu & Turner, 1996, pp. 236–239; Lukoff, Lu & Turner, 1995, p. 475; Turner et al., 1995, pp. 439–441.

related issues of differential diagnosis (Peteet et al., 2011a, pp. xvii-xviii). A Spiritual-ity White Paper Group was subsequently established (Lukoff et al., 2010, p. 424) and they published the findings and decisions of the symposium in a book titled *Religious and Spiritual Issues in Psychiatric Diagnosis: A Research Agenda for DSM-V* (Peteet et al., 2011b). In this book, Lukoff et al. (2011, p. 192) proposed an updated V62.89 defini-tion that reflects "current peer-reviewed research on religious or spiritual problems by including mention of the additional types of problems identified in the literature". Their proposed definition essentially reiterated the DSM original, though with the added specification of several spiritual problems:

> This category can be used when the focus of clinical attention is a religious or spiri-tual problem. Examples include distressing experiences that involve loss or ques-tioning of faith; *changes in membership practices, and beliefs (including conversion); New Religious Movements and cults; and life threatening terminal illness. Examples of spiritual problems include mystical experiences, near-death experiences, psychic experiences, alien abduction experiences, meditation and spiritual practice-related experiences, possession experiences, and* questioning of other spiritual values which may not necessarily be related to an organized church or religious institution. (ibid)

This definition, again, endorses a category that recognises the existence of non-psychopathological, psychotic-like, psychospiritual experiences, and enables clinical scope for considering these in diagnostic practice. Lukoff and company (2010, p. 441) further recommended that in DSM-5 "research is needed to answer remaining questions about the complex relationship between religion/spirituality and psychi-atric disorders", particularly when considering "the value laden and culturally con-ditioned nature of psychiatric diagnosis". In their view, such research necessitates critically examining "a variety of unusual experiences which appear to challenge our understanding of the world, such as mystical experiences" (ibid., p. 426). These recommendations called upon psychiatry to extend its philosophical and epistemo-logical bounds to enable the serious consideration of transpersonal phenomena in psychiatric diagnostics, particularly in the context of discerning between psychotic and psychospiritual experiences.

Despite the considerable body of literature substantiating the existence of psy-chospiritual realities, and noting the importance for psychiatry to investigate them in order to better understand the complexity of states of human consciousness, it appears the DSM-5 task force was reticent, or unable, to seriously adopt such consid-erations into its worldview. Although the category of 'Religious or spiritual problem' was included in DSM-5 (APA, 2013, p. 725), the appeal by Lukoff and colleagues to upgrade its definition so as to represent a wide array of psychospiritual phenom-ena and experiences was largely unsuccessful. For instance, the present DSM-5 definition is a verbatim replication of that in DSM-IV, but is now placed in a sub-section titled "Problems Related to Other Psychosocial, Personal, and Environmental

Circumstances" (ibid.). This clearly construes 'Religious or spiritual problem' dynamics as being circumstantial to psychosocial, personal, and environmental factors and, therefore, is a representation far removed from the original transpersonal meaning intended by Lukoff and colleagues.

Intriguingly, however, the words 'spiritual' and 'spirituality' are used prolifically throughout the DSM-5 manual, despite the task force's apparent reticence to invest this category with a broader scope of transpersonal meaning and application. This is a particularly noteworthy event, for it is the first time the word 'spirituality' has appeared within the DSM manuals. It ostensibly signifies a small but significant step towards the formal acknowledgment by mainstream psychiatry of a psychospiritual domain of being human. These particular usages, however, are conceptually and diagnostically unrelated to the 'Religious or spiritual problem' category, for they appear only in the manual's revised Cultural Formulation chapter (pp. 749–759) where they denote an aspect of "cultural identity" (pp. 749, 753), and their application is restricted to cultural diagnostic considerations. For example, the text advises that patients may proffer a "spiritual reason" as the cause of their problem and that "cultural variation in symptoms and in explanatory models associated with these cultural concepts may lead clinicians to misjudge the severity of a problem or assign the wrong diagnosis (e.g., unfamiliar spiritual explanations may be misunderstood as psychosis)" (pp. 752, 758–759). This is a fascinating development. For one, it demonstrates that mainstream psychiatry can incorporate psychospiritual considerations into its conceptual and operational framework. Also, the engagement with spiritual matters in the Cultural Formulation chapter seemingly reflects the transpersonal thinking expressed by Lukoff and colleagues in their V-Code proposal, which begs the questions: Why did the task force include psychospiritual considerations, within the context of psychosis, in the DSM-5 Cultural Formulation chapter, when approval of essentially the same in the proposed 'Religious or spiritual problem' category has been denied since the early 1990s? Is it because psychospiritual determinants in psychosis can be acknowledged for psychiatric patients from 'other' cultures, but not for mainstream Western patient populations? If so, why can unfamiliar spiritual explanations be misdiagnosed as psychosis in 'other' cultural contexts, but not in a Western cultural context? This question reflects the psychiatric 'cross-cultural conundrum' that I further examine in Chapter Twelve, Section 12.1.

Overall, Lukoff and company's V-Code proposal, and the subsequent introduction of a 'Religious or spiritual problem' category into the psychiatric lexicon, has seen psychospiritual matters invested with some clinical legitimacy, albeit limited. Although the essential transpersonal meaning of their original proposal has been edited from the final DSM product, the fact that this category has been accepted into the DSM series at all constitutes additional evidence that psychiatry can engage psychospiritual realities within its remit. Indeed, as is evidenced in the ensuing section, this attention to psychospiritual matters within mainstream psychiatry appears to be a growing phenomenon.

7.2 Contemporary outlooks on psychospiritual matters in global psychiatry

Since the 1990s, and particularly over the past decade, emergent pockets of attention to psychospiritual areas of human life have occurred within global mainstream psychiatry. For instance, in an American context, psychiatrist John Peteet, chair of the APA's Corresponding Committee on Religion, Spirituality and Psychiatry, claims that "recognition of the value of religious and spiritual beliefs and practices in mental health treatment has grown in recent years" (Moran, 2007, p. 10). The Committee's code of commitments states that "psychiatrists should foster recovery by making treatment decisions with patients in ways that respect and take into meaningful consideration their cultural, religious/spiritual, and personal ideals" (APA, 2006). Similarly, Stoddard (2012, p. 544), an APA Board of Trustees member, affirms that "there is increased recognition in clinical care and in research in psychiatry of the importance of religion and spirituality in our patients' lives". Additionally, the APA's *Position Statement on Diversity* upholds that "the American Psychiatric Association supports the development of cultural diversity among its membership and within the field of psychiatry", which includes issues regarding "religious/spiritual beliefs" (APA, 1999). In fact, the aforementioned book titled *Religious and Spiritual Issues in Psychiatric Diagnosis* (Peteet et al., 2011b) is a psychiatric text dedicated entirely to considering, and making clinical recommendations about, psychospiritual and religious matters in relation to key diagnostic categories such as depression, schizophrenia and psychotic disorders, substance use disorders, anxiety related disorders, post-traumatic stress, personality disorders, and child and adolescent psychopathology. These developments within American psychiatry represent initial but significant steps in extending its epistemological horizons to enable the investigation of possible psychospiritual determinants in psychopathology and psychosis.

There has also been a recent emergence of psychiatric interest in psychospiritual matters in other contexts. For instance, there have been attempts by some psychiatrists within the fields of neuroscience and neurotheology to understand human spiritual experience in light of medical science. There has also been an endeavour by some psychiatrists to examine mystical and metaphysical occurrences as ontological realities. These promising developments are examined below in more detail.

7.2.1 Neuroscience and neurotheology

Within the field of medicine there has been a longstanding and entrenched resistance to studying phenomena beyond the theoretical bounds set by empirical science. Research is restricted to that which is objective, observable, measurable, and replicable, while subjective experiences and states of consciousness, whether apparently normal or abnormal, are relegated to the dubious status of 'anecdotal'. As neuropsychiatrist Peter Fenwick (2009, p. 170) wryly observes, "science puts its fingers to its lips and is largely silent when the question of consciousness arises ... The peep show of the private world of the individual's mind should not be included in our theories".

Despite this reticence, the fields of neuroscience and neurotheology have made some preliminary headway in the scientific study of religion and spirituality.

7.2.1.1 Neuroscience and psychiatry

Neuroscience, as a medical discipline, generally endorses the materialist understanding that consciousness is epiphenomenal to the brain and physical body. Ipso facto, states of psychospiritual consciousness, if accepted as real, are generally also overlooked by neuroscience. Recently, however, there has been some interest in investigating this subject, though in keeping with the fundamental premise that "religious experience is brain-based" (Saver & Rabin, 1997, p. 195). Therefore, through the use of technology such as neuroimaging, it is theoretically possible to identify and measure changes in brain activity that correlate with subjective reports made by people about spiritual experiences, particularly in structured practices such as prayer or meditation (Fenwick, 2011, pp. 2, 4). According to Fenwick (ibid., p. 7), the empirical verification of such correlative brain activity constitutes "the beginning of a definite neuroscience of spirituality and spiritual experience". Although such neuroscientific thinking is couched in the language of reductive materialism, it does acknowledge the veracity of psychospiritual experience and, in so doing, brings it into the fold of legitimate scientific research.

Neuropsychiatry, as a branch of neuroscientific research, has also opened its scope of investigation to include psychospiritual considerations. Essentially, in this context, the envisioned task for neuropsychiatry is to "delineate the distinctive neural substrates of religious experience and their alteration in brain disorders" and to "review data that have been collected on religious experience in normal individuals and in different neurologic and neuropsychiatric syndromes" so that "a preliminary unifying model of the brain basis of religious experience may be constructed" (Saver & Rabin, 1997, p. 195). Hence, in order to refine diagnostic practices, neuropsychiatry aims to identify discrete neurological activity that corresponds with reported religio-psychospiritual and psychopathological experiences. For instance, Perroud (2009, p. 48) has proposed the idea of measuring neurotransmitter concentrations to ascertain whether "seritonergic and dopaminergic systems" flux in association with psychospiritual experiences, and maintains that such research "could help to understand the complex link between psychiatric disorders and spirituality". Fenwick (2009, p. 185) also observes that neuroscience has not only established a correlation between spiritual practices and neurological activity, but that these practices also have a beneficial impact on "brain function" and in fostering "an improvement in mental and physical health". This suggests the therapeutic value of such research and, arguably, substantiates Dean's assertion thirty years beforehand regarding the potential mental health benefits associated with the study and practice of metapsychiatry. Further, such neuropsychiatric investigation of psychospiritual matters may enable new insights into the nature of both mystic and psychotic states of consciousness.

7.2.1.2 Neurotheology and psychiatry

Neurotheology is a neuroscience adjunct which practices the biological investigation of metaphysical experiences. Beauregard & O'Leary (2007, p. 208) succinctly define "neurotheology" as a discipline that "analyses the biological basis of spirituality", while Newberg (2010, p. 1) defines it as "a unique field of scholarship that seeks to understand the relationship specifically between the brain and theology, and more broadly between the mind and religion". According to Miller (2001), neurotheology is a multidisciplinary body of research that includes "medicine, psychiatry, psychology, physics, complexity, chemistry, biology, philosophy, mathematics, computer science, genetics, theology, consciousness studies and several social sciences", while Beauregard & Paquette (2006, p. 186) refer to it as "spiritual neuroscience", which they describe as "a field of scientific investigation at the crossroads of psychology, religion and spirituality, and neuroscience". Fundamentally, then, neurotheology aims to ascertain if spiritual experience is centred in the brain and is intrinsic to human nature. As Newberg et al. (2002, p. 176) hypothesise:

> All human beings have a brain, and all of these brains work in a very similar fashion. So if we are ever going to get a sense of the universal aspects of religion, then the brain might be the best place to start.

Therefore, on the whole, it is a discipline that endorses what Muller (2008) refers to as a "bottom up" approach, whereby "explanations for religious belief and spirituality offered by neurotheologians ... derive from a science that sees our lives as being largely determined by biological factors". As in standard neuroscience, neurotheological research involves using brain scanning technology[67] to ascertain whether correlations exist between spiritual experiences and localised brain activity. This not only includes an examination of mystical, shamanic, and religious experiences, but also specific trance induction practices such as meditation, prayer, yoga, relaxation, dancing, chanting, hyperventilation (Horgan, 2004, p. 74). Although Cohen (2005, p. 134) derisively refers to neurotheology as "robing religion in the raiment of science", in a positive sense it represents an attempt by science to take spirituality seriously, albeit by reducing the spiritual experience to measurable pockets of brain activity.

As a relatively new discipline, it appears that neurotheology has not yet been adopted into the body of psychiatric and neuropsychiatric research. However, as Miller (2001) notes above, psychiatry is included within its multidisciplinary remit, and it appears that neurotheological research is indeed of some relevance to psychiatry. For example, findings in the field indicate that religious or spiritual matters and occurrences "are based not on delusional ideas but on experiences that are neurologically real" (Newberg et al., 2002, p. 126). Also, d'Aquili & Newberg (1999, p. 207) envisage

---

[67] Neurotheological research instruments include electroencephalography (EEG), positron emission tomography (PET), single photon emission computed tomography (SPECT), and functional magnetic resonance imaging (fMRI) (Newberg, 2010, pp. 122–123).

that through neurotheological research "it is possible ... mystical experiences may finally be clearly differentiated from any type of psychopathology". Hence, there is apparent scope for neurotheology to be extended into the field of psychiatric research to assist in better understanding the nature of psychospiritual matters in relation to psychotic experiences, to redress the apparent problem of discerning psychospiritual from psychopathological experiences, and to reduce the incidence of misdiagnosis.

An intriguing development within neurotheology, which is of profound relevance to psychiatry, is the questioning of the axiomatic materialist assumption as to the physical primacy of reality. Despite the materialist basis of neuroscientific and neurotheological thinking, there are some researchers in these fields who have stepped beyond this premise to pose the question: Are psychospiritual experiences caused by, or the cause of, brain changes? As Newberg (2010, p. 126) acknowledges, a conundrum in neurotheological research is whether brain scan results show "the brain creating an experience or responding to one?". Further to this, Newberg & Lee (2005, p. 481) caution that "care must be taken to avoid ... reducing spiritual experiences only to neurophysiological mechanisms", while Cunningham (2011b, p. 227) maintains that "religious experience ... cannot be anchored to an anatomically separate area of the brain". Newberg & Lee (2005, p. 484) raise the same issue in the context of God: "If the brain activity changes during a mystical communion with God, it is not clear whether the brain activity caused that experience or responded to that experience". Indeed, in their book *The Spiritual Brain: A Neuroscientist's Case for the Existence of the Soul*, Beauregard & O'Leary (2007, pp. 289–295) dedicate a chapter to exploring the research question: "Did God Create the Brain or Does the Brain Create God?". Here, they propose:

1. The need for "a new scientific frame of reference" with a research compass reaching beyond the limits of "dogmatic materialist scientism" (ibid., p. 294).
2. That such scientific research considers the possibility that "mystical experience from various spiritual traditions indicates that the nature of mind, consciousness, and reality as well as the meaning of life can be apprehended through an intuitive, unitive, and experiential form of knowing" (ibid.).

This is a radical proposal, for it repositions the locus of scientific investigation into subjective realms that have traditionally been perceived as unscientific. It also infers the possibility of psychospiritual primacy, and therefore represents a tentative step in scientific research to reconcile the tension between materialist and metaphysical thinking. In fact, Cook (2004, p. 150) describes neurotheology as a field of research that aims to understand "the functioning of the mind/brain in relation to God or *ultimate reality*" (italics added), which clearly accords primacy to the psychospiritual domain. This idea of the brain responding to rather than causing psychospiritual experiences, challenges the basic tenets of conventional science. By extrapolation, it also opens to the possibility that, as a state of consciousness, psychosis may likewise be the product of psychospiritual determinants, and that brain activity patterns observed in psychotic patients by neuropsychiatry may be of a correlational and not a causal nature.

7.2.2 Psychospiritual ventures within mainstream psychiatry

Since the 1994 advent of DSM-IV, there have been several attempts by psychiatrists to incorporate psychospiritual considerations into psychiatric thinking and practice. These ventures have all been driven by the view that an investigation of psycho-spiritual matters by psychiatry is important. An overview of some of these further demonstrates that, despite the predominant biogenic predisposition of contemporary mainstream psychiatry, it is possible to seriously consider psychospiritual matters in clinical thinking and practice, for many psychiatrists have done so. In fact, this appears to be an emergent trend rather than a collection of sporadic and anomalous incidents.

7.2.2.1 International association for spiritual psychiatry

Despite the DSM-IV task force's inability to fully accept Lukoff and colleagues' transpersonal V-Code category, psychiatrists elsewhere in the world were evidently able to embrace such psychospiritual ideas. A salient case in point was the establishment of the International Association for Spiritual Psychiatry (IASP) in 1994. IASP was founded by French psychiatrist Jean-Marc Mantel and its guiding maxim was "psychiatry, medicine of the soul" (IASP, 2005). Horopciuc & Petrea (1994) define the IASP notion of 'spiritual psychiatry' as a practice that "foresees mental pathology as an opportune junction of human spirituality with a full study of the self". The association began with a global membership of 250 clinicians who endorsed the aims of promoting "the integration of the spiritual dimension into modern medicine, psychology and psychiatry" and participating in "the creation of a psycho-spiritual medicine integrating scientific thought and mystical insight" (ibid.). In pragmatic terms, Mantel (2004, pp. 5, 6) depicted the spiritual psychiatrist as a spiritual practitioner-cum-clinician, who endorsed the moderate use of medication as an adjunct to psychotherapeutic guidance, and who aimed not only to remedy a presenting psychiatric problem, but ultimately, to foster a person's spiritual development. He aspired to instigate "the advent of a psychiatry which places the psychic crisis in a wider context, that of man in search of himself" and foresaw that "psychiatry will then be able to fully inhabit its function, that of an awakener of consciousness and an artisan of peace" (ibid., p. 6). As utopian and farfetched as this may seem from the perspective of orthodox psychiatry, such an approach has been exemplified in Tibetan psychiatry whereby the entire therapeutic system is founded upon the psychospiritual knowledge and maturity of practitioners.[68]

IASP disbanded in 2002. However, its outcomes were quite substantial during its eight years of operation. For example, it published a biannual journal and conducted a variety of activities, including "conferences, lectures, workshops, creation

---

[68] Chapter Thirteen provides a comprehensive critical investigation of Tibetan psychiatry and its understanding of psychosis.

of psycho-spiritual medicine centers, forum Internet [sic] on spiritual approaches to medicine, psychology and psychiatry, cooperation with other associations, etc." (IASP, 2005). Hence, as a modality of 'spiritual psychiatry' it demonstrated the feasibility of incorporating psychospiritual understandings into researching and therapeutically responding to instances of psychosis. My investigation throughout Focal Settings Three and Four very much supports this idea.

7.2.2.2 Spirituality and psychiatry special interest group

Another significant development in 'spiritual psychiatry' was the 1999 inauguration of the Royal College of Psychiatrists' Spirituality and Psychiatry Special Interest Group (SPSIG). Whereas IASP constituted an independent body of clinicians, SPSIG is affiliated with, and endorsed by, the Royal College of Psychiatrists (RCP) which is "the professional and educational body for psychiatrists in the United Kingdom" (Royal College of Psychiatrists, 2021). The growth of SPSIG's membership since then indicates a definitive professional interest in the interface between psychiatry and spirituality. For instance, in 2005 there were about 900 SPSIG members (Eagger, 2006), but by 2012 this had increased to a membership of 3000 (Cook, 2012), which represents about eighteen per cent of the total 16,321 RCP members for that year (Cameron, 2012, p. 15).[69] Subsequently, Dein et al. (2010, p. 64) have asserted that:

> the burgeoning interest in this field, from within the profession and from service users alike, supports our view that an understanding of the relationship of spirituality and religion to mental health, far from being an optional extra, should be counted as essential to good clinical practice.

Whereas Lukoff struggled in vain to see mystical concepts introduced into the American DSM manuals, these are being explored openly within UK psychiatry.

The SPSIG research scope is broad and eclectic. It includes mental health issues relating to "the problem of good and evil and a wide range of specific experiences invested with spiritual meaning including birth, death and near-death, mystical and trance states and varieties of religious experience" (SPSIG, 2013). Indeed, the website archive page features about two hundred papers submitted by members and guests that discuss a vast range of psychospiritual-related issues. For instance, Crowley (2007) notes the need to differentiate psychotic from mystical experiences and spiritual emergencies. Mitchell (2010, p. 4) correspondingly highlights the problematic point that it is "impossible to differentiate between mystical experiences and psychosis solely on the basis of phenomenological description", while Randal & Argyle (2005) address both of these issues. Other topics examined, which are normally pathologised or ignored by psychiatry, are: parapsychology (Pandarakalam, 2007), prayer (Raji, 2004; Fenwick, 2004), transpersonal psychiatry (Read, 2007), kundalini (Sourial, 2007;

---

[69] SPSIG (2021) currently has 3,600 members (as of May 2021).

Coghlan, 2007),[70] God (Coghlan, 2003; Lawrence, 2002), meditation (Sharma, 2008), "regression in the service of transcendence" (Read, 2011, p. 11), and spirit possession (Sanderson, 2012, 2003; Loewenthal, 2012).[71] All of these, when seriously considered, represent domains or states of experience and consciousness that ostensibly challenge medical psychiatry to reconsider its worldview for understanding, discerning, diagnosing, and treating psychotic disorders, and indeed, for defining mental illness.

As indicated above, a principal area of research and commentary for SPSIG is the relationship between spirituality and psychosis, and how this may shape psychiatric epistemology and diagnostic practices. The following list of article titles provides a snapshot of some key SPSIG research topics in relation to this:

- "Symptoms of spiritual crisis and the therapeusis of healing" (Brandon, 2010).
- "Spiritual aspects of psychosis and recovery" (Mitchell, 2010).
- "What proportion of psychiatrists take a spiritual history?" (Nazir, 2010).
- "Lack of spiritual practice—an important risk factor for suffering from distress" (Kohls & Walach, 2008).
- "Personal religious or spiritual beliefs, and the experience of hearing voices, having strong beliefs, or other experiences affecting mental wellbeing and general functioning" (Marriot, 2008).
- "Furthering the spiritual dimension of psychiatry in the United Kingdom" (Powell, 2007).
- "Psychosis and spirituality: The journey of an idea" (Clarke, 2006).
- "Psychosis or spiritual emergence?—Consideration of the transpersonal perspective within psychiatry" (Crowley, 2006).
- "'Spiritual emergency'—a useful explanatory model? A literature review and discussion paper" (Randal & Argyle, 2005).
- "Telepathy, parapsychology and psychiatry" (Beddow, 2004).
- "Mysterious ways: Spirituality and British psychiatry in the 20th century" (Sims, 2003).
- "Examining our spiritual spectacles: Dangers and pitfalls" (Raheja, 2001).

The view that spirituality should be central, rather than peripheral, to psychiatric thinking, training, and practice is also emphasised in a recommendation made in the SPSIG position statement: "Religion and spirituality and their relationship to the diagnosis, aetiology and treatment of psychiatric disorders should be considered as essential components of both psychiatric training and continuing professional development" (Cook, 2011, p. 10). This proposal is also affirmed verbatim in the official "statement on spirituality and religion in psychiatry" formulated by the World

---

[70] Definitions of kundalini vary significantly among commentators on this phenomenon. However, it generally refers to a psychospiritual force that can emerge within the body, and in some instances, create symptoms that mimic those of psychosis.

[71] The phenomenon of spiritual possession in the context of psychotic experience is thoroughly examined in Chapters Twelve and Thirteen.

Psychiatric Association Section on Religion, Spirituality and Psychiatry (Verhagen & Cook, 2010, p. 630). Overall, the SPSIG exemplifies the capacity for mainstream psychiatry to seriously investigate psychospiritual matters in relation to psychopathology and psychosis. The robust example set by this mainstream psychiatric entity dispels the prevailing clinical view that psychospiritual matters are beyond the investigative remit of medical psychiatry.

7.2.2.3 Further examples of psychospiritual interests in psychiatry

Contemporary psychiatric interest in psychospiritual matters is not only confined to groups such as IASP and SPSIG. A considerable and growing body of literature indicates that psychiatrists worldwide are considering this issue. The views expressed largely fall into two broad camps: one, that psychiatry as a discipline is deficient if psychospiritual experiences and concerns are not included in its remit; and two, that there is a subsequent need for psychospiritual materials to be included in psychiatric training.

In regard to the first idea, psychiatry is seen as deficient in several ways. For instance, Fabrega Jr (2000) describes contemporary medical psychiatry as the product "of a non-spiritual worldview" that consequently endorses "a secular, reductionistic credo of diagnosis and practice". Additionally, he maintains its excessive reliance on pharmaceutical interventions results in a failure to consider "the essential cultural, religious and spiritual meanings that are integral to the experience and diagnosis of psychopathology" (ibid.). Similarly, Dein et al. (2010, p. 64) submit that a spiritually sensitive model of psychiatric assessment should include "an enquiry into meaning" rather than simply check-listing symptoms. Huguelet et al. (2006, p. 371) consider doing so to be essential because, in their view, understanding people's religious and psychospiritual beliefs is often vital for helping them contend with psychotic beliefs and experiences. Keks & D'Souza (2003, pp. 170, 171) likewise assert that it is "essential that spirituality be taken seriously in the supportive management of patients with psychoses. Spirituality can be used constructively to help recovery and reintegration from psychosis". The views of such commentators arguably indicate that medical psychiatry's poor comprehension of psychospiritual matters not only impedes the delivery of optimal therapeutic support, but may also result in misguided and harmful interventions. Other commentators have expressed the view that the reductive model of medical psychiatry fails to recognise the interconnectivity between all aspects of life, including psychopathology. From this perspective, mental health and mental illness are not discrete states of being, but holistically interpenetrate each other. For example, Kingdon et al. (2010, pp. 246, 242) propose that "a continuum exists between psychoticism, normality and spirituality" and, therefore, "the experience of hallucinations, visual or auditory or both, can be among the most interesting areas where spirituality and psychosis merge". Combined, these views suggest that the instigation of psychiatric practice that is sensitive to psychospiritual issues calls for more than the incidental consideration of a 'Religious or spiritual problem' category. It necessitates a major paradigm shift.

Finally, in regard to the second idea, several commentators draw attention to the urgent need for psychospiritual skills and training in psychiatry. For example, Ng (2007, p. 65) notes that, at present, "psychiatrists in general are probably not well placed to assess religious and spiritual beliefs". Similarly, Yang et al. (2006, p. 173) report that "clinicians increasingly acknowledge that they need to take patients' lives and spiritual experiences into account, yet few have been trained in assessing or working with spiritual issues". In light of this situation, D'souza & George (2006, p. 409) suggest that effective clinical assessment and support practices must consider all aspects of the holistic body-mind-spirit matrix of human nature and that "clinicians should employ a variety of spiritually informed therapeutic tools to facilitate the patient's coping ability, thus enhancing well-being and recovery". Indeed, they recommend that "all medical students and graduates should be trained to take a spiritual history as part of history taking", including those studying psychiatry (ibid., p. 410). In this regard, the RCP have taken a proactive step by offering an online continuing professional development module titled *Exploring Spirituality with People Who Use Mental Health Services*,[72] which states:

> This module will help you to develop your awareness of patients' spiritual health needs. We aim to provide an outline of the current thinking and literature on this topic, and motivate you to incorporate this aspect of care into your practice. The module will also enable you to consider your own spiritual development, and will provide some helpful tools to assist you in taking a spiritual history. (Eagger & Ferdinando, 2013)

This is a progressive development, for it not only demonstrates the feasibility of implementing psychospiritual training within mainstream psychiatry, which, thirty-five years earlier, Stanley Dean called for as a metapsychiatry adjunct, but also addresses the notion that the effectiveness of this in psychiatric practice is relative to a clinician's own level of psychospiritual development. Indeed, some psychiatrists believe that the discipline's continuation is dependent on such developments. For instance, D'souza & George (2006, p. 411) envisage that the investigation of psychospiritual matters "in time may well come to be seen as the salvation of biomedicine". Regardless of the validity of such prediction, and the prevailing aversion within mainstream psychiatry to ascribing clinical importance to psychospiritual matters, there evidently exists within the discipline an emergent interest in the potential clinical relevance of such matters.

---

[72] This training program appears to be the culmination of a series of publications in the UK regarding the value and necessity of incorporating 'spirituality' into the thinking and practices of the mental health sector. For example, see: *Taken Seriously: Report of the Somerset Spirituality Project* (Mental Health Foundation, 2002); *Inspiring Hope: Recognising the Importance of Spirituality in a Whole Person Approach to Mental Health* (Gilbert et al., 2003); *Spirituality, Values and Mental Health: Jewels for the Journey* (Coyte et al., 2007).

7.3 Conclusion

In light of psychiatry's perennial disregard of psychospiritual determinants in psycho-pathology and psychosis research, my primary aim in Focal Setting Two has been to demonstrate the existence and *feasibility* of such research within psychiatry. Arguably, in identifying many such significant instances, this objective has been fulfilled. Indeed, the ground for continuing such research has already been established by Bucke, Dean, Lukoff, neuroscientific studies, and psychiatric special interest groups. Focal Setting Three goes a step further to propose the seeming *necessity* of such research, when considering the manifest similarities between psychospiritual and psychotic experiences.

FOCAL SETTING THREE

UNDERSTANDING PSYCHOSIS: DISCERNING PSYCHOSPIRITUAL FROM PSYCHOPATHOLOGICAL

Focal Setting Three critically investigates the problem of discerning psychotic from non-psychopathological psychotic-like psychospiritual experiences and questions whether such differentiation is possible.

CHAPTER 8

Psychopathological or psychospiritual: early to present models

8.0 Introduction

This chapter delves more deeply into the matter of psychotic-like features occurring in psychospiritual experiences. An introductory overview of literature pertaining to this issue is provided and an examination of the first comprehensive attempts to elicit a list of differentiating factors is undertaken. As Cunningham (2015) notes, psychiatry "does not recognize the difference between mystical and psychotic experiences". Hence, this chapter demonstrates how psychospiritual knowledge can offer potential new ways to understand psychosis and challenges psychiatry's materialist-based assumptions regarding the nature of psychopathology.

8.1 Discerning psychospiritual from psychopathological

The issue of discerning psychopathological from psychospiritual experiences in psychiatric practice has already been touched upon in Focal Setting Two. Bucke, Dean, the GAP authors, and Lukoff and company have all addressed this within a psychiatric context. However, the recognition of parallels and differences between psychopathological and psychospiritual states of consciousness is not new. Indeed, a wealth of texts exist in which authors have wrestled with the question of mapping convergences and divergences between psychopathological (psychotic) and psychospiritual (psychotic-like) experiences. For example, in ancient Greek literature, Socrates (in Plato's *Phaedrus*) claimed that "there is a divine as well as a human madness" (Long & Macleane, 1868, p. 40). However, while many contemporary investigators also note similarities and differences between psychotic and psychospiritual experiences, they mostly hold the common assumption that these are discrete phenomena.[73] This is exemplified by Douglas-Smith (1971, pp. 553–554) who concludes, after conducting an empirical study on religious mysticism, that the mystical experience "appears to be *sui generis*" and, therefore, distinct from psychotic disorders. Dodds (1951, p. 68) similarly notes that "the dividing line between common insanity and prophetic madness is ... hard to draw", thus inferring there is a dividing line despite the difficulty in discerning it.

The notion of differentiating psychotic from psychospiritual experiences, and the difficulty in doing so, constitutes a significant challenge to accepted psychiatric assumptions about the nature of 'psychopathology'. For instance, it is assumed that psychopathology (mental illness) stands in contradistinction to normalcy (mental health), and it is the job of psychiatry to identify and remedy the former. If, however, the existence of anomalous, non-psychopathological, psychotic-like mystical experiences is accepted, then this adds a problematic variable to the diagnostic formula, for such experiences are neither normal nor insane. A vexing question raised by this new dynamic is: If it seems like madness, but is not, then what, exactly, defines madness in contradistinction to non-madness? There appears to be no definitive answer to this question. Hence, the introduction of psychospiritual considerations into the diagnostic mix renders the fundamental psychiatric notion of psychopathology obscure and difficult to operationalise. This may partially explain why conventional psychiatry has generally eschewed the question and the difficulty of distinguishing psychopathological from psychospiritual experiences. To do so would likely unveil a host of intractable complexities that may destabilise accepted clinical and diagnostic views as to what is and is not psychotic. Such potential epistemological problems, however, do not justify avoiding the conundrums and ambiguities that invariably arise from trying to discriminate between psychotic and spiritual experiences. Rather, they present potential opportunities to better understand the enigma of psychosis by bringing to light new ideas for consideration, and alternative ways to consider traditional viewpoints. My later investigations throughout Chapters Nine and Ten support this line of thinking.

8.2 The Grofs' notion of spiritual emergency

Comprehensive attempts to formulate diagnostic criteria to differentiate between psychopathological and psychospiritual experiences is a relatively recent occurrence. Two pioneers in this field of investigation are the American psychiatrist Stanislav Grof and psychotherapist Christina Grof. Their extensive research into spiritual emergencies constitutes a significant challenge for psychiatry to reconsider its basic epistemological assumptions about the nature of reality and psychopathology. They coined the term "spiritual emergency" to designate apparently non-psychotic, psychospiritual experiences (Grof & Grof, 1995, p. 18), but also referred to these as a "transpersonal crisis" (Grof, 1983, p. 32) and a "psychospiritual crisis" (Grof, 2008a, 2000). It is their view that, rather than maintain the common psychiatric practice of equating mystical

---

[73] A content analysis of this body of literature is undertaken in Chapter Nine.

experiences with madness, there is a need to "reevaluate the relationship between psychiatry, spirituality, and psychosis" (Grof & Grof, 1989, p. xii). Hence, they believe it is imperative for psychiatry to differentiate between non-psychopathological spiritual emergencies and genuine psychotic experiences.

Stanislav Grof's conceptualisation of the notion of 'spiritual emergency' was directly influenced by three factors. First, his involvement in research over a twenty-year period (1950s to 1970s) on the metaphysical similarities between psychotic experiences and those precipitated by ingesting the hallucinogen LSD, in which a differentiation was made between "model psychosis" (i.e., LSD-induced hallucinogenic experiences) and "naturally occurring psychoses" (Grof, 1972; 1975, p. 1). Second, Maslow's (1963, 1962) idea of peak experiences. And third, the work of Italian psychiatrist and transpersonal practitioner Roberto Assagioli (1965, pp. 40–42) who developed a therapeutic approach called "psychosynthesis", which included the notion of a potential "crises" attendant to "spiritual awakening" that may be mistakenly identified as psychotic. It is unclear, however, when the term 'spiritual emergency' was first coined. Christina Grof states that she and Stanislav referred to a psychotic-like episode she experienced in 1976 as a "spiritual emergency" (Grof & Grof, 1995, p. 18). Whether or not this infers the term was created by both of them is not elucidated. Nor is it clear if it was fashioned at the time of this incident, or later, in retrospect.[74]

The notion of spiritual development is common to many, if not all, global cultures. According to Grof & Grof (1989, p. x), this can occur in two general forms; either as a benign "spiritual emergence" or the more dangerous "spiritual emergency". In their view, 'spiritual emergence' is a natural human evolutionary and developmental process, which they define as:

> the movement of an individual to a more expanded way of being that involves enhanced emotional and psychosomatic health, greater freedom of personal choices, and a sense of deeper connection with other people, nature and the cosmos. An important part of this development is an increasing awareness of the spiritual dimension in one's life and in the universal scheme of things. (Grof & Grof, 1995, pp. 40–41)

They explain that spiritual emergences often occur in an unobtrusive way and are easily integrated by a person into the flow and fabric of his or her everyday life. However, they can also emerge in a manner that is sudden, intense, and overwhelming, and in such instances, a spiritual emergence can become a spiritual emergency (see Table 4):

> People who are in such a crisis are bombarded with inner experiences that abruptly challenge their old beliefs and ways of existing, and their relationship with reality

---

[74] The earliest reference to the term's usage I can find is an unpublished 1977 mimeographed manuscript titled: "The concept of spiritual emergency: Understanding and treatment of transpersonal crises" (Grof & Grof, 1977). My attempt to procure a copy of this document from the authors was unsuccessful.

shifts very rapidly. Suddenly they feel uncomfortable in the formerly familiar world and may find it difficult to meet the demands of everyday life. They can have great problems distinguishing their inner visionary world from the external world of daily reality. (Grof & Grof, 1995, pp. 42–43)

Table 4. The Grofs' typology of differences between spiritual emergence and spiritual emergency.

Spiritual emergence	Spiritual emergency
Inner experiences are fluid, mild, easy to integrate.	Inner experiences are dynamic, jarring, difficult to integrate.
New spiritual insights are welcome, desirable, expansive.	New spiritual insights may be philosophically challenging and threatening.
Gradual infusion of ideas and insights into life.	Overwhelming influx of experiences and insights.
Experiences of energy that are contained and are easily manageable.	Experiences of jolting tremors, shaking, energy disruptive to daily life.
Easy differentiation between internal and external experience, and transition from one to other.	Sometimes difficult to distinguish between internal and external experiences, or simultaneous occurrence of both.
Ease in incorporating non-ordinary states of consciousness into daily life.	Inner experiences interrupt and disturb daily life.
Slow, gradual change in awareness of self and world.	Abrupt, rapid shift in perception of self and world.
Excitement about inner experiences as they arise and willingness and ability to co-operate with them.	Ambivalence toward inner experiences, and unwillingness or inability to co-operate with them using guidance.
Accepting attitude toward change.	Resistance to change.
Ease in giving up control.	Need to be in control.
Trust in process.	Dislike, mistrust in process.
Difficult experiences treated as opportunities for change.	Difficult experiences are overwhelming, often unwelcome.
Positive experiences accepted as gifts.	Positive experiences are difficult to accept, seem undeserved, can be painful.
Infrequent need to discuss experiences.	Frequent urgent need to discuss experiences.
Discriminating when communicating about process (when, how, with whom).	Indiscriminate communication about process (when, how, with whom).

Source: Grof & Grof, 1995, p. 45.

A spiritual emergency, then, is an extreme form of spiritual emergence that appears to mimic psychosis, but is actually a potential process for spiritual development. Indeed, in fashioning the term 'spiritual emergency' the Grofs (1989, p. x) intended that it denote both a "crisis and an opportunity". In other words, although it constitutes a crisis situation, it is not, ipso facto, psychopathological.

The Grofs highlighted the critical importance of understanding spiritual emergencies and discerning them from psychoses in psychiatric practice. They asserted that:

> episodes of nonordinary states of consciousness cover a very wide spectrum, from purely spiritual states without any pathological features to conditions that are clearly biological in nature and require medical treatment. It is extremely important to take a balanced approach and to be able to differentiate spiritual emergencies from genuine psychoses. (Grof & Grof, 1989, p. xiii)

Furthermore, they maintain that, in failing to make this differentiation, psychiatry has been inadvertently pathologising and thwarting potential transformative processes through the inappropriate use of medical treatments (Grof & Grof, 1995, p. 52). If so, it seems that such misdiagnosis and misplaced treatment can ironically have the iatrogenic effect of turning a spiritual emergency into a state of psychopathology.

To address the issue of ambiguity between psychopathology and spiritual emergency, and the related likelihood of misdiagnosis, the Grofs proposed that a balanced approach be adopted. They identified and described ten forms of spiritual emergency (see Table 5).

Table 5. Types of spiritual emergency as identified by the Grofs.

Type of spiritual emergency	Description
Shamanic crisis	During initiation throughout many cultures, neophyte shamans experience "a dramatic involuntary visionary state" in which they "typically undergo a journey into the underworld, the realm of the dead, where they are attacked by demons and exposed to horrendous tortures and ordeals". Similar experiences can occur in Western settings and may be a form of "psychospiritual crisis" rather than psychopathological.
Awakening of kundalini	In Indian mystical tradition, kundalini "is the generative cosmic energy, feminine in nature, that is responsible for the creation of the cosmos". It lays latent in the human "subtle or energetic body" and can be

(Continued)

Table 5. (Continued)

Type of spiritual emergency	Description
	activated via spiritual practices or occur spontaneously. This can result in an array of bodily events such as "intense sensations of energy and heat streaming up the spine", shaking, spasms, phantom pains; emotional symptoms such as "powerful waves of … anxiety, anger, sadness, or joy and ecstatic rapture"; and psychospiritual experiences such as "visions of brilliant light or various archetypal beings and a variety of internally perceived sounds … [and] powerful experiences of what seem to be memories from past lives".
Episodes of unitive consciousness ('peak experiences')	Maslow's mystical states of consciousness or 'peak experiences' in which people "have a sense of overcoming the usual fragmentation of the mind and body and feel that we have reached a state of unity and wholeness".
Psychological renewal through return to the centre	American psychiatrist John Weir Perry (1999) coined the term "renewal process". This designates a crisis situation in which people "experience their psyche as a colossal battlefield where a cosmic combat is being played out between the forces of Good and Evil, or Light and Darkness". This renewal process can manifest in a host of bizarre ways that look like, and are often identified as, psychotic phenomena.
Crisis of psychic opening	"An increase in intuitive abilities and the occurrence of psychic or paranormal phenomena are very common during spiritual emergencies of all kinds. However, in some instances, the influx of information from nonordinary sources, such as precognition, telepathy, or clairvoyance, becomes so overwhelming and confusing that it dominates the picture and constitutes a major problem, in and of itself".

(Continued)

Table 5. (Continued)

Type of spiritual emergency	Description
Past-life experiences	"Past-life experiences can complicate life in several different ways. Before their content emerges fully into consciousness and reveals itself, one can be haunted in everyday life by strange emotions, physical feelings, and visions without knowing where these are coming from or what they mean. Experienced out of context, these experiences naturally appear incomprehensible and irrational".
Communication with spirit guides and 'channeling'	Spirit guides "are usually perceived as discarnate humans, suprahuman entities, or deities existing on higher planes of consciousness and endowed with extraordinary wisdom". In 'channeling' a person "transmits to others messages received from a source that appears to be external … Experiences of channeling can precipitate a serious psychological and spiritual crisis. One possibility is that the individual involved can interpret the experience as an indication of beginning insanity. This is particularly likely if the channeling involves hearing voices, a well-known symptom of paranoid schizophrenia".
Near-death experiences (NDEs)	NDEs occur when a person is near death, or pronounced dead, yet recovers to report an experience that may include: floating above the scene in a conscious yet disembodied form, "a review of their entire lives … [and/or] passing through a dark tunnel or funnel toward a divine light of supernatural brilliance and beauty … Near-death experiences very frequently lead to spiritual emergencies … [and] can radically undermine the worldview of the people involved, because it catapults them abruptly and without warning into a reality that is diametrically different".

(Continued)

Table 5. (Continued)

Type of spiritual emergency	Description
Close encounters with UFOs and alien abduction experiences	"The experiences of encounters with extra-terrestrial spacecrafts and of abduction by alien beings can often precipitate serious emotional and intellectual crises that have much in common with spiritual emergencies ... C.G. Jung ... suggested that these phenomena might be archetypal visions originating in the collective unconscious of humanity, rather than psychotic hallucinations or visits by extraterrestrials from distant civilizations".
Possession states	"People in this type of transpersonal crisis have a distinct feeling that their psyche and body have been invaded and that they are being controlled by an evil entity or energy with personal characteristics. They perceive it as coming from outside their own personality and as being hostile and disturbing ... The problem manifests as serious psychopathology ... This condition clearly belongs in the category of 'spiritual emergency' in spite of the fact that it involves negative energies and is associated with many objectionable forms of behaviour".

Source: Grof, 2000.[75]

It is very likely that a person would be presumed psychotic if he or she reported any of the above experiences in a clinical setting, especially if distressed. However, in positing the possibility of non-psychopathological psychotic-like phenomena, the Grofs' notion of spiritual emergency challenges the traditional diagnostic picture of psychosis. Although they acknowledge the existence of psychopathology, they also suggest that its presenting signs and symptoms may, in fact, be indicative

---

[75] The description for each type of spiritual emergency in the above table is a composite of my quoting, paraphrasing, and summarising Grof's description of the same in his book *Psychology of the Future: Lessons from Modern Consciousness Research* (Grof, 2000). These types of spiritual emergency have also been listed and discussed elsewhere in the literature (for example, see: Grof, 2008a; Grof & Grof, 1995, 1989; Bragdon, 1990). Also, Park (1991) overviews them in his doctoral dissertation, with a specific focus on kundalini, while Goretzki (2007) provides a thoroughgoing description and appraisal of each in her doctoral dissertation.

of a psychospiritual occurrence in the form of spiritual emergency. This raises the obvious question: How can a psychiatrist differentiate between instances of spiritual emergence or emergency and psychopathology if the symptoms of both are so similar?

In response to this pressing question, the Grofs fashioned an observation-based taxonomy of factors that differentiate a psychiatric disorder from a spiritual emergence (see Table 6). They structured this to address both medical and psychological considerations.

Table 6. The Grofs' differentiation taxonomy between spiritual emergence and psychiatric disorders.

Psychiatric disorder	Spiritual Emergence (SE)[76]
Characteristics of the process indicating need for medical approach to the problem.	Characteristics of the process suggesting that the strategy for SE might work.[77]
Criteria of a medical nature	
Clinical examination and laboratory tests detect a physical disease that causes psychological changes.	Negative results of clinical examination and laboratory tests for a physical disease.
Clinical examination and laboratory tests detect a disease process of the brain that causes psychological changes (neurological reflexes, cerebrospinal fluid, X ray, etc.).	Negative results of clinical examinations and laboratory tests for pathological process afflicting the brain.
Specific psychological tests indicate organic impairment of the brain.	Negative results of psychological tests for organic impairment.
Impairment of intellect and memory, clouded consciousness, problems with basic orientation (name, time, place), poor co-ordination.	Intellect and memory qualitatively challenged but intact, consciousness usually clear, good basic orientation, co-ordination not seriously impaired.
Confusion, disorganization, and defective intellectual functioning interfere with communication and co-operation.	Ability to communicate and co-operate (occasional deep involvement in the inner process might be a problem).

(Continued)

---

[76] The Grofs appear to have used the term 'spiritual emergence' here to infer both spiritual emergences and spiritual emergencies.
[77] Therapeutic approaches for spiritual emergences are generally of a holistic and psychosocial nature (see, for example—Grof, 2008a; Grof & Grof, c2007; Lukoff, 2007; Grof, 1994; Bragdon, 1990).

Table 6. (Continued)

Psychiatric disorder	Spiritual Emergence (SE)
Criteria of a psychological nature	
Personal history shows serious difficulties in interpersonal relationships since childhood, inability to make friends and have intimate sexual relationships, poor social adjustment, usually long history of psychiatric problems.	Adequate pre-episode functioning as evidenced by interpersonal skills, some success in school and vocation, network of friends, and ability to have sexual relationships; no serious psychiatric history.
Poorly organized and defined content of the process, unqualified changes of emotions and behaviour, unspecific organization of psychological functions, lack of meaning of any kind, no indication of direction development, loosening of associations, incoherence.	Sequences of biographical memories, themes of birth and death, transpersonal experiences, possible insight that the process is healing or spiritual in nature, change and development of themes, often definable progression, incidence of true synchronicities (evident to others).
Autistic withdrawal, aggressivity, or controlling and manipulative behaviour interferes with a good working relationship and makes co-operation impossible.	Ability to relate and co-operate, often even during episodes of dramatic experiences that occur spontaneously or in the course of psychotherapeutic work.
Inability to see the process as an intrapsychic affair, confusion between the inner experiences and the outer world, excessive use of projection and blaming, 'acting out'.	Awareness of the intrapsychic nature of the process, satisfactory ability to distinguish between the inner and the outer, 'owning' the process, ability to keep it internalized.
Basic mistrust, perception of the world and all people as hostile, delusions of persecution, acoustic hallucinations of enemies ('voices') with a very unpleasant content.	Sufficient trust to accept help and co-operate; persecutory delusions and 'voices' absent.
Violations of basic rules of therapy ('not to hurt oneself or anyone else, not to destroy property'), destructive and self-destructive (suicidal or self-mutilating) impulses and a tendency to act on them without warning.	Ability to honour basic rules of therapy, absence of destructive or self-destructive ideas and tendencies, or ability to talk about them and to accept precautionary measures.
Behaviour endangering health and causing serious concerns (refusal to eat or drink for prolonged periods of time, neglect of basic hygienic rules).	Good co-operation in things related to physical health, basic maintenance, and hygienic rules.

Source: Grof & Grof, 1995, pp. 314–315.

While others have made similar attempts to identify points of differentiation between psychotic and psychospiritual experiences,[78] the Grofs' taxonomy was marked by its comprehensive diagnostic detail, informed by Stanislav's psychiatric expertise. Such thinking by a psychiatrist was uncommon because, apart from some simple issues pertaining to religious or cultural belief, mainstream psychiatry generally viewed the full psychospiritual gamut as suspect.

The Grofs also identified an inherent and critical limitation to this project. In contradistinction to their key objective of identifying differential criteria, they paradoxically acknowledged the ultimate impossibility of doing so. Although they asserted the necessity for psychiatry to recognise the phenomenon of spiritual emergencies in order to prevent mistaken diagnoses, they also recognised that such a task was impossible for the discipline in its extant form. For instance, they noted that "the term *psychosis* is not accurately and objectively defined in contemporary psychiatry. Until that happens, it will be impossible to offer a sharper delineation between the two conditions" (Grof & Grof, 1995, p. 53). Psychiatry's inability to delineate the clinical boundaries of psychosis has been an enduring problem; however, this is amplified by the idea of discerning psychotic from psychospiritual experiences for it raises difficult questions that seemingly have no ready solutions. How might psychotic instances be differentiated from manifold other types of anomalous, yet non-psychopathological, states of consciousness? Indeed, is it possible to absolutely differentiate them, and if not, does the use of diagnostic categories and criteria actually detract from better understanding the perplexing phenomenon of so-called psychosis? The emergence of such questions is intrinsic to introducing psychospiritual considerations into the field of psychiatric research, and while it is understandable that their challenge to psychiatry's basic assumptions and practices may cause consternation, such a challenge can equally be seen as an opportunity to develop new ways of understanding the enigma of psychosis and the unknown depths of human consciousness.

A related issue of 'impossibility', raised by the Grofs, concerns the conceptual foundations upon which mainstream psychiatry rests. In responding to inquiries from "many mental health professionals" about how to make a definitive differential diagnosis in clinical practice, Grof (2008b) acknowledged that "it is in principle impossible to make such differentiation according to the standards used in somatic medicine". This conclusion pertains to the dichotomy in psychiatry between organic and functional psychoses. Organic psychoses result from proven anatomical causes such as "encephalitis, brain tumors, or dementias" (Grof, 2008b) and subsequently belong "unquestionably in the domain of medicine" (Grof & Grof, 1989, p. 3). By contrast,

---

[78] For instance, see Lukoff's diagnostic flow chart in Section 8.3 of this chapter. Also, in Appendix Six, I provide a collation of tabled models for discerning psychotic from psychospiritual experiences proposed by twelve of the authors from my Chapter Nine content analysis. These tabled models demonstrate the diversity of ideas in, and the complexity of the task of, striving to identify psychotic versus psychospiritual characteristic features.

functional psychoses, which constitute the predominant form of psychotic states, are disorders for which "no medical explanation has been found in spite of the focused efforts of generations of researchers from various fields" (ibid., pp. 3–4). Yet, rather than accepting the aetiological obscurity of functional psychoses, or considering their possible psychological aetiology, psychiatry instead assumes "a pathological process in the brain yet to be discovered by future research" (Grof, 2008b). However, Grof (ibid.) maintains that "functional psychoses are not defined medically but psychologically", and consequently "it is impossible to provide a rigorous differential diagnosis between psychospiritual crisis ('spiritual emergency') and psychosis in the way it is done in medical practice in relation to different forms of encephalitis, brain tumors, or dementias". Indeed, he asserts that in the absence of establishing clear aetiology in functional psychoses, "there is no reason to refer to these conditions as 'mental diseases'" (ibid.). This proposition effectively refutes psychiatry's core understanding of functional psychosis as being intrinsically psychopathological. In light of this seemingly intractable dilemma, Grof (ibid.) has proposed that his taxonomy of differential criteria be used *not* for making absolute clinical distinctions between psychopathological and psychospiritual experiences, but for generally determining whether the optimal therapeutic approach is to support, or pharmacologically suppress, the symptoms.

In sum, it appears the Grofs' work has made an important contribution to the venture of better understanding the manifold anomalous states of consciousness that are generally (mis)diagnosed as psychoses. Importantly, they have called into question standard psychiatric perceptions of psychosis through their work on the apparent need to discern psychospiritual from psychopathological experiences. Articulating the close phenomenological parallels between the two clearly challenges psychiatry to revisit its primary assumptions about the nature and aetiology of psychosis. Indeed, the materialist belief regarding the biological aetiology of all psychoses effectively precludes the serious consideration by medical psychiatry of possible psychospiritual determinants in psychosis. Yet, accepting the psychogenesis of psychosis is also problematic. Because functional psychoses and spiritual emergencies are both ostensibly psychic phenomena, it seems the quest to demarcate them is inherently impossible. Arguably, these conundrums indicate the need for psychiatry to relinquish old convictions about the bio-pathological nature of psychosis, and to accept the seeming reality that such enigmatic experiences are square pegs that cannot be hammered into the round holes of materialist ideology. As Jung (1960, p. 158) maintained over a century ago, "only beyond the brain, beyond the anatomical substrate, do we reach what is important for us—the psyche; as indefinable as ever, still eluding all explanation, no matter how ingenious".[79] From this perspective it seems pathways to better understanding psychosis may be initiated *not* via pathology-based differential

---

[79] Although this quotation appears in the 1960 version of Jung's *Collected Works*, he originally made the comment in 1908 at an academic lecture in Zurich.

diagnosis, but by an open-ended phenomenological investigation of 'psychotic' and psychotic-like experiences.

8.3 David Lukoff and MEPF

David Lukoff also made a ground-breaking attempt to create a system for discerning psychospiritual from psychotic experiences. An examination of his notion of Mystical Experiences with Psychotic Features (MEPF) has already been undertaken in Chapter Seven. However, in addition to formulating this proposed diagnostic category, Lukoff (1985, pp. 162–163) created a flow chart (see Figure 2) for diagnostically differentiating "mystical experiences from psychotic disorders". Although his notion of MEPF was informed and inspired by the Grofs' work on discerning spiritual emergencies from psychoses, his model differed significantly from theirs in that it sought to establish a rapprochement between traditional psychiatric and transpersonal approaches to diagnosing anomalous psychic experiences. Whereas the Grofs fashioned a binary taxonomy that generally mirrored the schism between materialist and transpersonal approaches to psychiatry, Lukoff created an operationalised system that mimicked the DSM diagnostic approach.

Lukoff's diagnostic flow chart represents the most sophisticated effort to date to create an operationalised system for differentiating psychoses from potentially 'growthful' psychospiritual experiences, while simultaneously attempting to establish a rapprochement between psychiatric and transpersonal modes of understanding. Additionally, he has endeavoured to formulate a spectrum of diagnostic entities to account for various mixed manifestations of psychotic and mystical experiences. Yet, in terms of limitations, his entire system, including the vital category of MEPF, does not account for the possibility of a purely mystical experience with no psychotic features. Also, despite his laudable attempt to reconcile the diagnostic problems inherent to discerning psychotic from psychospiritual experiences, an essential core question seemingly remains unresolved: If non-psychotic psychospiritual experiences mimic symptoms essential for diagnosing psychotic disorders, how is it possible, or *is* it possible, to distinguish the two? Chapters Nine and Ten further explore this conundrum to demonstrate and conclude that such differentiation is seemingly not possible.

Figure 2 – Lukoff's MEPF diagnostic flowchart

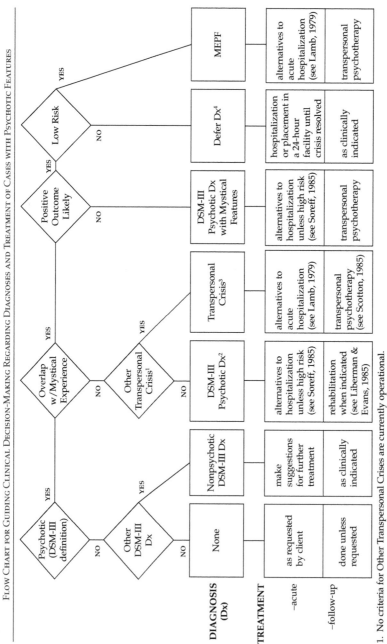

FLOW CHART FOR GUIDING CLINICAL DECISION-MAKING REGARDING DIAGNOSES AND TREATMENT OF CASES WITH PSYCHOTIC FEATURES

1. No criteria for Other Transpersonal Crises are currently operational.
2. DSM-III psychotic Dx's include: Pervasive Developmental Disorders, Schizophrenic and Paranoid Disorders, Some Organic Mental Disorders, some Affective Disorders, and Psychotic Disorders Not Elsewhere Classified.
3. See Grof & Grof (1985) for a discussion of other possible transpersonal crises.
4. Allow for a resolution of crisis. Then reassess risk and diagnosis.

(Source – Lukoff, 1985, p. 163)

Figure 2. Lukoff's MEPF diagnostic flowchart.

8.4 Conclusion

The common occurrence of psychotic-like features in psychospiritual experiences posits a significant challenge to psychiatry, as it calls for better understanding of both psychotic and psychospiritual instances, in order to discern them. While psychiatry's recognition of this issue is limited to simply considering cross-cultural factors, the Grofs and Lukoff recognised the necessity to formulate differential diagnostic criteria to avoid misdiagnosis. Each subsequently created a proposed differential diagnostic system for psychiatric use based on robust psychospiritual research. However, their work is not unique. My ensuing Chapter Nine content analysis illustrates the widespread existence of such thinking, and the complexity of discerning psychotic from psychospiritual experiences.

CHAPTER 9

Content analysis: discerning psychosis from psychospiritual experiences

9.0 Introduction

Here, I undertake a comprehensive content analysis of literature wherein commentators have discussed prospective criteria for discerning between psychotic and psychotic-like psychospiritual experiences. My study, which is based loosely on de Menezes Junior & Moreira-Almeida's (2009)[80] meta-analysis, aims to identify the top nine differentiation criteria identified by authors within this research field. However, while their study aimed to formulate a prospective list of differential diagnostic criteria, my study additionally aims to contest the psychopathological validity of each identified criterion. Doing so works to further challenge psychiatry's prescriptive, diagnostic, and psychopathology-based approach for construing and understanding psychosis.

9.1 The de Menezes Junior & Moreira-Almeida (2009) study

The work of de Menezes Junior & Moreira-Almeida (2009) represents the most comprehensive meta-analysis of literature published to date in the field of discerning psychotic from psychospiritual experiences. Their endeavour aimed to "identify criteria to allow the elaboration of a differential diagnosis between spiritual experiences and psychotic and dissociative disorders" (ibid., p. 75). This included a review of the work of Grof, Lukoff, and many other key commentators from this field of research. Their analysis of these materials elicited a number of criteria "that could indicate an

---

appropriate distinction between spiritual experiences and psychotic and dissociative disorders" (ibid.). From these, the topmost nine criteria identified by authors as being indicative of a psychospiritual rather than a psychotic experience, were listed in descending order of incidence. These were (pp. 80–81):

1. Lack of suffering (thirteen authors).
2. Lack of functional impairment (eleven authors).
3. The experience has a short duration and occurs sporadically (ten authors).
4. A critical attitude exists regarding the objective reality of the experience (nine authors).
5. Compatibility with the patient's cultural background (eight authors).
6. Absence of comorbidities (five authors).
7. Control over the experience (five authors).
8. The experience promotes personal growth over time (five authors).
9. The experience is directed towards others (three authors).

Hence, according to de Menezes Junior & Moreira-Almeida's findings, an absence of suffering and functional impairment, concomitant with short, sporadic duration of an anomalous experience, is highly indicative of a psychospiritual experience. Conversely, an anomalous experience of long duration, involving suffering, and functional impairment, is highly indicative of a psychopathological or psychotic experience.

Due to its comprehensive and current nature, de Menezes Junior & Moreira-Almeida's meta-analysis represents a significant and laudable development in the quest to understand the similarities and differences between psychospiritual and psychotic experiences. In particular, it steps beyond the traditional psychiatric practice of viewing psychospiritual experiences as either psychotic or psychopathologically suspect, and instead considers them as valid human experiences. However, despite these advancements, their adoption of a psychopathology-based diagnostic approach is arguably flawed, for this presumes that psychotic and psychotic-like experiences can be cleanly differentiated. It is my proposition, however, that such differentiation is ultimately not possible. Hence, despite the progressive merits of de Menezes Junior & Moreira-Almeida's research, in the bigger picture it arguably works to obscure, rather than facilitate, a better understanding of anomalous states of human consciousness. To support this claim, I have conducted my own comprehensive content analysis that challenges the veracity of the psychopathology-based diagnostic approach adopted by de Menezes Junior & Moreira-Almeida, and many others, in this field of inquiry.

9.2 Content analysis: psychotic versus psychospiritual experiences

While the general endeavour by commentators to discern psychotic from psychospiritual experiences has been a progressive development, an apparent fundamental flaw is that such research has adopted and replicated psychiatry's approach of diagnostic dualism, which assumes that psychopathology is discernible from mental health. Ipso facto, it is assumed that psychosis can be differentiated from psychotic-like psychospiritual experiences. Therefore, while the aim of my content analysis mirrors that of de Menezes Junior & Moreira-Almeida in that it endeavours to elicit a list of key differentiation criteria, beyond this it differs markedly. For instance, whereas they compiled a list of nine key *psychospiritual* criteria, I have compiled a list of nine key *psychotic* criteria (see Table 7 below). And while they adopted their criteria as a proposed diagnostic tool for use in discerning psychotic from psychospiritual experiences, my study challenges the veracity of the criteria identified by authors to demonstrate their diagnostic invalidity. By critiquing each criterion in turn, I aim to show that none are absolute indicators of psychopathology, hence, none work to discern psychotic from psychospiritual experiences. Doing so contests the soundness of psychiatry's psychopathology-based diagnostic practices and raises questions that point to potential new psychosis research pathways. If the notion of psychopathology is shown to be essentially dubious, then how is it possible to use a psychopathology-based diagnostic approach to discern psychotic from psychospiritual experiences? Would the use of a heuristic approach, that eschews assumptions of psychopathology, open new pathways to better understanding psychosis and psychotic-like psychospiritual experiences? This research initiative sets the stage for Focal Setting Four which further argues that absolute differentiation is not possible.

9.2.1 Methodological overview

My research has entailed undertaking a content analysis of texts that engage the issue of discerning psychospiritual from psychotic experiences and eliciting from these a list of the topmost nine key differentiation criteria identified by authors. I used an open-ended and process-oriented approach to elicit a corpus of literature for appraisal. By adopting this approach, and not limiting my resource pool to items obtained through a targeted keyword-search, I aimed to establish a broader spectrum of findings for analysis than did de Menezes Junior & Moreira-Almeida's study. This enabled me to garner seventy texts that identified possible characteristics for differentiating psychospiritual from psychotic experiences.[81] My subsequent content analysis of these texts identifies and discusses the topmost nine psychotic criteria, and then critically disputes the diagnostic validity of each to demonstrate that clinically discerning psychotic from psychospiritual experiences is apparently not possible. This critical

---

[81] To avoid duplication, I chose only items wherein commentators proffered their own views on the issue of differentiation and excluded articles which simply reiterated the findings of others. My inclusion of the work of de Menezes Junior & Moreira-Almeida is an exception for it represents the most comprehensive literature review in this research field. Table A2 in Appendix Five lists the citations for all seventy texts examined.

process also calls to question the validity of the diagnostic criteria formulated by psychiatry for identifying psychosis.

9.2.2 General findings

In total, an examination of the seventy texts elicited 193 criteria identified by authors as being psychopathologically indicative of a psychotic rather than psychospiritual experiences. My study, therefore, seems to corroborate Jackson & Fulford's (1997, p. 60) expectation that attempts to phenomenologically discern psychopathological from psychospiritual experiences will likely elicit "a bewildering variety of forms". This kaleidoscopic body of viewpoints arguably indicates the high degree of ambiguity that exists within the field of psychosis research.

The preponderance (about ninety per cent) of criteria identified by authors mirrored the picture of psychosis as understood by traditional psychiatry. For example, ten authors indicated that DSM or ICD diagnostic criteria generally served to differentiate psychotic from psychospiritual experiences, while others specifically identified differentiators as the presence of paranoia (n=9), negative affect (n=9), poor insight (n=8), and risk of harm to self or others (n=8). The psychogenic thinking of psychoanalytic psychiatry/psychology also featured among criteria, with some authors positing that a psychotic rather than a psychospiritual experience is indicated by the presence of unresolved stress, trauma, and tension. These findings arguably indicate the high degree to which the research field of discerning psychotic from psychospiritual experiences has been influenced by the psychiatric modus operandi of identifying diagnostic signs and symptoms of psychopathology.

Despite this trend toward replicating a traditional psychiatric model of understanding, a considerable number of authors identified differentiation criteria of a metaphysical nature. For instance, seventeen authors (about twenty-five per cent) suggested that the absence of psychospiritual skills and/or teachers was indicative of a psychotic rather than a psychospiritual experience.[82] This criterion exemplifies the challenge that psychospiritual considerations can proffer to the materialist-based binary thinking of psychiatry, for it ostensibly implies that psychosis is not psychopathological per se, nor stands in psychopathological contradistinction to psychospiritual experiences. Rather, it can be seen as a psychospiritual event gone awry due to an absence of the requisite skills and teachers that may otherwise enable people to understand and integrate their anomalous and dynamic psychic experiences.

---

[82] The notion of 'psychospiritual teachers' generally infers psychospiritual adepts who have the expertise to provide guidance for people undergoing psychotic-like spiritual emergence experiences. For example, transpersonal-oriented clinicians and therapists, religious counsellors, shamanic practitioners, monks, nuns, mystics, etc. This criterion is further examined below in Section 9.3.6, while other significant items of a metaphysical nature identified by authors are examined in Chapter Ten.

9.2.3 Top nine criteria identified by authors

As explained above, my content analysis of seventy texts entailed a process of eliciting the top nine criteria that authors identified as being characteristic of psychotic experiences, in contradistinction to psychospiritual experiences. These are listed below, in descending sequence of incidence (see Table 7).[83]

Table 7. Top nine psychosis criteria identified by authors.

Ranking	Psychosis criteria	#
1	Loss of agency or control	33
2	Social dysfunction	23
3	Ego-related issues	23
4	Experience lacks a developmental nature	22
5	Culturally or religiously aberrant beliefs and experiences	19
6	Absence of psychospiritual skills and/or teachers	17
7	Hearing voices	16
8	Social isolation	16
9	Generally negative experience	12

Note: # = frequency of identification of a criterion by authors.

Seven of these items correspond with the signs and symptoms of psychosis described in mainstream psychiatric literature. In decreasing order of frequency, these are: loss of agency or control (n=33); social dysfunction (n=23); ego-related issues (n=23); culturally or religiously aberrant beliefs and experiences (n=19); hearing voices (n=16); social isolation (n=16); and generally negative experience (n=12). Two of these nine psychotic differentiators do not feature in psychiatric descriptions of psychosis, namely, that the experience lacks a developmental nature (n=22), and that the experience results from an absence of psychospiritual skills and/or teachers (n=17). These two latter items are of particular interest, and are critically examined in Section 9.3, as they open potential new vistas for better understanding the nature of psychosis.

In terms of comparison between the findings of my and de Menezes Junior & Moreira-Almeida's study, all but one of their nine psychospiritual indicators also appear in my study, albeit as psychopathological counterpoints (see Table 8). By 'psychopathological counterpoint' I mean incidents whereby a psychospiritual criterion in their findings inversely correlates with a psychotic criterion in my findings. For example, the psychospiritual indicator of 'lack of suffering' in their study inversely

---

[83] Of the seventy articles, twelve include a proposed typology for differentiating psychotic from psychospiritual experiences. (See: DeHoff, 2012; Watkins, 2010; Eeles et al., 2003; Greenwell, 2002; Chadwick, 2001; Jackson, 2001; Kemp, 2000; Austin, 1998; Grof & Grof, 1995; Nelson, 1994; Siegler et al., 1969; Siglag, 1986.) These typologies are collated in Appendix Six. However, the Grofs' typology is excluded from the appendix as it already appears above in Chapter Eight, Section 8.2, Table 4.

correlates with the psychotic indicator of 'generally negative experience' in my study, their 'lack of functional impairment' with my 'social dysfunction', their 'control' with my 'loss of control', and so on.

Table 8. Comparative topmost nine criteria by de Menezes Junior & Moreira-Almeida and Spittles.

Ranking	de Menezes Junior & Moreira-Almeida (Psychospiritual criteria)	Spittles (Psychosis criteria)	Ranking
1	Lack of suffering	Generally negative experience	9
2	Lack of functional impairment	Social dysfunction	2
3	The experience has a short duration and occurs sporadically	Long duration of experience	*
4	A critical attitude exists regarding the objective reality of the experience	Lacking insight	*
5	Compatibility with the patient's cultural background	Culturally or religiously aberrant beliefs	5
6	Absence of comorbidities	N/A	*
7	Control over the experience	Loss of agency or control	1
8	The experience promotes personal growth over time	Experience lacks a developmental nature	4
9	The experience is directed towards others	Egocentric experience (focus on 'me', not others)	*

Note: * = does not appear in my topmost nine criteria
      N/A = not applicable. Does not appear in my findings.

While our respective studies have utilised different approaches for sourcing materials (i.e., targeted versus open-ended), and have focussed on divergent differentiation criteria (i.e., psychospiritual verses psychotic), they have elicited markedly similar results. Overall, then, it appears the findings of my study largely parallel their findings.

The correlation in our respective findings seemingly supports the notion that psychotic and psychospiritual experiences are discrete occurrences that should be diagnostically differentiated. However, the ensuing critical examination of my study's topmost nine 'psychotic' criteria disputes this, for an examination of the literature reveals that *all* of these criteria also appear within psychospiritual contexts. Therefore, *none* are ultimately effective for diagnostic differentiation purposes. This suggests that psychotic and psychospiritual experiences are not discrete, but are inextricably interconnected and indiscernible. If so, this challenges the idea that psychosis is a pure form of psychopathology that can be diagnostically distinguished from non-psychopathological psychospiritual experiences. It correspondingly proffers a challenge to psychiatry's fundamental modus operandi of psychopathology-seeking, for if there are no absolute criteria for discerning psychotic from psychospiritual instances, how can the same criteria identify 'psychosis' as a form of psychopathology?

9.3 Elucidating and challenging the top nine criteria

Whereas de Menezes Junior & Moreira-Almeida's response to the issue of discerning psychotic from psychospiritual experiences was to conduct a meta-analysis in order to identify nine differentiation criteria, my response has been to elicit and challenge the veracity of nine differentiation criteria and, in so doing, concomitantly challenge the efficacy of using a differential diagnostic approach to resolve this issue. Throughout this section, then, a twofold examination of each of the topmost nine criteria is undertaken. First, each criterion is elucidated and discussed in the context of its identification by authors as signifying psychotic rather than psychospiritual experiences. While doing so seems to corroborate claims by authors as to the psychopathological nature of each criterion, this is countered by then identifying instances of the same criterion being used in psychospiritual contexts. Doing so does not negate the apparent parallels between psychotic and psychospiritual experiences, but demonstrates a fundamental flaw in utilising the psychiatric differential diagnosis approach to redress this issue. Demonstrating that all the criteria identified by authors can occur within both psychotic and psychospiritual contexts negates their validity as proposed psychopathological indicators. *Overall, this works to support my proposal that using a heuristic approach, which eschews psychiatry's approach of psychopathology-seeking, may open research pathways that enable a better understanding of psychosis and other anomalous human states of consciousness.*

9.3.1 Criterion one findings: general loss of agency or control

The loss of personal agency refers to anomalous experiences that are seemingly outside a person's conscious control. The terms 'agency' and 'control' were used variously and interchangeably by authors. For the sake of simplicity, I have hyphenated the two as 'agency-control' throughout this section. About forty-seven per cent of authors identified this as indicative of psychotic rather than psychospiritual experiences. Jackson & Fulford (1997, p. 55) exemplify this in their observation that "in the case of *pathological* psychotic phenomena, there is a radical *failure* of action. In the case of *spiritual* psychotic phenomena, action is radically *enhanced*".[84] Here, psychopathology is evidenced by agency incapacitation, as opposed to psychospiritual experiences whereby such agency is not only accessible but heightened. Other authors

---

[84] Jackson & Fulford's unusual idea of non-pathological psychosis (i.e., psychospiritual experience as benign 'psychosis') is discussed in Chapter Ten, Section 10.5.2.

proffered similar views. For instance, the earliest reference to loss of agency-control as a psychopathological indicator was by John Perceval (1840, p. 274), who, in reflection on his own psychosis, speaks of "his imagination not being under his own control". Likewise, Arieti (1961, p. 20) refers to the "passive agent" of schizophrenic states, Noll (1983, p. 450) observes that psychotic experiences "are clearly beyond the control of the experiencer", and Jackson (2001, p. 170) holds that the content of psychosis is "involitional". The general thinking here is that people are passive victims of psychopathology, as opposed to their being able to exercise agency-control in psychospiritual instances.

Some authors identified loss of agency-control as the transpersonal crux of diagnostic differentiation. For instance, Stephen & Suryani (2000, p. 6) note that a lack of agency-control in exercising "autonomous imagination" delineates the schizophrenic from the shaman. The notion of 'autonomous imagination' is defined by Stephen (1997, pp. 337–338) as "a continuous stream-of-imagery thought taking place in the mind, although mostly outside conscious awareness. At regular intervals, it spontaneously enters consciousness in the form of sleep dreams; and under certain conditions … may result in waking visions and other hallucinations". She maintains that, while hallucinatory forms of autonomous imagination are mostly involuntary, it is possible with "special training", as in the case of shamanism, to establish intentional access to and control of these states of consciousness (ibid., p. 338). This is akin to Robbins' (2011) notion of primordial mental activity (PMA).[85] He argues that florid psychosis occurs when PMA is uncontrolled and "comes to have a life of its own", and that the acquisition of skills to navigate this domain of consciousness can make the difference between psychopathological and healthy outcomes (ibid., pp. 129–130, 111). Several other authors also identified the inability to enter anomalous states of consciousness at will as discerning the psychotic person from the shamanic or spiritual adept (McGhee, 2002, p. 346; Noll, 1983, p. 450; Wapnick, 1969, p. 65). Indeed, Noll (1983) maintains that the presence or absence of such controlled mastery is the ultimate defining feature separating psychotic from shamanic experience.

One author identified the Zen Buddhist notion of 'nen'[86] as being centrally pertinent to the loss of agency-control in psychosis. From a Zen Buddhist perspective, the nature

---

[85] Michael Robbins' hypothesis of PMA represents a merging of anthropological and psychoanalytic thinking. He defines PMA as:

> a normal way that mind works both in learning and expression that is qualitatively different from rational realistic self-reflective thought. It appears to have a distinctive neurological circuitry and to be present from the onset of life. It is driven by somatic sensation and affect, it is enactive and concrete, holistic and de-centered, and produces states of belief and actualization that disregard time and logical causality and does not distinguish internal from external reality. (Robbins, 2012, p. 258)

He maintains that this modality of human consciousness has a broad scope of expression, including dreaming, creativity, infancy, psychospiritual experiences and psychosis (ibid., p. 259).

[86] The notion of 'nen' is highly complex and is discussed at length, and in its myriad permutations, by Zen master Katsuki Sekida in his book *Zen Training* (1985). According to Sekida (ibid., p. 17), the Japanese word 'nen' cannot be translated literally into English, but loosely denotes a specific type of mind-action or

and degree of individual agency-control is pivotal to differentiating psychospiritual experience from psychosis. In terms of the former, Sekida (1985, p. 113) maintains that spiritual enlightenment, or "one-eon nen", occurs when "the student induces the steady succession of first nen-actions, with no reflecting upon them in the form of second nen, and no self-consciousness in the form of third nen". Hence, in advanced meditative practice, the third and second nen are intentionally rendered dormant so that "the first nen receives stimuli from the external world without restriction ... Everything is direct, fresh, impressive, and overwhelmingly abundant" (ibid., p. 179). However, as Sekida (ibid.) further explains, for people experiencing psychosis the integrating role of third nen is somehow rendered dysfunctional. Consequently, the first nen is:

> overwhelmed with stimuli ... Thronging ideas, the kind of religious devotion in which one feels overcome by the love of God, cases of mental confusion in which the patient experiences so much stimulation that he cannot respond to it all—these are all symptomatic of the uncontrolled release of the first nen.[87]

According to this phenomenological description from Zen tradition, while the Zen enlightenment experience results from a deliberate and systematic eclipsing of the third and second nen, psychotic experience results from an involuntary malfunction in all three nen, beginning with the collapse, or fracturing, of the third nen due to unbearable internal stressors, or other impinging factors, then psychopathologically transferring to the second and first nen (pp. 179–182). In other words, the inadvertent occurrence of nen malfunction in psychosis psychopathologically differentiates it from the conscious and controlled actions leading to psychospiritual illumination.[88] Here, again, it is the loss of personal agency-control, and not the psychotic-like nature of the experience per se, which discerns it as being psychopathological. This examination of

---

"thought impulse". He explains that nen is composed of three interrelated stages of nen-action that "alternate with each other, from moment to moment, and we may feel as if they were arising simultaneously" (p. 108). Hence, upon closer inspection, that which appears to be a single mind-action is actually comprised of three actions in rapid 'simultaneous' succession:

1. the unconscious, outward-looking, non-reflective "pure sensation" (the first nen);
2. the unconscious, inward-looking, reflective recognition of the first nen (the second nen); and
3. the consolidation of these two actions into a single act of perception and understanding via the "recognition of ourselves becoming aware of the observation" (the third nen) (pp. 109–114).

The ongoing systemic networking of multitudes of nen-actions, then, constitutes the basis of the human capacity for perception, subjectivity, and reality-making.

[87] The dynamics of psychotic experience in relation to nen is further discussed in the context of the subject of 'issues of ontology' in Chapter Ten, Section 10.2.

[88] The relationship between psychotic-like experiences and the intentional acquisition of psychospiritual skills represents an important body of knowledge that lies beyond psychiatry's epistemological bounds. This is discussed below in more detail in Section 9.3.6.

nen also provides a sophisticated example of how human cognition and psychosis can be understood beyond the investigative scope of Western medical psychiatry.

9.3.1.1 Criterion one rebuttal

The above examples seem to corroborate the idea that a loss of agency-control constitutes a valid criterion for discerning psychotic from psychospiritual experiences. However, commentators within and beyond my body of critical analysis texts have made the counter observation that the activation of agency-control is integral to psychotic experience whereas psychospiritual experiences are characterised by a loss of agency-control. For example, Pahnke & Richards (1966, pp. 188, 190) refer to the "spontaneously-occurring experiences recorded in the literature of mysticism" and maintain that these can devolve into psychotic paranoia "when one attempts to control the experience instead of passively yielding to whatever develops". Hence, from this perspective, *it is not the absence, but the application, of agency-control which can turn a psychospiritual experience into a psychotic experience.* Other research also proposes that agency-control may play an active role in psychotic formation. For instance, in their recent investigation into the role of agency in psychosis, Jones, Shattell et al. (2016, p. 332) describe "multiple ways in which participants experienced themselves as actively involved in the onset and subsequent development and elaboration of (positive) psychotic symptoms". Contrary to the prevailing view that psychosis is marked by a loss of agency-control, this research suggests that it may play an integral role in psychotic process and formations.

Conversely, some commentators speak of the involuntary nature of psychospiritual experiences. This is evident in Grof's (2000) observation that people experiencing spiritual emergency possession states can have "a distinct feeling that their psyche and body have been invaded and that they are being controlled by an evil entity or energy with personal characteristics. They perceive it as coming from outside their own personality and as being hostile and disturbing". Here, a loss of agency and control is identified as common to spiritual emergencies. Indeed, references to unbidden and uncontrollable spiritual experiences abound within the mystical literature. For example, James (1905, p. 382) identifies passivity as a defining characteristic of mystic experience, whereby "the mystic feels as if his own will were in abeyance". Similarly, Laibelman (2004, p. 396) refers to the "uncontrollable mystical encounter", while Underhill (1912, p. 458) speaks of the "uncontrollable psychic and spiritual states" that may be experienced on the mystic path.[89] Hence, it appears that loss or presence of agency can occur in both psychotic and psychospiritual experience.

In sum, it appears that 'loss of agency and control' is a dubious criterion for differentiating psychopathology from psychospirituality. Despite the fact that this criterion was most frequently identified by the authors in my study as being indicative

---

[89] I have engaged this issue earlier in my appraisal of the GAP report. See Section 6.3.3 for further examples of the perceived involuntary nature of mystical experiences.

of psychosis, there are numerous examples in the literature that counter its veracity. Indeed, different commentators have incongruously observed that loss of agency-control is inherent to both psychotic and psychospiritual experiences. In light of this paradoxical mix of views, it consequently appears that the experience of 'loss of agency and control' is not uniquely psychopathological and is therefore invalid as a criterion for discerning psychotic from psychospiritual experiences.

9.3.2 Criterion two findings: social dysfunction

About one third of authors in my study identified social dysfunction as differentiating psychotic from psychospiritual instances. Essentially, this criterion reflects the view that social dysfunction is a key gauge of psychopathology. In mainstream psychiatry it is seen as a principal adverse consequence and defining feature of psychotic disorders, particularly schizophrenia (APA, 2013, pp. 98, 104). My use of the term here, however, refers only to the inability of persons to maintain their usual vocational and recreational activities (i.e., work, studies, hobbies, interests, etc.).[90] One of the earliest examples is by Boisen (1936, p. 160), who notes that "the case is hopeless" (i.e., psychotic rather than psychospiritual) if a person is unable to uphold economic and social concerns. Lukoff (1985, pp. 165–166) also espouses the view that people "meet the criteria for a psychotic state" when showing "widespread deficiencies in handling the everyday commonsense tasks involved in independent living". Zaehner (1961, p. 89), proffers the more relative assessment that "the difference, it would appear, is only one of degree, not of kind". Hence, in his understanding, social dysfunction resulting from altered states of consciousness is not psychopathological per se, but only if the experience, and attendant social dysfunction, is protracted. However, most authors who identified this as a differentiation criterion seemed to reflect the psychiatric understanding that social dysfunction is typically indicative of psychosis when co-occurring with other particular anomalous symptoms.

9.3.2.1 Criterion two rebuttal

Despite the prevailing identification of social dysfunction as a key differentiation criterion by authors, it is seemingly not an unequivocal indicator of psychopathology, for both long and short bouts of social incapacitation have been recognised in mystical literature as commonplace along the path of spiritual development. In fact, Grof & Grof (1995, p. 45) maintain that the disruption of "daily life" is a common feature of spiritual emergencies. This is corroborated by Ho (2016, p. 185), a clinical psychologist, who has observed from his own experiences of apparent 'psychotic mania' that "psychiatric symptoms have indeed incurred occupational and social costs", but he

---

[90] I have separated social dysfunction (i.e., everyday normal activities) from social isolation (i.e., inability to maintain normal social relationships). Although they overlap, they generally represent two different expressions of apparent psychopathology.

further explains that this was a temporary aspect of a larger transformative process resulting in "gains in creativity, literary-artistic-esthetic sensibilities, and capacity to enjoy life; and in health, physical, mental, and spiritual". He maintains that "spirituality and madness coexist in a dialectical relationship" and understands his experiences to be inextricable expressions of both madness and spirituality (ibid., p. 183). As such, while his social function has been compromised in one context of understanding, it is ultimately enriched in another.[91] Hence, it appears the differentiation criterion of 'social dysfunction' is not a universal signifier of psychopathology, for it is common to both psychotic and psychospiritual experiences. Even if, as Zaehner suggests, duration of social dysfunction is adopted as a relative differentiator, then the questions still remain—Beyond what extent of social dysfunction is psychopathology deemed to be diagnosable? Why is this so? And how does one decide whether an experience is psychotic or psychospiritual *prior* to this ambiguous time juncture?

9.3.3 Criterion three findings: ego-related issues

The general reasoning behind this criterion is that certain forms of ego-related issues can discern psychotic from transformative psychospiritual experiences. This was identified as a differentiator in assorted psychopathological contexts by about one third of authors. Some earlier versions of this were understood in terms of ego fragmentation. For instance, Siegler et al. (1969, p. 956) depicts a simple binary model of differentiation which contrasts the transpersonal experience of the "feeling of being at one with the world" to the psychotic experience of "no-self ego fragmentation". Wapnick (1969, p. 64) endorses a similar dualistic view of fragmentation but adds an element of complexity via the metaphor of "shell attachment and transcendence". He maintains that, while the schizophrenic is rendered dysfunctional when his or her *"protective shell has been suddenly and prematurely broken"*, the mystic "through his long training process, is able to slough the shell off gradually" (ibid.). Again, this depicts psychosis as something that can occur in the absence of psychospiritual skills and training, which is an understanding utterly absent from psychiatric thinking.

Several other authors identified ego weakness as a criterion for discerning psychopathology. Proponents of this view generally seemed to believe that psychotic collapse results from a fundamental weakness in ego integrity. For instance, Meher Baba (1988, p. 3) refers to the "inherent psychic weakness ... of the mind in ordinary madness", while Carroll (2007, p. 242) maintains that "the difference between a mystic and a mentally ill person revolves around the basic state of health of their ego". The thinking here is that people exhibiting ego weakness are unable to integrate or withstand the psychic intensity of mystic experiences and consequently descend into madness. For example, Greeley (1974, p. 81) holds that for "a personality that is weak or badly integrated ... a mystical experience may be enough to unhinge it

---

[91] The idea of psychosis being an intrinsic or potentially beneficent developmental process is discussed below in Section 9.3.4 and in Chapter Ten, Sections 10.5 and 10.6.

completely". Similarly, Siglag (1986, p. 74) explains that a "strong ego is reported as being present preceding the mystical experience, but the etiology of schizophrenia indicates a weakened or poorly developed ego as leading to that type of experience". More recently, Goretzki et al. (2009, p. 91) have concluded that a possible "difference between people having psychosis and people having only spiritual emergency" is that the latter possesses a "strong ego-complex". From a developmental perspective, these views strongly parallel those of the above ego fragmentation criterion, as both suggest that psychosis can result from not being able to withstand or integrate psychospiritual experiences due to ego weakness, whereas having a strong ego can result in a positive experience of personal growth.

From another perspective, some authors maintained that the presence of ego inflation differentiates psychotic from psychospiritual instances. Here, contrary to notions of ego *breakdown*, psychopathology is envisaged as dysfunctional ego *expansion*. Authors subscribing to this view claimed that, whereas healthy psychospiritual experiences are marked by a person exhibiting equanimity and humility, psychosis is marked by the presence of ego inflation. For example, Zaehner (1961, p. 100) maintains that, in contrast to mystical experience, which "deposes the mere ego from its previous supremacy", people in psychosis can "exhibit a limitless expansion of the ego". Similarly, Watkins (2010, p. 216) observes that the humility of the mystic stands in contradistinction to the egocentric psychotic who displays "an inflated or grossly exaggerated sense of self-importance that culminates in development of grandiose delusional beliefs". This reflects conventional psychiatric thinking, for DSM-5 identifies grandiose delusions as "one of the key features that define the psychotic disorders" (APA, 2013, p. 87). Hence, it represents another instance whereby authors from my study have selected a classic psychiatric psychotic indicator as a differentiation criterion.

Two further forms of ego-related issues identified by authors as discerning psychotic from psychospiritual occurrences were egocentricity and ego grasping. In terms of egocentricity, several authors maintained that, whereas psychospiritual experience is other-oriented, a person experiencing psychosis is self-absorbed. For example, Brown (2005, p. 56) posits that "in the mystical states the intuitions appeared to emerge from the self towards the world, whereas in the psychotic states the intuitions tended to revolve around the intents of the world towards the self". Jackson (2001, p. 170) also distinguishes the "humility" and "altruism" of spiritual experience from the "self-centredness" of psychotic experience, and Watson (2010, pp. 216, 218) contrasts psychospiritual "humility" and "selflessness" with psychotic "self-importance" and "narcissistically constricted 'all about me' attitude". In terms of ego grasping, several authors saw this as indicative of psychopathology, in contradistinction to the letting go of ego in psychospiritual experiences. For example, Nelson (1994, p. 349) states that the schizophrenic "desperately clutches his ego", while Stifler et al. (1993, p. 371) concludes in their empirical study on "psychotics and contemplatives" that "the most striking difference between these two groups was their respective levels of 'ego-grasping orientation'" and that "a clear relationship between ego grasping and psychosis is demonstrated". This view is presumably based on the prevailing wisdom in mystical literature that the achievement of spiritual enlightenment entails relinquishing one's ego grasp on life and surrendering to the deeper self. Regardless, the overall idea of ego-related issues was seen by many authors in my study as central to discerning psychotic from psychospiritual experiences.

9.3.3.1 Criterion three rebuttal

While the above correlation of 'ego-related issues' with psychopathology appears to have merit, this criterion ultimately fails in that such issues also occur in context of psychospiritual experiences. Consider, for example, the experience of spiritual emergence or emergency. As already mentioned above, the Grofs depict such experiences as processes of potential personal development and transformation, hence it stands to reason that they may naturally involve egocentric manifestations of fragmentation, weakness, inflation, grasping, or defence. Indeed, Assagioli (1989, p. 35) maintains that the initial phase of a spiritual awakening process may often entail "self-centeredness … and inflating the personal ego", though this gradually passes as the experience is integrated. It therefore appears that, for many people, the transition from a lower to a higher state of consciousness may entail various dynamics of ego disruption. For instance, Varga (2011, p. 281) observes that contending with "ego inflation" is a stage that many people must pass through when integrating kundalini experiences. In terms of shamanic processes, Rock et al. (2008, p. 63) note that people with weaker or "thinner" ego-boundaries are inherently more susceptible to trance induction via "shamanic-like stimulus" than those who have stronger or "thicker" ego boundaries. In context of spirit possession in traditional initiation processes, Prince (1974, p. 324) similarly speaks of the "ego dissolution" that precedes an eventual "growing up". Hence, it appears that the criterion of 'ego-related issues' is not intrinsically psychotic because ego upheaval and confusion can also commonly occur in psychospiritual experiences and transformative processes.

9.3.4 Criterion four findings: the experience lacks a developmental nature

The idea that anomalous or psychotic-like experiences may reflect a positive developmental process is absent from the epistemology of medical psychiatry. Hence, it is particularly pertinent that this notion featured as the fourth highest indicator of psychosis in my study and was identified by about thirty-one per cent of authors. Indeed, its counterpart that 'the experience promotes personal growth over time' also appears among de Menezes Junior & Moreira-Almeida's top criteria of psychospiritual experiences. Arguably, the high incidence of this item in both studies indicates both the potential and importance for psychiatrists to look beyond the limited purview of diagnostic psychopathology and to incorporate psychospiritual knowledge into their epistemology.

All authors who identified this differentiator concurred that psychosis is indicated by an absence of personal development. However, this was generally, and intriguingly, identified in the context of the outcome of an experience. That is, a good outcome reflects personal development, and is thus a psychospiritual experience, while a bad outcome reflects an absence of personal development, and is thus a psychotic experience. For instance, in one of the earliest expressions of this view, Boisen (1936, p. ix) states quite simply that "the difference lies in the outcome. Where the attempt is successful and some degree of victory is won, it is commonly recognised as religious experience. Where it is unsuccessful or indeterminate, it is commonly spoken of as 'insanity'". Sims (1997, p. 81) likewise identifies the absence of personal development as "a crucial difference" between psychotic and psychospiritual experiences. Watkins (2010, pp. 216–220) adopts Boisen's developmental idea as a benchmark for formulating a typology of seven criteria to clinically discern psychospiritual from psychotic experiences, namely: peace versus agitation; growth versus stagnation; humility versus inflation; balance versus preoccupation; free will versus compulsion; legitimacy versus eccentricity; and inclusiveness versus isolation.[92] From his perspective, all psychoses represent "potentially transformative psychospiritual crises", hence he counsels that "sufficient time should be allowed for the initial impact of a crisis to subside since episodes which eventually prove spiritually enriching or transformative are sometimes marked by agitation, preoccupation, and inflation during the early phases" (ibid., pp. xiii, 215). Similarly, Brett (2002, p. 322) sees the absence of a developmental outcome as the ultimate differentiating factor, but also notes that an essential commonality between psychospiritual and psychotic experiences is that each constitutes a state "in which the form of experience is altered from normal consciousness". She consequently concludes that "phenomena occurring in a spiritual context may be identical to those traditionally viewed as symptoms of psychosis, but cannot be seen as psychotic in themselves" (ibid.). In other words, this suggests that psychopathology is not identifiable in the form or content of an anomalous experience, but in the outcome. Finally, (Carroll, 2007) understands such development in evolutionary terms, whereby psychosis represents non-developmental psychopathology as opposed to the evolutionary advancement inherent in psychospiritual experiences. Again, this depicts the outcome of an anomalous experience as the ultimate criterion for differentiation purposes.

This criterion proffers an intrinsic challenge to conventional psychiatric thinking and practice. For one, the notion that differentiation is dependent on outcome seemingly renders diagnostic practice tentative and relatively obsolete, as psychopathology cannot be identified until after an *unspecified* period of observation. At what point, and why, can an experience be identified as psychopathological? There is no answer to this question as the timeline and nature of each person's prospective developmental process is unique. However, in light of this conundrum, Jackson (2010, pp. 152–153) maintains that the nature of the outcome is not inherent, but strongly dependent on whether or not a host of internal and external stressors and dynamics are redressed. He subsequently warns that "this indicates the potential for clinical interventions

---

[92] See Appendix Six, Table A14 for an explication on each of these binary items.

which increase stress, either through invalidating the individual's experience, or through sometimes unavoidable measures such as compulsory hospitalisation, to be iatrogenic" (ibid.). This thinking reflects the Grofs' (1995, p. 52) concern that, in circumstances of spiritual emergency, psychiatric treatment interventions, based on pathologising rather than seeking to better understand anomalous experiences, may not only result in misdiagnosis, but may inadvertently curtail the developmental process and *cause* a psychotic outcome.

The idea that psychiatric intervention, based on a poor understanding of psychospiritual matters, may precipitate a psychopathological outcome, arguably supports the necessity for creating an effective differential diagnosis system. Indeed, research conducted by Brett et al. (2007) demonstrates a significant correlation between the way in which an anomalous experience is understood (by the person having the experience, and others) and consequent clinical outcomes. Their research shows "the potential to elicit information that may clarify the nature of the continuum of psychotic and psychotic-like experiences" (ibid., p. s29). Subsequent similar research conducted by Brett (2010, p. 162) found that "anomaly-related distress" in participants was reduced through "appraising anomalies within a 'spiritual' framework" and through having "a higher level of perceived social support and/or understanding regarding the anomalies". Hence, most participants held that investing their respective anomalous experiences with value and meaning was very important. As one person stated, "the one thing that is really important ... is to have faith in something that is unbelievable ... I've got to cling to the view that it is a positive experience, when I'm being told everyday by doctors and nurses that I should feel sorry for myself" (p. 163). Interestingly, Brett (p. 173) concludes that this finding "undermines the utility of distinguishing transformative crisis from other forms of psychotic experience". She maintains that the therapeutic benefit people may derive from appreciating the "purposeful" aspect of an anomalous experience is undermined if such experiences are labelled as psychopathological (ibid.). In such instances the experience would appear to lack a developmental nature and, according to many authors in my study, would be grounds for diagnosing psychosis. This begs the question: to what degree does the act of psychopathology-seeking create the psychopathology it is looking for?

9.3.4.1 Criterion four rebuttal

The idea that psychopathology is identifiable via the absence of a developmental outcome is both promising and problematic. In terms of promise, the idea of beneficent and transformative psychotic-like experiences opens to new ways of understanding and therapeutically responding to psychosis. As Watkins suggests above, it may be that most, if not all, psychoses represent a transformative psychospiritual experience in potential. If so, then the optimal psychiatric task is, arguably, not to differentiate and diagnose psychopathology, but rather, to identify and foster latent developmental potentialities via a deeper understanding of anomalous and psychospiritual phenomena, and to circumvent deleterious clinical outcomes that may stem from lack of supportive understanding.

While the notion of considering the developmental nature of psychotic-like experiences has apparent merit, its validity as a differentiation criterion is dubious and problematic. For one, it is impractical in terms of application because a diagnostic decision cannot be made until the nature of the outcome is ascertained. This constitutes a situation whereby outcome is antecedent to diagnosis, which is contrary to standard diagnostic practices. Furthermore, this problem is compounded by the aforementioned issue of duration, for it raises the question: at what point in time can the developmental potential of a psychotic-like episode be deemed to have failed and thus enable the diagnosis of psychosis to be made? The duration of a psychospiritual developmental process is not fixed and, in some instances, such a process can last for years.[93] Hence, the designation of any time frame beyond which psychopathology is indicated is unavoidably arbitrary and runs the risk of misdiagnosis. It also risks stemming the developmental potential of the process and inadvertently precipitating psychosis.

Therefore, it appears the tautological idea that a psychotic-like experience which lacks a developmental nature is ipso facto psychotic is unfeasible as a differentiation criterion because the developmental duration of the process cannot be known until a developmental outcome occurs. If, however, psychotic-like experiences are viewed as psychospiritual development processes in potential, then the notion of discernment and related diagnostic dilemmas become redundant. A suggested alternative is to put aside notions of psychopathology and differential diagnostics to adopt an inquisitive phenomenological approach which may elicit insights that lead to a better understanding of the complex and enigmatic nature of the deeper human psyche.

9.3.5 Criterion five findings: culturally or religiously aberrant beliefs and experiences

This criterion sits squarely within the diagnostic rubric of conventional psychiatric thinking. DSM-III inaugurated the inclusion of cultural concerns in diagnostic practices and interest in this has advanced with each updated edition. For instance, the recently published DSM-5 explains that "the boundaries between normality and pathology vary across cultures ... Hence, the level at which an experience becomes problematic or pathological will differ ... [and] awareness of the significance of culture may correct mistaken interpretations of psychopathology" (APA, 2013, p. 14). In terms of schizophrenia, the diagnosing clinician is advised to be aware that "ideas that appear to be delusional in one culture (e.g. witchcraft) may be commonly held in

---

[93] Ten per cent of authors in my content analysis suggested that psychosis is indicated by an anomalous experience of long duration (for example, see: de Menezes Junior & Moreira-Almeida, 2009; Jackson, 2001; Wulff, 2000; Lacan, 1993; Buckley, 1981; Zaehner, 1961; James, 1905). The validity of duration of experience as a criterion for discerning psychotic from psychospiritual occurrences is further explored in Chapter Twelve, Section 12.3.2.

another. In some cultures, visual or auditory hallucinations with a religious content (e.g. hearing God's voice) are a normal part of religious experience" (ibid., p. 103). Bizarre delusions, however, are conceptualised as culturally errant. DSM-5 states that "delusions are deemed bizarre if they are clearly implausible and not understandable to same-culture peers" (p. 87). Similarly, the diagnostic criteria listed for Schizotypal Personality Disorder include phenomena that transgress the basic laws of materialism; namely the presence of "odd beliefs or magical thinking that influences behavior and is inconsistent with subcultural norms (e.g., superstitiousness, belief in clairvoyance, telepathy, or 'sixth sense')" (p. 655). In DSM-5, magical thinking is defined as "the erroneous belief that one's thoughts, words, or actions will cause or prevent a specific outcome in some way that defies commonly understood laws of cause and effect" (p. 824). Hence, while cultural sensitivity is endorsed by psychiatry, it is also made clear that experiences and beliefs that significantly deviate from religious, cultural, social, and materialist norms are deemed indicative of psychopathology.

The above psychiatric thinking was generally mirrored by commentators within my literature review. Consideration of the extent to which an experience deviates from cultural norms was identified by about twenty-seven per cent of authors as a criterion for differentiating psychotic from psychospiritual experiences. For example, Johnson & Friedman (2008, p. 523) suggest that clinicians "compare idiosyncratic behavior and beliefs to normative practices in religious/spiritual community" when making a differential diagnosis between psychotic and "Religious/Spiritual/Transpersonal" experiences. Similarly, Siddle et al. (2002, p. 132) propose asking the diagnostic question: "Are any religious ideas expressed likely to be unacceptable to the patient's peers? Would nonpsychotic churchgoing religious people also find these ideas unacceptable?". Watkins (2010, p. 218) observes that psychoses "are often highly idiosyncratic, eccentric, or bizarre and diverge substantially from generally accepted standards", while Noll (1983, p. 452) identifies "magical thinking" as a culturally deviant indicator of psychopathology. It therefore appears that psychiatry's notion of exercising cultural sensitivity in diagnostic considerations has generally been adopted by many commentators attempting to discern psychotic from psychospiritual experiences.

9.3.5.1 Criterion five rebuttal

Although exercising cultural discernment is evidently a progressive development in discerning madness from normalcy, and psychotic from transpersonal experiences, particularly in terms of reducing the risk of mistaken diagnoses, this practice is not without its logical problems. For example, medical psychiatry considers experiences such as hallucinations, spirit possession, and various types of magical thinking (e.g. telepathy, clairvoyance, etc.) to be psychopathological misapprehensions of reality. From a materialist stance, which medical psychiatry represents, such experiences defy 'commonly understood laws of cause and effect' and are, therefore, psychopathological. The tenets of materialism reflect a physical view regarding the nature and laws of reality, whereby beliefs and experiences of a metaphysical nature are considered intrinsically delusory and/or psychopathological because they transgress the laws of reality. It therefore seems counterintuitive, in a cultural context, to suggest such experiences are not psychopathological *per se*, but only so if deviating from the norms of a given cultural milieu. This is exemplified in the *DSM-5 Guidebook's* diagnostic suggestion for Brief Psychotic Disorder that:

> The diagnosis does not apply when the psychotic symptoms appear to have developed in response to culturally sanctioned activities, such as *Qigong*, a Chinese health-enhancing practice that can reportedly lead to transient psychosis. This is an important consideration, because psychotic-like phenomena are reported to occur during extended religious or ceremonial rituals in several non-Western cultures. (Black & Grant, 2014, p. 69)

Arguably, this instruction tacitly suggests that madness is ultimately defined more by cultural considerations than biological or psychological malfunction, as culture seems to be a key point of clinical reference when deciding what is mad and what is not. While psychiatry obviously does not intend this meaning, its cultural relativism seemingly runs counter to its materialist and deterministic model for diagnosing psychopathology. A further problem with this criterion is that its proponents do not explain why deviance from culturally sanctioned psychospiritual norms is psychopathological. What, exactly, defines such purported psychopathology? This was not explained by the authors in my study who maintained this differentiating view and nor has it been explicated or substantiated by DSM authors.

The veracity of this criterion is also challenged by descriptions within psychospiritual research texts of culturally or religiously aberrant beliefs and experiences occurring in a non-psychopathological context. Take, for example, the phenomenon of hearing voices. The literature is replete with reports of so-called auditory hallucinations being experienced by psychiatric patients, religious adherents, and many 'normal' people within mainstream modern society.[94] What, then, specifically denotes voice hearing as psychopathological when it is common in psychiatric, cross-cultural, and secular contexts? Indeed, the heterogeneous nature of voice hearing is evident in a multifaceted study of anomalous experiences conducted by Brett (2010, p. 166), which found that symptoms of ostensible psychopathology occurred "across the clinical-non-clinical spectrum". Subsequently, she concludes that "externalising appraisals do not define psychotic disorder" (ibid.). If voice hearing is common within and beyond culturally or religiously sanctioned circumstances, then proposing that it is psychopathological, except in culturally normative instances, is seemingly unsound.

The same principle applies to the phenomenon of extrasensory perception. Although the DSM-5 authors consider reported experiences by patients of extrasensory perception to be psychopathological 'magical thinking', such experiences are

---

[94] For example, see: Romme et al., 2009; Watkins, 1998; Tien, 1991; Sidgwick et al., 1894; Gurney et al., 1886a; Gurney et al., 1886b. Chapter Eleven, Section 11.1 discusses this issue in more detail.

actually heterogeneous across the sociocultural spectrum. This is evidenced in the work of several authors examined above who identified extrasensory perception as a legitimate psychospiritual phenomenon.[95] Hence, in considering these examples, it seems conjectural to propose that a behaviour or belief is psychotic, rather than psychospiritual, merely on the grounds that it is not culturally normative.

9.3.6 Criterion six findings: absence of psychospiritual skills and/or teachers

The notion that a paucity of psychospiritual skills and teaching differentiates psychotic from psychospiritual outcomes was identified by about twenty-four per cent of authors in my study. This criterion was identified in two broad contexts: namely, guided social support and unguided personal experimentation. In terms of the former, the view is that people can become psychotic due to a lack of cultural support and understanding and/or through not receiving the requisite guidance and training from a spiritual teacher or adept. For instance, Wilber (1975, p. 122) notes that "some individuals diagnosed as schizophrenic may indeed be psychologically lost ... for want of an adequate guide", while Greyson (1993, p. 46) warns that "kundalini should only be awakened by a gradual process under the guidance of someone who has first-hand experience with it; otherwise, a kundalini awakening in a body and soul not properly prepared can produce negative effects, including psychosis". From a sociological perspective, Greeley (1974, p. 87) sees the absence of spiritually-informed understanding and guidance within a cultural milieu as a form of ignorance that can result in the creation of madness. He poses the question: "If a person is told he's a 'nut' or 'crazy' for having such an interlude, could he not in fact become mentally disturbed within that context of conflict and judgement?" (ibid.). Hence, he suggests that some instances of mental illness can be precipitated via suggestion, whereby a person experiencing a psychotic-like episode is rendered mentally ill through psychiatric labelling and the stigmatisation and distress that this can cause.

Similarly, from an anthropological perspective, Silverman (1967, p. 29) observes that a person experiencing a shamanic crisis in a traditional society is culturally bolstered by "emotional supports and the modes of collective solutions", while, conversely, "supports are all too often completely unavailable to the schizophrenic in our culture". Interestingly, he further argues that it is not the absence of guidance and support per se that can tip a shamanic crisis into a psychosis, but rather, the overwhelming "pervasiveness of the anxiety" that may result from such absence (ibid.). This is an intriguing observation that warrants further investigation and lends credence to my argument that a better understanding of psychosis may be gained through the consideration of a diversity of psychospiritual views. Are some instances of psychosis precipitated by the intense anxiety generated in not having access to the psychospiritual knowledge, guidance, and social support that might enable a person to navigate

---

[95] For example, Dean's metapsychiatry (Chapter Six, Section 6.2.2), Grof's spiritual emergence (Chapter Eight, Section 8.2), and Lukoff's Mystical Experiences with Psychotic Features (Chapter Eight, Section 8.3).

through stormy transpersonal experiences? This question conceptually shifts the essential locus of psychopathology from the individual to the social body in which he or she lives. From this perspective, psychopathology may be the result of a person experiencing transpersonal states of consciousness within a society that offers little in terms of supportive psychospiritual knowledge and guidance.

Some authors in my study also depicted this criterion in the context of personal experimentation independent of spiritual teachers or guidance. The earliest instance of this was by the philosopher Immanuel Kant (1964 [1798], p. 17) in his book *The Classification of Mental Disorders*, in which he alludes to a practice whereby researchers wilfully induce an altered state of consciousness that "approaches derangement" in order to study and better understand psychopathology via first-hand experience. He warns that in such experiments "an artificial insanity can easily become a real one" (ibid.). Although he does not explicitly say that an absence of psychospiritual training can result in madness, he does infer that the careless or unskilled engagement in such practices can lead to insanity. This suggests that insanity may be caused not only by an absence of psychospiritual orientation skills, but also by the inept and uncontrolled application of the same. Another exemplary instance is evident in Jung's (1968, p. 49) experimentation with a method of self-exploration he called *active imagination*, which he describes as "a sequence of fantasies produced by deliberate concentration". After sixteen years (1914–1930) of such experimentation, Jung (2009, p. 360) concluded that "to the superficial observer, it will appear like madness. It would also have developed into one, had I not been able to absorb the overpowering force of the original experiences". And, indeed, in the light of Western standards of normalcy, Jung's (2009) record of his forays into the realms of active imagination throughout his book *Liber Novus* do read like madness. However, he maintained sanity through his capacity to employ a framework of self-composed meditative practices that enabled him to absorb, rather than be absorbed by, the mythic content of his active imaginations. For him, this was the difference between facilitating a transformative experience and sliding into psychosis.

This criterion is of particular significance because it brings to light a concept that is utterly absent from the thinking and practice of mainstream psychiatry. The idea that acquiring and applying psychospiritual skills can fundamentally determine psychosis outcomes is far removed from prevailing psychiatric thinking, which generally endorses the notion of biological causality. In identifying this criterion, authors do not attribute causality to the presence of a putative anatomical dysfunction or anomaly, but rather, to the absence of particular psychospiritual abilities and tutelage. Hence, psychopathology is not seen as implicit and biologically embedded, but as relative to the presence or absence of a framework of psychospiritual understanding, skills, knowledge, and support. Ostensibly, the presence of such a framework may enable a person to navigate, and indeed, flourish through anomalous states of consciousness. Conversely, the absence of the same may default into psychopathology.

The idea that inadequate psychospiritual guidance and skills procurement can ostensibly result in a psychotic outcome is typified in Campbell's (1972) metaphorical depiction of psychotic 'drowning' versus psychospiritual 'swimming'. He maintains that "our schizophrenic patient is actually experiencing inadvertently that same beatific ocean deep which the yogi and saint are ever striving to enjoy: except that, whereas they are swimming in it, he is drowning" (ibid., pp. 219–220). Elsewhere, he highlights the pivotal importance of psychospiritual teachers and skills acquisition by explaining that "the mystic, endowed by native talents ... and following, stage by stage, the instructions of a master, enters the waters and finds he can swim; whereas the schizophrenic, unprepared, unguided, and ungifted, has fallen or has intentionally plunged, and is drowning" (p. 209). Essentially, these metaphorical statements speak of whether or not a person has acquired the techniques of transcendence to enable him or her to integrate and navigate metaphysical domains of reality. As such, psychosis is not depicted as a form of psychopathology per se, but as an experiential anomaly resulting from the absence of adequate psychospiritual 'swimming lessons'. This poses intriguing new possible pathways to better understanding the metaphysical depths that ostensibly underlie the relationship between psychotic and psychospiritual experiences.

Some commentators have referred to such transcendence techniques as 'technologies of consciousness', a term denoting the practical techniques used for fostering psychospiritual development, which are fundamental to the cultural epistemologies of many societies. For instance, Wheelwell (1997, p. 536) states that "spiritual practices, like insight (vipashyana) meditation and (zen) koans, are ... technologies of consciousness, designed to access the road towards freedom", while Stutchbury (2004, p. 77) holds that "cutting edge mind-science research draws on the dialogue developing between western scientific neuroscience and the 'technologies of consciousness' of Tibetan Buddhism". Indeed, Wilber (1984, p. 20) asserts that such practices constitute a form of scientific pursuit, as does Sri Aurobindo (1999, p. 7) who explains that Yogic methods, "like the operations of Science, are formed upon a knowledge developed and confirmed by regular experiment, practical analysis and constant result". Furthermore, Rao (2005a, p. 15) explains that "mental technologies like meditation and spiritual counseling are tools for spiritual development, which have measurable effects on one's life and wellness", including issues pertaining to "mental illness and psychopathology" (2005b, p. 36). Apart from some emergent forms of transpersonal psychology, such technologies are all but absent from Western psychological and psychiatric practices.

It therefore appears that psychospiritual training practices are of considerable pertinence to better understanding psychosis. In fact, Sekida (1985, p. 126) refers to Zen Buddhist meditation as a structured "self-operated psychiatric method" that simultaneously facilitates self-actualisation while circumventing psychopathology. To what degree, then, does the general absence of such knowledge, skills, and guidance within industrialised societies, and mainstream psychiatry, result in psychotic states that may have been prevented? Is there scope for psychiatry to place more emphasis on preventing psychotic episodes by drawing on knowledge from psychospiritual traditions and practices? This issue arguably proffers a challenge and opportunity to psychiatry. The challenge is to consider the possibility that psychiatry's failure to better understand and incorporate psychospiritual knowledge into its epistemology can ironically result in iatrogenic outcomes, whereby ill-informed remedial measures cause, rather than prevent, psychosis. The opportunity is for psychiatry to broaden its worldview to incorporate ancient and well-tested psychospiritual knowledge systems into its understanding of, and therapeutic responses to, psychosis.

9.3.6.1 Criterion six rebuttal

Although it is evident that the absence of psychospiritual skills and/or teachers can result in psychosis, this is not to say it constitutes a diagnostic criterion for discerning psychotic from psychotic-like psychospiritual experiences. In fact, psychospiritual adherents within many training modalities commonly become, or appear to become, psychotic, in the presence of skills and/or teachers. For instance, Dyga & Stupak (2015, p. 51) report that in a survey conducted with Buddhist meditation teachers it was acknowledged that "psychosis can develop at either the initial or the advanced stages of practice". Indeed, as already noted above, the *DSM-5 Guidebook* recognises that psychotic-like episodes can result from the practice of Qigong; a view which is supported by Ng's (1999) research into the phenomenon of "Qigong-induced psychoses" occurring amongst Qigong students. It therefore appears that instances of psychosis can occur regardless of the absence, or presence, of psychospiritual skills or teachers. Furthermore, to suggest that the absence of psychospiritual skills and/or teachers can be diagnostically indicative of psychosis, inversely suggests that non-psychotic anomalous experiences occur only in the presence of such aptitude and tutelage. However, as already discussed in Chapter Eight, eruptive psychotic-like psychospiritual experiences, or spiritual emergencies, can occur spontaneously in the absence of psychospiritual skills and/or teachers. Overall, then, it is evident that while the absence of psychospiritual aptitude and tutelage can play a role in precipitating psychotic experiences, this is not universal and consequently refutes its status as a differential diagnostic criterion.

9.3.7 Criterion seven findings: hearing voices

This criterion, which was identified by about twenty-three per cent of authors, reflects the thinking of classic textbook psychiatry. However, eleven (about sixteen per cent) of these maintained that only hostile voices evidenced psychosis. The view that hearing voices, or having auditory hallucinations, constitutes a key diagnostic indicator of psychotic disorders has prevailed throughout DSM editions since the manual's inception. In DSM-5 it continues to feature as a primary diagnostic criterion in all psychotic disorders, except catatonia (APA, 2013, pp. 87–122). When considering the centrality of this criterion to diagnosing psychotic disorders, it is significant that about seventy-seven per cent of authors *did not* identify it as a differentiator. This is possibly because they saw the phenomenon as common to both psychotic and psychospiritual experiences, and therefore not as a clear item of differentiation. Although none of the authors inferred that voice hearing per se is invariably psychotic, they all mirrored psychiatric thinking in identifying it as a general criterion of psychopathology.

Interestingly, most authors in my study contrasted this criterion against the visual hallucinations of psychospiritual experiences (i.e. psychotic auditory hallucinations versus non-psychopathological visual hallucinations).[96] For instance, Austin (1998, p. 31) describes the mystical path as including hallucinatory phenomena which are "in general, more visual; not threatening" compared to schizophrenic process where such phenomena are "in general, more auditory; can be threatening", while Jackson (2001, p. 170) contrasts the "benign" and visual "pseudo hallucinations" of psychospiritual experience with the "malignant" and auditory "true hallucinations" of psychotic experience. This juxtaposition of psychotic auditory hallucinations against non-psychotic visual hallucinations constitutes a step beyond psychiatry's general view that, minus cultural exceptions, all hallucinatory experience is ostensibly psychotic. The notion of a non-psychotic hallucination poses a conceptual and semantic quandary because, in the psychiatric domain, the term 'hallucination' essentially infers an experience of being psychopathologically out of touch with consensus reality. If, for argument's sake, psychiatry was to accept the veracity of this particular distinction it would subsequently require a significant redrafting of the definition of 'hallucination'. It would also command an explanation as to why hearing a voice, or voices, that nobody else can hear is psychopathological, while seeing something that nobody else can see, is not? This question also holds for the authors from my study cited above because, despite their diagnostic assertions, none have provided such an explanation.

Other authors suggested that it is not the nature of the hallucination, but the nature of the voice, which differentiates psychopathological from psychospiritual experiences. This occurred in four contexts. First, was the view that critical voices are psychotic while benevolent voices are psychospiritual. For example, Noll (1983, p. 453) notes that, in contrast to "the nagging, accusatory, and intrusive 'voices' that plague the schizophrenic", the shaman hears voices that are "usually of a positive, helpful, healing nature".[97] Second, and similar to the first, is the view that command voices are psychotic while non-command, or instructive, voices are psychospiritual. Nelson (1994, p. 249) explicates this clearly in comparing schizophrenic states to instances of "regression in the service of transcendence" (RIST),[98] in which "hallucinated voices that sometimes accompany RIST are of the higher order, and though they may advise, they never command". In other words, psychopathology here pivots on whether the voice represents coercion or counsel. Third, was the view that a psychospiritual

---

[96] There was one exception to this common view. In his schema of "comparison between the healthy, mystic and psychotic person" Kemp (2000, p. 162) lists both visions and voices as being indicative of psychotic experience.

[97] For similar views, see: Clarke, 2000, p. 14; Stephen & Suryani, 2000, p. 23.

[98] Nelson (1994, p. 247) defines RIST as "a natural healing process that lowers defences against confronting unresolved impediments to higher consciousness" through which "the outcome can be madness as well as enlightenment". This and related notions are examined in Chapter Ten, Section 10.6.

experience of voices involves some degree of control whereas a psychotic experience of voices does not (Watkins, 2010, p. 217; Noll, 1983, p. 453). This is similar to the first differentiation criterion of agency-control discussed above in Section 9.3.1. Finally, three authors posited differentiation as being external versus internal voices; the former symptomatic of psychosis, and the latter, of kundalini experiences (Greenwell, 2002; Greyson, 1993, p. 48; Sannella, 1987, p. 109). Again, none of these views are bolstered by an explanation as to why one form of voice hearing is psychopathological and the other is not.

9.3.7.1 Criterion seven rebuttal

While this mix of perspectives work to shine an edifying light on the complex nature of the phenomenon of voice hearing, it simultaneously casts a cloud of perplexity over the clinical endeavour (be it psychiatric or otherwise) to definitively discern psychopathology from normalcy. It also portrays a clear fallibility in attempting to understand psychosis through the limited, and limiting, conceptual lens of binary diagnostics and psychopathology. Indeed, there are many contexts of voice hearing that challenge psychiatry's designation of auditory hallucinations as a primary psychotic diagnostic criterion. A broader examination of this issue in Chapter Eleven demonstrates the difficultly, if not the impossibility, of delineating the psychopathological parameters of voice hearing and/or psychosis.

9.3.8 Criterion eight findings: social isolation

As noted above in Section 9.3.2, social isolation is adjunct to social dysfunction in psychiatric diagnostics. A common characteristic of intense anomalous experiences is that they can result in social isolation. About twenty-three per cent of authors in my study identified this as differentiating psychotic from psychospiritual experiences. For instance, Siegler et al. (1969, p. 956) fashioned a typology for differentiating psychedelic from psychotic experiences[99] and note that with the former there is typically a "feeling that one can join the company of other enlightened people", while with the latter there is a "feeling that one is less and less human, more and more isolated". Similarly, in his doctoral research on mystical versus schizophrenic experience, Siglag (1986, p. 74) found that, for most people, a mystical experience "enhances their ability to contribute to the community" while those diagnosed with schizophrenia tend to "withdraw from relationships with other people". Most commentators in my study proffered a similar such picture of differentiation.

---

[99] In their research, the authors conducted a detailed analysis of psychiatrist R. D. Laing's book *The Politics of Experience* (1967), from which they fashioned their typology. See Appendix Six, Table A12 for a copy of this typology.

9.3.8.1 Criterion eight rebuttal

Despite the common view that social isolation differentiates psychotic from psycho-spiritual experiences, this is arguably not an unequivocal sign of psychopathology. For instance, in his study of mystic versus psychotic experiences, Wapnick (1969) conducted a comparative analysis of two personal accounts of anomalous experiences; one, the diary of the sixteenth-century Spanish mystic St. Teresa of Avila, and the other, the diary of a 1940s psychiatric patient, Lara Jefferson. He subsequently observed that, unlike Lara, "Teresa was able to maintain some degree of social contact, though living in a cloister. Moreover, her decisions to isolate herself were within her conscious control" (ibid., p. 63). This seemingly indicates that, in Wapnick's view, it is not social isolation per se that denotes psychopathology, but the loss of agency that makes it so. It also appears that social isolation, by choice or default, may feature in psychospiritual experiences. For instance, Cashwell et al. (2007, pp. 141, 144) list "social isolation" as a defining feature of what they call "spiritual bypass", which is a term denoting an attempt to "resolve a spiritual emergency at the spiritual level only". Further to spiritual emergency, Randal & Argyle (2005, p. 8) observe that rather than being a definitive outcome of psychotic experiences, social isolation can often be the product of stigmatisation stemming from a psychospiritual experience being misdiagnosed as psychotic. Each of these views arguably challenges the suggestion that social isolation is a definitive criterion for differentiating psychotic from psychospiritual experiences.

9.3.9 Criterion nine findings: generally negative experience

This criterion, which was posited by about seventeen per cent of authors, represents the view that psychotic and psychospiritual experiences are generally discernible in that the former is negative in nature, and the latter is positive. For instance, in contrast to the professed positive nature of psychospiritual experiences, Johnson & Friedman (2008, p. 523) claim that "psychopathology is often characterized by greater ... terror", while Siegler et al. (1969, p. 956) portray psychotic experience as one where "the future is the realm of anxiety and danger". In terms of schizophrenia, Hunt (2007, p. 216) describes a "painful sense of deletion of presence and inner vitality", Nelson (1994, p. 348) holds that schizophrenic persons are distressingly confronted with "an incomprehensible universe", and Siglag (1986, p. 138) observes that they "experience terror, fear, depression, and a sense of insecurity". These depict various negative outcomes as being emblematic of psychotic experience.

9.3.9.1 Criterion nine rebuttal

Although this criterion may appear to be plausible, it seems ultimately to be a value judgment as the literature is rife with examples of protracted periods of negative experience in a psychospiritual context. For example, a pervasive aspect of the transformation process in mysticism is aptly referred to as "the dark night of the soul"

(Underhill, 1912), while Krishna's (1977) autobiographical account of his transformative kundalini process involved many lengthy bouts of severe physical and psychic suffering, over a twenty-year period, before he was finally able to integrate the experience. Hence, it seems simplistic to suggest that negative experience is indicative of psychopathology in contrast to the supposed positive effect of a psychospiritual experience. Negative and positive experiences, of long and short duration, commonly feature in both psychospiritual and psychotic events.

9.4 Conclusion

The task of discerning psychotic from psychotic-like psychospiritual experiences is complex and seemingly impossible. Indeed, I have demonstrated that each of the topmost nine criteria identified by authors as characteristically psychotic are conversely identified by others as typically psychospiritual. Arguably, this impasse shows the inaptness of employing psychiatry's psychopathology-seeking approach in the field of psychospiritual research. Rather than trying to discern psychotic from psychospiritual experiences, adopting an open-ended phenomenological approach that aims to better understand their commonalities may be a more fruitful investigative path. Chapter Ten examines seven further themes elicited from my content analysis that support this contention.

CHAPTER 10

Content analysis:
new conceptual pathways

10.0 Introduction

This chapter continues my content analysis in examining seven themes identified by authors that extend beyond classical psychiatric thinking and ostensibly offer new conceptual pathways to better understanding psychosis. This includes the idea that it ultimately appears impossible to differentiate psychotic from psychotic-like psychospiritual experiences. Hence, this chapter also works to conceptually segue into Focal Setting Four, which challenges the veracity of adopting psychiatry's binary model of differential diagnosis and psychopathology-seeking as an investigative approach for understanding psychosis in light of psychospiritual considerations.

10.1 The validity problem

A common issue authors alluded to throughout my content analysis was that which I have called 'the validity problem'. Essentially, the validity problem is characterised by the question: What substantiates the asserted psychopathology of differentiation criteria identified by various commentators? Several authors in my study spoke to this question. This is exemplified in Kemp's (2000, p. 58) critical view that: "If neither psychosis nor mysticism can be pinned down and defined, how is it possible to equate the two? To verify the equation of two variables, they must both be instantiated". Other authors in my study proffered similar viewpoints. For instance, Ortolf (1994, p. 10) argues that "effective differential criteria require clear, well-substantiated operationalizations" in order to better understand, and discern between, psychotic and mystic phenomena. In their study, de Menezes Junior & Moreira-Almeida (2009, p. 80) also note that "there is a scarcity of empirical studies that prospectively test the differentiating criteria of what would be a spiritual experience and what would be a mental disorder". Likewise, Johnson & Friedman (2008, p. 513) allude to the "lack of empirical support" for "diagnostic suggestions" within the literature pertaining to discerning psychotic from mystical experiences and suggest that "it would be useful to develop sound empirical approaches" (ibid., p. 522), while Jackson & Fulford (1997, p. 60, fn. 2) highlight the issue of ambiguous definition in their observation that "the clinical concept of 'psychosis' is notoriously broad in scope, so much so that psychiatrists have sometimes sought to abandon it altogether … There is no agreement, either, on the criteria for the genuinely mystical". Such views seemingly constitute a significant challenge to diagnostic practices because they legitimately point out that, in the absence of empirical substantiation, proposed psychopathological differentiation criteria are rendered speculative and provisional. It therefore appears that Johnson & Friedman's suggestion regarding the need to formulate sound empirical approaches within this field of diagnostics is prudent.

As demonstrated throughout Chapter Nine, however, seeking to establish empirically valid diagnostic criteria for discerning psychotic from psychospiritual experiences is seemingly an impossible task because all such criteria can appear in both types of experiences. This arguably suggests that the two states of consciousness share a common psychic ground and that an open-ended approach of phenomenological investigation, which sidesteps the practice of pinpointing psychopathology, might lead to an epistemic breakthrough in this field of research. Indeed, the entire differentiation enterprise is modelled on psychiatry's a priori acceptance of the unsubstantiated notion that distinct forms of psychopathology exist. Ironically, then, the materialist approach of bifurcating diagnostics, when applied to the field of psychic disturbances and anomalies, is seemingly rendered invalid at the outset, for it fails to substantiate the psychopathology of the criteria used as differential measures. In other words, such criteria reflect axiomatic suppositions that have not been empirically validated. American neuroscientist Steven Hyman (2010, p. 157) derisively refers to this type of thinking as "an unintended epistemic prison" and remonstrates that it has been "palpably impeding scientific progress" in American psychiatric research since the 1980 inauguration of a DSM-III medical model. He further maintains that the reified nature of diagnostic entities has "controlled the research questions [investigators] could ask, and perhaps, even imagine" (ibid.). It could equally be proposed that reductive psychiatry's epistemic prison impedes a better understanding of psychosis by proscribing the asking, and even the imagining, of investigative research questions regarding possible psychospiritual considerations.

It is evident throughout Chapter Nine that even when psychospiritual considerations are included in clinical diagnostics, the scope of understanding generally reflects, and is limited by, unsubstantiated axiomatic assumptions regarding psychopathology that guide conventional psychiatric practice. Such an approach assumes, without validation, that psychotic experiences are psychopathologically distinct from psychospiritual experiences. Consequently, it precludes investigation of the possibility that the two experiences are not essentially different, but share common roots and are therefore indistinguishable.

10.2 Issues of ontology

In my study a variety of issues pertaining to the experience of ontological distress and distortion were identified as a differentiation criterion by authors.[100] For instance, psychotic experience is described as marked by "estrangement from self" (Siegler et al., 1969, p. 956), "a sense of insecurity" of self (Siglag, 1986, p. 138), and "the experience of feeling as though one is separated from the world by a thick, glass wall, being trapped in a silent, unreal room" (Pahnke & Richards, 1966, p. 188). Similarly, Clarke (2000, p. 14) proposes that the "well-foundedness or otherwise of the self of the individual undergoing the experience" discerns whether an experience becomes psychotic or not. Examples of other proffered ontological psychosis differentiators are:

- Withdrawal from the external world into the self (Stephen & Suryani, 2000, p. 26; Grof & Grof, 1995, p. 315; Nelson, 1994, p. 249).
- Being unable to discern outer from inner reality (Grof & Grof, 1995, p. 315; Noll, 1983, p. 452).
- The experience of outer and inner reality being sundered (Austin, 1998, p. 31; Wapnick, 1966, p. 69).
- Impairment to time-space orientation (Grof & Grof, 1995, p. 315).
- Monocular focus (Cantlie, 2014, p. 109).[101]
- A "situation of ontological insecurity" due to an upheaval of a person's "urdoxa" (Brett, 2002, p. 327).[102]

All of these criteria ostensibly reflect the general notion that the psychotic process is evidenced by the experience of ontological distress and distortion.

In the field of psychosis research, a key and original thinker along these lines is the Scottish psychiatrist Ronald Laing who adapted the works of existential philosophers to formulate the idea that psychotic experience is fundamentally one of what he called "ontological insecurity" (1990, p. 42). According to Laing (ibid.), in a state of ontological insecurity:

---

[100] In total, about forty-four per cent of authors discussed an ontological-type psychotic manifestation. However, these were diverse in nature so I sub-categorised them into eighteen different criteria. In other words, I did not identify 'issues of ontology' as a criterion in itself, but as an umbrella category composed of multiple criteria.

[101] Cantlie (2014, p. 109) maintains that the Indian sadhu can be discerned from "the ordinary madman" in that "the sadhus are aware both of the life they left and the life that, for whatever motives, they have now decided to adopt. Their focus is binocular". Extrapolating from this, I coined the term 'monocular focus' to designate the psychotic person's ostensible conflation of past and present experience.

[102] Brett (2002, p. 325) defines ordoxa as "a primordial, unshakeable certainty in the fundamental features or dimensions of the world and myself", which, when shaken, or ill-formed, can result in a person feeling dislocated from his or her 'self'.

> the individual … may feel more unreal than real; in a literal sense, more dead than
> alive; precariously differentiated from the rest of the world, so that his identity and
> autonomy are always in question. He may lack the experience of his own temporal
> continuity. He may not possess an over-riding sense of personal consistency or
> cohesiveness. He may feel more insubstantial than substantial, and unable to
> assume that the stuff he is made of is genuine, good, valuable. And he may feel his
> self as partially divorced from his body.

Hence, his notion of ontological insecurity denotes an extensive impairment to a person's fundamental ground of being. He further maintains that the key to understanding "how certain psychoses can develop" lay in comprehending the dynamics of the respective existential states of ontological security and insecurity (ibid.).[103] He therefore depicts the phenomenon of ontological insecurity as fundamental to understanding and defining psychotic experience.

Issues and questions of ontology in psychosis research, then, clearly open to different ways of understanding than those which guide medical psychiatry's inquiry into the nature of psychosis. For instance, medical psychiatry aims to objectively identify psychopathological symptoms and configure these into psychotic diagnostic criteria. Such an approach generally deems a psychotic person's subjective and transpersonal experiences as incidental and therefore not pertinent to examination. With ontological considerations, however, the investigative gaze turns inwards to question the nature of subjective experience. Doing so raises questions that probe beyond the limited objective scope of psychiatric observation and inquiry. What is the generic nature of human ontology and of the different cultural ontologies therein? What is the nature of the different states of being that appear to exist within the psychotic 'world'? What is the relationship between the subjective and physical self in psychotic experience? Can psychosis be understood merely as the presence of a psychopathological 'brokenness', or may it possibly be the consequence of an absence of the psycho-social-spiritual skills, capacities, instruction, and understanding required for optimal mental health?

Such questions and thinking are alien to medical materialism yet they do exist within the worldviews of other cultures and traditions. For example, this is exemplified in Sekida's (1985, p. 183) phenomenological description of how psychosis is precipitated by nen malfunction.

---

[103] Laing (1990, pp. 41–42) describes the state of ontological security as follows:

> The individual, then, may experience his own being as real, alive, whole; as differentiated from the rest
> of the world in ordinary circumstances so clearly that his identity and autonomy are never in question; as
> a continuum in time; as having an inner consistency, substantiality, genuineness, and worth; as spatially
> coextensive with the body; and, usually, as having begun in or around birth and liable to extinction with
> death. He thus has a firm core of ontological security.

A more detailed examination of Laing's work is undertaken later in Section 10.6.3 below.

In the case of the psychotic person, the sequence of three nen actions ... is deranged because of the malfunction or fatigue of the reflecting action, especially that of the third nen. This must necessarily be followed by the third nen's failure to perform normally its identifying function, and by the progressive isolation of the nen from each other. The first nen, especially, becomes isolated in this way. Hence, the psychotic often fails to identify his own sensations, perceptions, and mood as his own and begins to feel alienated from himself.

This is not to say that the Zen notion of nen function is the final word on the cause and nature of psychosis, but it certainly demonstrates a worldview that offers conceptual avenues for better understanding psychosis beyond psychiatry's reductive psychopathology-seeking, and related assumptions of biological aetiology and incomprehensibility. Additionally, and importantly, an understanding of the effective role of nen in shaping human perception and cognition is the product of close subjective investigation, as is the view that psychosis is caused by nen malfunction. This exemplifies how research into the phenomenological nuances of human subjectivity can foster a better understanding of the apparent connection between psychotic and psychospiritual experiences.

10.3 Anomalies of the mythic/subliminal domain

The mythic domain denotes the deeper realm of human consciousness. Although there is a considerable body of literature in which authors attempt to better understand the nature of psychosis from a mythic perspective, the focus here is primarily on observations made by Jung and other authors in my study who addressed this issue in terms of differentiating psychotic from psychospiritual experiences. Jung (1966, p. 66) broadly refers to this domain as the "collective unconscious" from which the myths of all cultures and religions have emerged. In his earlier work he defined the unconscious as "the foundation on which consciousness is built" and "the sum of all psychic processes below the threshold of consciousness" (Jung, 1914, p. 964). Thus, it represents the primordial source of the human psyche. Later, he coined the term "collective unconscious" to denote the domain of consciousness shared by all humanity, which is comprised of "subliminal perceptions, thoughts feelings ... subliminal vestiges of archaic functions that exist *a priori* ... [and] subliminal combinations in symbolic form, not yet capable of becoming conscious" (Jung, 1966, pp. 303–304). For Jung, this is an actual domain of reality—"It too is a world, but a world of images" (ibid., p. 298). He subsequently chose the term "archetype" to infer "archaic or ... primordial types, that is, with universal images that have existed since the remotest times" (Jung, 1968, pp. 4–5). Hence, his notion of the collective unconscious essentially speaks of the psychospiritual realm of human consciousness.

Unlike the psychotic-versus-mystical binary envisioned by most commentators in my study, from a Jungian perspective, psychosis does not stand in contradistinction to mystical experience, but represents the psychopathological outcome of individuals' unsound or ruptured relationships with their psychospiritual depths. Jung (1969, p. 69) maintains that the difference between the normal person and the psychotic person is that the former is psychically anchored within "the directness and directedness of the conscious mind", while the latter is "under the direct influence of the unconscious". Elsewhere he explains that "if the unconscious simply rides roughshod over the conscious mind, a psychotic condition develops" (Jung, 1966, p. 162). This depicts psychosis as an uncontrolled irruption of unconscious archetypal content into the conscious mind. Further to this, Jung (1968, p. 39) suggests that, for people predisposed towards psychosis, it may happen that "the archetypal images, which are endowed with a certain autonomy anyway on account of their natural numinosity, will escape from conscious control altogether and become completely independent, thus producing the phenomena of possession". Indeed, he holds that "they undoubtedly belong to the material that comes to light in schizophrenia" (ibid., p. 287). In further reference to schizophrenia, he proposes that,

> the unconscious usurps the reality function [of the conscious mind] and substitutes its own reality. Unconscious thoughts become audible as voices, or are perceived as visions or body-hallucinations, or they manifest themselves in senseless, unshakable judgments upheld in the face of reality. (Jung, 1966, pp. 282–283)

Hence, what mainstream psychiatry sees as the diagnostic symptoms of psychosis, Jung depicts as unconscious archetypal forms or forces that have flooded and supplanted the conscious mind. This fundamentally represents a psychospiritual understanding of the nature and cause of psychosis.

In light of this viewpoint, the difference between psychotic and psychospiritual experience lies in the nature of a person's relationship with his or her irruptive unconscious materials. A person experiencing psychosis is overwhelmed by this influx and mistakenly attempts to translate it literally via his or her framework of conscious reality. Conversely, in psychospiritual instances, a person is able to maintain a measure of psychic equanimity and, in recognising it as an experience of the unconscious, attempts to grasp its meaning symbolically. Subsequently, Jung (1966, pp. 217, 283) exhorts that "we must not concretize our fantasies" and explains that "it would be real insanity only if the contents of the unconscious became a reality that took the place of conscious reality; in other words, if they were to be believed without reserve". Other authors in my study also identified such concretisation as evidencing psychosis. For instance, Hunt (2007, p. 217) perceives "the literalization of metaphoric understanding" to be a form of "pathological hyperreflexivity", while Goretzki et al. (2009, p. 91) observe that psychotic persons act literally on the "powerful archetypal forces that swamp" them. Interestingly, over a half century before Jung, Perceval (1840, p. 274) discussed this phenomenon in reflecting on his own psychotic experience. He reported that:

> the spirit speaks poetically, but the man understands it literally. Thus you will hear one lunatic declare that he is made of iron, and that nothing can break him …

The meaning of the spirit is, that this man is strong as iron ... but the lunatic takes the literal sense.

Like Jung, Perceval understood psychopathology to be *not* in the form of the experience itself (i.e. delusional ideation), but in the misinterpretation of the content of subliminal ideas or imagery. From this perspective, psychotic interpretations of reality can generally be understood to reflect the inability, or unpreparedness, to discern between conscious and unconscious mental material.

Jung's mythological take on psychotic experience also brings to light potential material for better understanding what Jaspers has called the 'ununderstandability' of psychosis.[104] For instance, on a 1956 internationally broadcasted radio symposium, Jung (1960, p. 250) stated that:

> In ... psychopathology, I feel that the most pressing need is a deeper and more comprehensive knowledge of the complex psychic structures which confront the psychotherapist. We know far too little about the contents and the meaning of pathological mental products ... This is particularly true of the psychology of schizophrenia. Our knowledge of this commonest of all mental diseases is still in a very unsatisfactory state.

This arguably suggests that the more clinicians are informed about the depths and dimensions of human psychic life, both conceptually and experientially, the less incomprehensible psychosis becomes. Is it possible that the attainment of a 'more comprehensive knowledge' about human psychic structures may change the present picture of psychopathology? For instance, are 'incomprehensible' psychotic symptoms such as delusions and hallucinations psychopathological per se, or are they normal and natural within their native domain of the unconscious mind? Rather than dismiss the content of delusions as 'incomprehensible' and clinically unimportant, might it be therapeutically more effective to attempt to engage and understand them as meaningful mythic or symbolic material? The later examination of Jungian psychiatrist John Weir Perry's work[105] indicates that this question can be answered in the affirmative.

Finally, and importantly, although Jung depicts psychosis as a form of psychopathology and differentiates between healthy and unhealthy engagement with unconscious content, it appears his model of understanding essentially undermines the binary logic that drives the whole enterprise of distinguishing between psychotic and psychospiritual experiences. There appears to be an underlying assumption in this field of research that, although psychotic and psychospiritual experiences share many similarities, they are ontologically distinct. Hence, the conceptual and diagnostic task is to identify and map differentiation criteria. But what if they are inextricably wedded

---

[104] In my study, eleven authors (about sixteen per cent) identified the presence of incomprehensible beliefs and behaviour as indicative of psychotic rather than psychospiritual experience.

[105] See Chapter Eleven, Section 11.3 for an elucidation on Perry's work concerning the meaningful and functional nature of 'psychotic delusions'. This further demonstrates how that which is ordinarily seen as incomprehensible may reveal meaning when investigated from a psychospiritual perspective.

and, ultimately, cannot be differentiated? As demonstrated throughout this section, it seems Jung's view leans away from strict binary and differential thinking to indicate a common source for both types of experience, for he depicts psychotic, mystic, and mythic manifestations as all stemming from the unconscious or subliminal mind. Consequently, the attempt to formulate differential diagnostic criteria seems a dubious enterprise, particularly when based on reductive and dualistic medical notions of psychopathology. Arguably, a non-pathologising approach of inquiry might be more effective in trying to better understand the nature and causes of psychosis, and to inform apposite, holistic, therapeutic practices.

10.4 Divine madness

References to the experience of divine madness, or God-intoxication, are replete throughout both secular and religious texts. In my content analysis this idea was posited by Meher Baba (1988, p. 9) who speaks of discerning between "ordinary madness" and "divine madness". From a psychiatric perspective, experiences of divine madness are likely to be diagnosed as grandiose type psychotic delusions (APA, 2013, p. 91). However, from a transpersonal perspective they are understood as reflecting a genuine, though often distorted, exposure to mystic states of consciousness. For instance, Nelson (1994, p. 349) refers to the "godlike" schizophrenic experience whereby a person "expresses his power over reality as the quintessence of madness: 'I'm God, but you're not!'". Jung (1966, pp. 274–275) also adopts the notion of 'godlikeness' from Goethe's *Faust* (2001) to denote situations whereby "the patient's condition consists in his attributing to himself qualities or values which obviously do not belong to him, for to be 'godlike' is to be like a spirit superior to the spirit of man". He describes this as a "serious misunderstanding" and a "question of inflation" that occurs when "the ego has appropriated something that does not belong to it ... Thus he becomes a superman, superior to all others, a demigod at the very least. 'I and the Father are one'" (ibid., pp. 228–229). Hence, in such situations it is not the 'delusional' belief per se that constitutes psychopathology, but the act of literal rather than symbolic interpretation that makes it so. Likewise, Assagioli (1965, p. 45) maintains that "the key to an understanding" of so-called grandiose delusions is to be aware that:

> The fatal error of all who fall victim to these illusions is to attribute to their personal ego or 'self' the qualities and powers of the Self. In philosophical terms, it is a case of confusion between an absolute and a relative truth, between the metaphysical and the empirical levels of reality; in religious terms, between God and the 'soul'.

In other words, the mystic experience of 'God being within me and all others' is mistakenly and egocentrically translated by a psychotic person as meaning 'I am God'. Here, the presumed cause of seeming disorder is not the presence of a biological aberration, but the absence of an ability to correctly interpret overwhelming influxes of mystic consciousness. This arguably suggests a psychospiritual aetiology of psychosis.

The transition from divine madness to mystic illumination is generally orchestrated through tutelage from a psychospiritual master in technologies of consciousness. For example, in speaking of his extensive experience working with God-intoxicated people called "masts", Meher Baba (1988, pp. 9, 11) explains that in instances of ordinary madness "the person can, through suitable treatment and healing, only return to the normality of the ordinary functioning of consciousness", whereas, a person in the thralls of divine madness, when aided by "the directive help of the Master", will eventually "emerge into a supra-normal state of new integration and harmony"; a state of "unimpeachable sanity". Hence, in his view, it is essential for psychotic-like instances of divine madness to be guided by an adept in technologies of consciousness so that they may fulfil their transformative potential. However, such support is impossible if psychospiritual considerations are not central to the epistemology of any given healing tradition. This is the case with mainstream Western psychology (and psychiatry). As Kiran Kumar et al. (2005, p. 108) explain, "in modern psychology due to non-recognition of the possibility of a transcendent Self, all the discussions on self terminate at the level of bio-psycho-social identity". Subsequently, the mainstream therapeutic trajectory of modern psychology is "self-actualisation", while for Indian psychology, it is "Self-realization" (ibid., p. 120). Whereas the former aims at maintaining secular normality the latter aims to transcend this (see Figure 3).

An item of particular interest here is the notion that the state of *normal* consciousness, from which some people psychotically stray and hopefully return to via therapeutic recovery practices, is seen from a mystic viewpoint as a dubious form of ego-based sanity (i.e. quasi-sanity), in that it fails to fully apprehend larger and deeper psycho-spiritual reality. This idea is commonly iterated throughout psychospiritual literature and has profound ramifications for better understanding psychosis. If psychosis is a form of psychopathology intrinsically characterised by a person being out of touch with normal reality, yet normal reality is likewise out of touch with a larger mystic reality, then what is the benchmark for identifying true psychopathology? Here, both

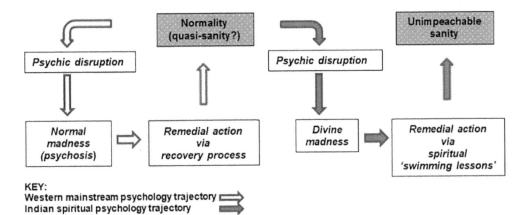

Figure 3. Comparative psychic disruption trajectories in Western and Indian psychology.

psychosis and normality are out of touch with reality in their unique, respective ways. Therefore, rather than perceiving ostensible psychopathology in purely negative terms (i.e., as a morbid departure from normality or sanity, to which one should be returned as soon as possible), it may also be viewed as a potentially positive indication (i.e., a prospective step towards transcending the limitations of normality to achieve a state of enhanced sanity). Indeed, there are manifold psychotic-like forms of transpersonal experience that manifest along a vast spectrum of human states of consciousness. Further research by psychiatry into the notion of divine madness may advance knowledge about the nature of psychosis, normality, and many other unknown or poorly understood transpersonal states of human consciousness.

10.5 Non-psychopathological psychotic experiences

Traditionally, the term 'psychosis' denotes a form of psychopathology. Even within fields of research that recognise the legitimacy of psychospiritual realities a strong trend exists towards discerning between benign transpersonal and psychopathological psychotic experiences. However, in my study two authors unconventionally referred to psychospiritual experiences as benign forms of psychosis. Although these are atypical instances, it is apposite to examine them as they demonstrate the complexity of attempting to understand psychosis in relation and contradistinction to psychotic-like psychospiritual experiences.

10.5.1 Carroll (2007) and benign psychosis

The first instance is Carroll's (2007) proposed model for discerning malignant from benign psychosis. Her model depicts a spectrum of altered states of consciousness (ASC) ranging from regressive and malignant psychotic states at one end, through to evolutionary and benign psychotic states at the other, with "average ego consciousness" midway between (ibid., p. 74, see Figure 4). She describes this as a model of "inner experiences that shed the light of consciousness on particular aspects of the unconscious mind" (p. 73).

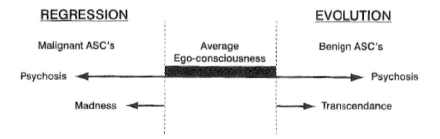

Figure 4. Carroll's spectrum of ASC from malignant to benign psychosis.
Source: Carroll, 2007, p. 74.

Intriguingly, she places the term 'psychosis' at both ends of the spectrum and explains that: "If we drew consciousness on a continuum, we would place the ASCs associated with common types of madness (regression and malignant psychosis) at one end of the spectrum and mystical (transcendence and benign psychosis) at the opposite end" (p. 74). Her use of the word 'psychosis' here to represent a 'mystical state' is puzzling, for commentators in this field of research predominantly use the two terms divergently to connote experiences on opposite sides of the insane-sane divide. Regarding this seeming anomaly Carroll explains that:

> I use the word 'psychosis' on both ends of the spectrum to mean inner chaos, a disconnect from consensual reality and/or a loss of personal identity ... the term 'malignant psychosis' refers to an ego that hasn't reached an average adult level of development and is therefore not well equipped to handle challenges thrown by unconscious forces ... Whereas a 'benign psychosis' refers to a temporary state of chaos experienced by a healthy, adult ego that has served the person well until the moment of overwhelm happened. (Carroll, 22/10/2014, personal communication)[106]

Hence, her 'benign psychosis' seems to correlate with the Grofs' 'spiritual emergency', whereby a person's ego is temporarily destabilised by an uncontrolled influx of transpersonal content. Interestingly, however, while the Grofs distinguish a psychosis from a spiritual emergency, Carroll depicts both as types of 'psychosis', with the former being frankly psychopathological (malignant) and the latter being quasi-psychopathological or problematic (benign). In a positive light, this potentially represents a 'loosening' of the strictly morbid meaning usually implied by the word 'psychosis', and might therefore be seen as a constructive step towards investing the word with a broader range of connotation (i.e., malignant to benign), which, in turn, may lead to a diminishment of the word's stigmatising effect. On the other hand, referring to an experience of spiritual emergency as a type of psychosis might work to invest the former with the inherent psychopathological status of the latter. Overall, then, Carroll's transposition of the term 'psychosis' into a psychospiritual context arguably works to obfuscate, more than clarify, a better understanding of the nature of both psychotic and psychospiritual phenomena.

10.5.2 Jackson & Fulford (1997) and benign psychosis

Jackson & Fulford (1997) also proffer the idea of "benign psychosis" in their seminal paper titled "Spiritual experience and psychopathology". Their context of meaning, however, differs significantly from Carroll's, who saw 'benign psychosis' as denoting chaotic, psychotic-like states of psychospiritual imbalance in contradistinction to classic psychosis. According to Jackson & Fulford (ibid., p. 43), a primary aim of their research was to determine whether "psychotic phenomena can occur

---

[106] I contacted the author, Marlyse Carroll, to seek clarification on this puzzling issue.

in the context of benign spiritual experiences, and if so, to explain the significance of this occurrence". This suggests that psychospiritual experiences can include the benign play of actual psychotic phenomena. Accordingly, their paper expounds on their observation that "phenomena which in a medical context would probably be diagnosed as psychotic *symptoms*, may occur in the context of non-pathological, and indeed essentially benign, spiritual experiences", which they call "'psychotic *phenomena*' as distinct from 'psychotic *symptoms*'" (p. 41).[107] Hence, their notion of "non-pathological psychotic experiences", which they also call "spiritual psychotic experiences" (pp. 41, 42), infers psychotic *phenomena* as opposed to classic psychotic *symptoms*. Further to this, they explain that while psychotic *symptoms* are the "proper object of medical treatment", psychotic *phenomena* are essentially a psychospiritual concern (p. 42). They subsequently argue that "pathological and spiritual psychotic phenomena cannot be distinguished" by using standard psychiatric descriptive, categorical, or diagnostic systems, but by discerning "the way in which psychotic phenomena themselves are embedded in the values and beliefs of the person concerned" (ibid.). Their depiction of values and beliefs as core differentiation focal points opens an intriguing new possible research door for understanding the psychosis-versus-psychospiritual conundrum.

In relation to the issue of values and beliefs, Jackson & Fulford (p. 55) make the astute observation that people experiencing psychotic-like phenomena can often maintain highly functional lives. Indeed, their functionality may be increased as a direct result of the experience. The authors note that "in the case of *pathological* psychotic phenomena, there is a radical *failure* of action … In the case of *spiritual* psychotic phenomena, action is radically *enhanced*" (p. 55).[108] Hence, it appears that in psychospiritual instances, people who exhibit classic psychotic symptoms can experience a gain, rather than loss, of functionality. This raises a challenging question: Is the sole evaluation of symptoms effective in discerning psychotic from psychospiritual experiences (if, indeed, such a distinction can ultimately be made)? Jackson & Fulford (p. 56) believe not and argue that "these phenomena *cannot* be distinguished by form and content alone, at least as these have traditionally been understood". They propose that the distinction pivots on whether a person's capacity for action fails, or is enhanced, in the face of anomalous beliefs and experiences. Whereas a failure of action indicates a psychopathological psychotic experience, action enhancement indicates a non-psychopathological (psychospiritual) psychotic experience (p. 55). They further hold that this capacity for action "is embedded in the individual's values and beliefs" (p. 57). Hence, it is not the psychotic form or content of a belief, but a failure to ascribe value to this belief, that indicates psychopathology. In the absence of such value, both action

---

[107] The findings in Jackson's (1991) doctoral dissertation, titled *A study of the relationship between psychotic and religious experience*, informed their formulation of this idea.

[108] Although I have already quoted this in Chapter Nine, Section 9.3.1, it bears repeating here in light of the discussion on values, beliefs, and functionality. The important subject of functionality is further examined in Chapter Eleven, Section 11.2.2 in the context of the apparently common situation whereby psychotic delusions serve a function-enhancing role in people's lives.

and functionality are undermined. Conversely, the capacity to ascribe value results in enhanced action and functionality.

To substantiate this idea Jackson & Fulford proffer the example of 'Simon', an undiagnosed participant in their study, who exhibited classic psychotic symptoms of religious delusions, paranoia, and thought insertion. Though apparently psychotic from a psychiatric framework of understanding, his delusional ideation actually enabled him

> to succeed as a high-achieving black person in a predominantly white, racist context. He had high self-esteem, firm moral convictions, and a strong sense of purpose in life. His beliefs then, whilst unusual in content, and psychotic in form, were essentially affirming, and if anything increased rather that [sic] detracted from his ability to function effectively. (p. 46)

This suggests that a deeper investigation into the nature of beliefs, values, capacity for action, and functionality in psychotic-like experiences may enable the development of potentially effective psychosocial and psychospiritual therapeutic responses that complement, or supersede, the prevailing biomedical treatment model.

10.5.3 The promise of the notion of non-psychopathological psychotic experiences

It appears that the notion of benign, psychospiritual, non-psychopathological 'psychosis' offers prospective new investigative avenues for understanding psychosis. Importantly, both Carroll and Jackson & Fulford depict benign psychosis as an anomalous experience, or state of being, that mimics the symptomatology of malignant psychosis, yet is non-psychopathological due to its developmental potential or action-enhancing nature. Although the use of the term 'psychosis' in a non-pathological context is fraught with conceptual and semantic ambiguities, and a more neutral term might be preferable, this does not alter the valuable essence of the idea that people can have anomalous experiences that are ostensibly indistinguishable from classic psychosis. Indeed, many of these people, as Jackson & Fulford demonstrate, thrive because of, and not despite, their apparent traits of psychopathology.

Despite Carroll's and Jackson & Fulford's intriguing insights and novel use of the word 'psychotic' in non-psychotic contexts, like other authors in my study they viewed mad and mystic experiences as separate states of being and ultimately sought to discern psychopathological (malignant) from psychospiritual (benign) experiences. However, according to Marzanski & Bratton (2002, p. 360) proponents of this differentiating view "presuppose rather than explain the distinction". In other words, although this clinical approach is commonplace, it is actually theoretical and unsubstantiated and fails to consider the possibility that instances of malignant and benign 'psychosis' may be intrinsically wedded and indistinguishable. Indeed, the ensuing section on the notion of 'regression in the service of transcendence' lends credence to this possibility.

10.6 Regression in the service of transcendence

A significant theme evident in my content analysis was the notion that psychosis may represent a disruptive but integral aspect of a larger developmental or healing process. Indeed, this is suggested by UK psychiatrist, Russell Razzaque (2014), in the title of his book *Breaking Down is Waking Up,* wherein he argues that there is seemingly "something positive and transformative" inherent to psychosis and other forms of mental illness. Accordingly, several key proponents of the idea of self-healing psychosis are investigated below, both within and beyond the scope of my content analysis.[109] While some of these endorse a model that seeks to discern psychosis proper from a psychosis-like healing process, others perceive all instances of psychosis as healing processes in potential. My aim here is to further demonstrate the edifying value of exploring psychospiritual understandings of psychosis and to segue into Focal Setting Four, which argues that psychotic and psychotic-like psychospiritual experiences are ultimately indistinguishable.

10.6.1 Nelson (1994) and psychotic regression in the service of transcendence

Within the scope of my critical analysis literature, Nelson (1994, p. 33) used the term "regression in the service of transcendence" (RIST) to represent the idea and possibility of psychosis being integral to a psychospiritual renewal process. He maintains that regression is a natural human psychic process that can manifest in various forms, including as a "necessary preparation for emergence into higher states of consciousness, including spiritual levels" (ibid.). Regression in such instances is in the service of transcendence whereby a person "symbolically *dies* to his old life, to be reborn to a higher mode of functioning that subsumes the lower mode" (p. 246). However, Nelson (ibid.) also claims that RIST may devolve into psychosis if the ego is overwhelmed by exposure to the contents of the deeper psyche in the form of "menacing hallucinations that render him unable to go on with ordinary life. It can destroy his ego and degenerate into malignant regression" (ibid.).[110] While he notes that hallucinatory experiences are common to RIST (p. 246), he also warns that "the outcome can be madness as well as enlightenment" (p. 247). According to Nelson, then, while *psychotic-like* experiences are integral to RIST, these are not necessarily representative of psychosis *per se*. He subsequently formulated a comprehensive list of criteria for discerning psychotic from psychotic-like RIST experiences (pp. 248–249).[111] He also

---

[109] While the work of Nelson and Jung featured in my content analysis, that of Washburn, Laing, and Perry did not.

[110] Although Nelson does not use the actual term 'psychosis' here, his reference to 'malignant regression' infers psychosis. Indeed, his book is replete with instances of such a construal. For instance, he refers to "malignant psychotic regressions that permanently submerge the self in primitive areas of the psyche" (Nelson, 1994, p. xx).

[111] See Appendix Six, Table A11.

cautions that "unless there is physical danger of harm, antipsychotic medicines should generally be avoided in RIST, for they can freeze the process at a partially regressed level and foster long term dependence on medicine" (p. 247). In other words, in some instances psychosis may result from, rather than be remedied or prevented by, the use of anti-psychotic medications. If true, this highlights the pragmatic importance for psychiatry to consider possible psychospiritual determinants in its interventions with psychotic-like occurrences, for failure to do so may unwittingly result in instigating cases of iatrogenic psychosis.

10.6.2 Washburn (1988) and psychotic regression in the service of transcendence

The term 'regression in the service of transcendence' did not originate with Nelson. It was first coined by transpersonal theorist Michael Washburn in his book *The Ego and the Dynamic Ground* (1988), which argues that:

> the ego early in life separates itself from the deep psyche (the Dynamic Ground) and, therefore, must later in life spiral back to the deep psyche if, reunited with the original bases of its being, it is to achieve higher, whole-psyche integration. (Washburn, 2003, p. ix)

However, both have used the term to reflect essentially the same meaning. Like Nelson, Washburn (ibid., p. 157) acknowledges that psychopathological psychosis often occurs independently of RIST, and also warns that RIST can lead to either psychosis or transcendence (2003, p. 82; 1988, p. 37). Both authors also note that RIST is marked by psychotic-like occurrences that can be mistaken for signs of psychopathology. On this point, Washburn (1988, p. 157) states that:

> typical among the tribulations of this period are ... (1) strange physical symptoms; (2) bizarre and morbid states of consciousness; (3) dread and estrangement (or strangeness) ... (4) disturbance of thought processes; (5) loss of control of personality; (6) eruption of the instincts; and (7) recurrence of the ego/Ground conflict, with danger of ego death.

However, whereas Nelson proffered a list of differentiation criteria in response to the issue of the marked similarity between features of RIST and psychosis, Washburn did not. Also, while Washburn generally remained within the scope of transpersonal theory, Nelson (1994, p. xxi), as a psychiatrist, wrote with the aim of "reintegrating spiritual psychologies with modern science". In building on Washburn's work, Nelson has demonstrated the capacity for transpersonal theory and considerations to be integrated into psychiatric epistemology and diagnostic practice.

10.6.3 Laing (1972) and the 'psychotic' metanoiac journey

Both Nelson's and Washburn's thinking were informed by the work of Laing who also endorses the notion of benign and/or transformative processes marked by psychotic-like features. Laing was a key exponent of the 1960s radical psychiatry movement, and his existential-phenomenological approach to understanding psychotic experience is profound and complex. Therefore, it is apposite to first examine some key aspects of this before continuing to explore his views on the regressive-transformative nature of psychosis. From an existential perspective, Laing (1972, pp. 11, 15) proffers the paradigm-changing hypothesis that schizophrenia "may itself be a resource a human being calls upon when all else seems impossible", and that for such people psychosis represents "a desperate strategy of liberation within the microsocial situation he finds himself". Indeed, while he acknowledges that the term 'schizophrenia' is a "social fact", in that it is a psychiatric construct for depicting an apparent form of psychopathology, he also maintains that "to be mad is not necessarily to be ill" (1967, pp. 100, 113). Elaborating on this point he explains that:

> 'schizophrenia' is a diagnosis, a label applied by some people to others. This does not prove that the labelled person is subject to an essentially pathological process, of unknown nature and origin, going on *in* his or her body … But it does establish as a social fact that the person labelled is one of Them. (p. 99)

He consequently concludes that "there is no such 'condition' as 'schizophrenia' but the label is a social fact and the social fact a *political event*" (p. 100). In his view, then, schizophrenia is not an actual form of psychopathology that occurs *in* people. Rather, it is a clinical construct based on the unsubstantiated aetiological assumption of "a subtle underlying organic process" (p. 87). Further to this he contends that "it is wrong to impute to someone a hypothetical disease of unknown etiology and undiscovered pathology unless *he* can prove otherwise" (p. 87), and elsewhere that "those people who make this set of attributions have to prove that it refers to something real. My summary of the evidence to date, is that they have not done so" (1972, p. 13). Ipso facto, schizophrenia as a social construct is not real in an ontological sense; only as a social fact and political event.

Laing further maintains that the existential phenomenon called 'schizophrenia' by psychiatry "has little to do with the clinical examination, diagnosis, prognosis and prescriptions for therapy" (1967, p. 107) and that "just about everything that can be known about the psychopathology of schizophrenia or of schizophrenia as a disease … are all ways of *not* understanding" the experience, or the person who is having it (1990, p. 33). For him, that which is called 'schizophrenia', or 'psychosis', may be better understood as a "natural *healing* process" (1967, p. 105). Hence, he did not view psychosis as psychopathological per se, but as a meaningful process which, under the right circumstances, may fulfil its natural healing potential.

Laing's view on the transformative potential of so-called 'psychosis' differs from the bifurcating view held by other commentators in this field of research. He refers to psychosis as a *"metanoiac voyage"*, which he understands to be "a potential healing process" and a "voyage of discovery into self of a potentially revolutionary nature and with a potentially liberating outcome" (Laing, 1972, p. 12). Hence, while other proponents of this view have sought to differentiate psychosis from potentially transformative psychotic-like psychospiritual experiences, Laing sees *all* psychotic experiences as intrinsic processes of potential renewal. In this light he asserts that "madness need not be all break*down*. It is also break*through*" (1965, p. 9). According to Thornton (2005, p. 8), Laing's term 'metanoia' is meant to connote "an intense experience that brings one as close to the edge of sanity as possible before emerging. It is a spiritual experience". Indeed, Laing (1967, pp. 108–109) explains that psychosis "may be judged to be invalidly mad or to be validly mystical … It is on the existential meaning of such unusual experience that I wish to focus". This arguably depicts metanoia as being 'validly mystical' and suggests that the various metanoiac manifestations of psychosis may be better understood via an existential-phenomenological lens of inquiry. Laing (1990, p. 34) explains that this approach aims to elicit a subjective "understanding of the patient's *existential position* … to know how the patient is experiencing himself and the world, including oneself". This is an act of trying to empathically understand a psychotic person, rather than viewing him or her in an objective, diagnostic, and clinical manner. Furthermore, he describes the psychotic person as one who "muddles ego with self, inner with outer, natural and supernatural. Nevertheless, he often can be to us, even through his profound wretchedness and disintegration, the hierophant of the sacred" (Laing, 1967, pp. 109–110). This also places psychotic metanoiac manifestations within the compass of 'the sacred' and arguably sets the conceptual stage for bringing psychiatric and psychospiritual worldviews together.

In the context of 'regression in the service of transcendence', Laing sees the psychotic metanoiac voyage as a dialectical process comprised of both regressive and transformative components. Hence, a period of regression is followed by *"neo-genesis, a new movement forward whose principles and regularities we know very little about"* (Laing, 1972, pp. 16, 18). As such, he maintains that psychosis ideally represents an inherent healing process whereby a person journeys into, and returns from, an "inner world" (1967, p. 103). He notes, however, that due to Western society's and psychiatry's poor understanding of such matters, the healing potential of this process is hampered by a lack of proficient guides (ibid.). Instead, in Laing's (p. 106) view, people experiencing psychosis are subjected by psychiatry to a *"degradation ceremonial"*, in contrast to the apposite therapeutic response of an *"initiation ceremonial through which the person will be guided with full social encouragement and sanction into inner space and time, by people who have been there and back again"*.[112] Subsequently,

---

[112] Laing (1967, pp. 101, 106) describes the differences between a degradation and initiation ceremonial as follows:

> *Degradation Ceremonial*—The 'committed' person labelled as patient, and specifically as 'schizophrenic', is degraded from full existential status as human agent and responsible person, no longer in possession of his own definition of himself, unable to retain his own possessions, precluded from the exercise of his discretion and whom he meets, what he does. His time is no longer his own and the space he occupies no longer

he proposes a "sequence of experiential stepping stones" (p. 107) for structuring an initiation ceremonial and guiding a person into and through psychosis.[113]

This is a ground-breaking idea in Western psychiatric epistemology. Especially coming from a psychiatrist, for it demonstrates how an existential-phenomenological approach to better understanding psychosis can elicit technologies of consciousness for use in new therapeutic approaches in psychiatry. Likewise, his proposal that people who have been into and through psychosis should act as guides for others experiencing the same, is seemingly an idea ahead of its time. Indeed, he makes the revolutionary observation that "schizophrenics have more to teach psychiatrists about the inner world than psychiatrists their patients" (1967, p. 91). Concomitant to this he argues that the role of the psychiatrist is to "assist the movement of what is called 'an acute schizophrenic episode' instead of arresting it" (Laing, 1972, p. 15). He also maintains, like Nelson, that pharmaceutical treatment can thwart the psychotic renewal process and, indeed, that *all* conventional psychiatric modalities of "'treating' the patient" reflect a gross misunderstanding of the psychotic process at hand (Laing, 1967, p. 102). He consequently asserts that conventional psychiatric practices are mostly counter-productive and often iatrogenic (ibid.). Overall, then, Laing's way of understanding psychosis proffers a root and branch challenge to psychiatric epistemology and practice, and also to proponents of the idea of diagnostically discerning between psychotic and psychotic-like psychospiritual experiences. If all instances of psychosis are healing journeys in potential, then it appears impossible to delineate the psychopathological markers necessary for differential diagnosis. Indeed, what is there to differentiate if the psychotic-like features are integral to the process of transformative upheaval?

10.6.4 Perry (1974) and the self-healing potential of 'psychosis'

The work of psychiatrist John Weir Perry, which builds on Jungian concepts and theories regarding the psychotic process, brings a unique perspective to potential ways of better understanding psychosis. This is particularly so regarding his insightful and

---

of his choosing. After being subjected to a degradation ceremonial known as psychiatric examination he is bereft of his civil liberties in being imprisoned in a total institution known as a 'mental hospital'. More completely, more radically than anywhere else in our society, he is invalidated as a human being.

Initiation Ceremonial—Instead of the degradation ceremonial of psychiatric examination, diagnosis and prognostication, we need, for those who are ready for it, an initiation ceremonial, through which the person will be guided with full social encouragement and sanction, into inner space and time, by people who have been there and back again. Psychiatrically, this would appear as ex-patients helping future patients to go mad.

[113] For Laing (1967, p. 106), the steps of an initiation ceremonial are:

i) a voyage from outer to inner; ii) from life to a kind of death; iii) from going forward to going back; iv) from temporal movement to temporal standstill; v) from mundane time to aeonic time; vi) from the ego to the self; vii) from being outside (post-birth) back into the womb of all things (pre-birth) ... and then subsequently a return voyage from ... 1) inner to outer; 2) from death to life; 3) from the movement back to a movement once more forward; 4) from immortality back to mortality; 5) from eternity back to time; 6) from self to a new ego; 7) from a cosmic foetalisation to an existential rebirth.

meaningful construal of delusions, which are supposedly incomprehensible. For Perry (1974, p. 21), psychosis is an archetypal "renewal process" that fundamentally aims to serve the function of precipitating self-healing and development. As he explains:

> the dynamics of the psychotic episode, as I see it, center upon the image of the self, of the way the individual experiences herself. When it is too limited, isolated, one-sided, or debased, this 'self-image' becomes due for a reorganization, and various compensatory mechanisms come into play. (ibid., p. 20)

He depicts this as occurring at different interrelated levels of being. For instance, at an ego level he sees the so-called 'psychotic'[114] process working to contend "with the pressing emotional issues to which the psyche needs to respond" in order to free-up a life damaged, retarded, or ossified by unresolved traumas and problems (p. 79). At a psychosocial level 'psychosis' represents an attempt by the psyche to "compensate the culture's biases" that can delimit the ego's innate creative capacity to the extent that it "suffers from a constricted consciousness that has been educated out of its needed contact with the natural elements of the psychic life" (pp. 107, 11). And at a psychospiritual level Perry (1999, p. vii) sees 'psychosis' as "nature's way of healing a restricted emotional development and of liberating certain vitally needed functions—in short, a spiritual awakening". He further notes that this functional capacity is inherent to both 'psychotic' and mystical experiences (p. 27). Hence, from this perspective, 'psychosis' is understood to be a natural, autonomous, and potentially remedial act by the deeper psyche which aims:

1. To reconcile and reconstitute a person's overly stultified and conflicted ego life.
2. To circumvent psychic blocks created by conservative cultural norms so as to enact latent human capacities.
3. To foster the evolutionary and spiritual development of individuals and societies.

In this, Perry's depiction of personal, social, and psychospiritual levels of renewal in 'psychotic' processes approximates Laing's thinking, but with a Jungian-transpersonal rather than an existential-political focus. Both views, however, make a valuable, albeit different, contribution to this field of research.

The idea of 'psychosis' being potentially remedial and essentially functional is antithetical to the psychopathological depiction of 'psychosis' endorsed by psychiatry. Yet, Perry (1974, p. 23) maintains that a 'psychotic' episode is not psychopathological per se, but represents a 'normal' personality that is "in profound need of reorganization". Here, contrary to psychiatric thinking, he identifies the 'normal'

---

[114] Perry generally places inverted commas around psychiatric words such as 'psychosis' and 'delusions' to highlight and rebut their inherent psychopathological meaning. He is in effect saying 'so-called psychosis or delusions'. In order to maintain congruency with his context of meaning and understanding I henceforth do the same throughout this section in which his views are appraised.

personality as the locus of affliction or psychopathological disorder, which 'psychosis', as a natural psychic function, aims to remediate. In other words, whereas a psychiatric treatment approach aims to bring 'psychotic' people back to 'normal', Perry sees 'psychosis' as innately striving to remediate and transcend a dysfunctional state of 'normal'. In this light he asserts that "certain psychic states, presently treated as acute 'psychotic' sickness, should instead be honoured as valid operations of the visionary mind playing its rightful part in the spiritual development of individuals and of cultures" (Perry, 1999, p. viii). Like aforementioned commentators, he also warns that without apposite social understanding and empathic therapeutic support a renewal process can become stuck in "the disruptiveness of a chaos without transformation" (pp. 108, 111). Indeed, the veracity and therapeutic efficacy of his views about 'psychosis' is seemingly supported by the effectiveness of his empathic approach in practice. For example, in reporting on therapeutic outcomes at his Diabasis facility,[115] Perry (p. 164) notes that "our most surprising finding in the cases of early acute episode was that grossly 'psychotic' clients have usually come into a coherent and reality-oriented state spontaneously within two to six days, without need for medications". Arguably, this outcome, combined with repeated warnings by other commentators regarding the capacity for traditional psychiatric interventions to thwart the healing potential in 'psychotic' processes, raises the question as to whether some, if not all, instances of psychosis, are innate and functional attempts at self-healing?

10.6.5 Jung (1969) and the transcendent function

Jung's conceptualisation of the transcendent function and his application of active imagination fundamentally informed his works. His years of experimentation with active imagination are described in his *Liber Novus* (2009, more commonly known as *The Red Book*) which, according to Shamdasani (2009, p. 221), is "nothing less than the central book in his oeuvre". Jung (1969, pp. 69, 82) defines the transcendent function as arising "from the union of conscious and unconscious contents" and as "the collaboration of conscious and unconscious data". He describes active imagination as "the hermeneutic treatment of creative fantasies" and asserts that his use of this in self-experimentation "resulted in a synthesis of the individual with the collective psyche" (Jung, 1966, p. 521). Indeed, for Jung (1965, pp. 178, 192), the use of active imagination

---

[115] Perry (1999, p. 159) describes Diabasis as:

> a residence facility that lived through three years and more of inpatient work with acute 'schizophrenic' episodes in young adults without the use of medications ... Its purpose was to provide a home in which the clients might have the opportunity to experience with full awareness their deepest processes during their intense turmoil.

It is beyond this book's scope to provide a fuller appraisal of the therapeutic efficacy of Perry's model for working with 'psychotic' people. For more on this, see: Cornwall, 2002; Perry, 1999, 1987; O'Callaghan, 1982. The chief aim here is to support my argument that it is possible to better understand psychosis beyond the views endorsed by medical psychiatry, especially through the lens of psychospiritual considerations.

was a "scientific experiment", and he maintains that "all my works, all my creativity, has come from those initial fantasies". Hence, it appears that active imagination formed the crucible from which Jung's voluminous and influential works emerged.

For Jung, active imagination was not an exercise in make-believe, but a foray into an extant domain of psychic existence. In addressing this issue, he asserts that "the scientific credo of our time has developed a superstitious phobia about fantasy. But the real is what works. The fantasies of the unconscious work—there can be no doubt about that" (Jung, 1966, p. 217). Further to this, when commenting on the parallels between active imagination and psychosis, he explains that "the reason why the involvement looks very much like a psychosis is that the patient is integrating the same fantasy-material to which the insane person falls victim because he cannot integrate it but is swallowed up by it" (Jung, 1970, p. 531). He proposes that initiating the transcendent function via active imagination is potentially "a third way" of contending with exposure to unconscious materials, other than the common and unbalanced responses of regression or inflation (Jung, 1966, p. 521). In other words, this suggests that, through engagement with and synthesis of unconscious material, the horizons of conscious awareness may be incrementally broadened. As such, what was once unconscious becomes integrated into the scope of ordinary cognisance, in an ongoing dialectical process of self-individuation.

This exemplifies the idea of psychotic and psychospiritual contents sharing the same source and substance. Phenomenologically, the only difference between the two is that psychosis occurs when a person fails to integrate unconscious materials, whereas transcendence occurs when such integration is successful. Indeed, Jung (1939, p. 1003) states that when exposed to unmediated unconscious content the person who becomes psychotic "is really drowned in a flood of insurmountably strong forces and thought forms". This is strikingly similar to Campbell's metaphor of swimming versus drowning.[116] In Jung's case, it is the effective application of innate skills that enables him to keep his head above the turbulent waters of the unconscious in which he found himself immersed when practising active imagination.

If Jung is correct, then the intrinsic similarities between psychotic and psychospiritual states of being mean that they cannot be distinguished in traditional diagnostic terms. From his experiential description it appears the line separating the two is very tenuous and blurry, if, indeed, it exists in any reified sense at all. For instance, in recollecting his own forays into the unconscious he explains that:

> One is assailed by the fear that perhaps this is madness. This is how madness begins, this *is* madness … You cannot get conscious of these unconscious facts without giving yourself to them. If you can overcome your fear of the unconscious and can let yourself go down, then these facts take on a life of their own. You can be gripped by these ideas so much that you really go mad, or nearly so. (Jung, 1970, p. 97)

---

[116] I discussed Campbell's metaphor of swimming versus drowning in Chapter Nine, Section 9.3.6.

This plainly portrays his personal struggle at the interface between integration and madness, where it seems madness and sanity are indistinguishable. A similar view is iterated by Jung's translator, Richard Hull, who, after reading Jung's *Liber Novus* commented that:

> there can be no doubt that Jung has gone through everything that an insane person goes through, and more ... The only difference between him and a regular inmate is his astounding capacity to stand off from the terrifying reality of his visions, to observe and understand what was happening, and to hammer out of his experience a system of therapy that works. But for this unique achievement he'd be as mad as a hatter. (Shamdasani quoting Hull, 2009, p. 221, fn. 257)

Hence, from a Jungian perspective, it appears that the contents of the unconscious are not psychotic per se. Rather, circumventing a psychotic outcome depends on a person having a particular fortitude and navigational skill set, or, as Jung (1939, p. 1004) puts it, "whether the individual can stand a certain panic, or the chronic strain of a psyche at war with itself". This paints a markedly different picture of psychosis than that posited by conventional psychiatry and psychology, and opens a vast and largely unexplored domain for possible future investigation into the enigmatic vicissitudes of 'psychotic' experience.

10.7 Psychosis as indistinguishable from psychotic-like renewal processes

To reiterate, a common approach by commentators in the field of researching psychotic and psychotic-like psychospiritual experiences has been to attempt to diagnostically differentiate between them. Jackson (2010, p. 140) refers to this as the *"spiritual-psychotic paradox"* and muses:

> How can two categories of experience, which are defined partly in terms of their opposite pragmatic effects, be so closely related as to suggest the presence of a common underlying process? What determines whether a particular individual's experience falls one side of the line or the other?

This line of inquiry is seemingly based on the materialist assumption that the two states are discrete, which logically leads to the question: How do we discern between that which is psychotic and that which looks psychotic but is not? This question, and the unsubstantiated assumption upon which it is based, arguably works to limit ways in which psychosis may be understood. Such binary thinking is an apparent extrapolation from psychiatry's belief that mental illness and mental health are separate states of being. Ipso facto, it can subsequently be concluded that psychosis and psychotic-like psychospiritual processes must also be different and differentiated. In terms of opening possible new ways for understanding Jackson's 'spiritual-psychotic paradox', it is arguably apposite to ask questions such as: Why do we need to discern between that which is psychotic and that which looks psychotic but is not? What is it, exactly, that substantiates the need to do so? Is it possible that they are integral to each other and cannot be differentiated? If psychosis can manifest as integral to a larger transformative process then how can it be psychopathological? Is such healing potential latent in all psychotic instances, or only some? Indeed, there are commentators on this issue who seem to suggest the impossibility of discerning a psychopathological state of psychosis from a healthful psychotic-like psychospiritual experience.

Several authors in my content analysis proffered views proposing that psychotic and psychospiritual experiences share an essentially common nature. Podvoll (1979, pp. 589, 586), for example, speaks of "the mystic and psychotic paths as converging" and his hyphenated reference to "a mystical-psychotic experience" clearly identifies the two as coterminous. He subsequently maintains that "a complete understanding of the psychotic experience must include knowledge of the desire and methods to transcend the ... pre-psychotic personality". Like Perry, he suggests that the ultimate psychotic trajectory is one which aims to transcend the normal ego-self. Arguably, then, the corresponding therapeutic task for clinicians is to help enable the fulfilment of this process. Indeed, Podvoll (ibid., p. 586) holds that "the important distinction is not between what is pathological and what is normal but ... what constitutes the difference between 'spiritual defeat and spiritual victory'". This depicts both incidents as essentially psychospiritual in nature, with psychosis as a form of spiritual defeat presumably resulting from a lack of spiritual guidance and/or skills. Boisen (1936, p. 298) similarly speaks of "a definite relationship between the mystical and the pathological". He perceives both as "nature's attempts ... to effect reorganization of the personality" and claims that the distinction is "to be drawn solely in terms of the results achieved" (ibid., pp. 81, 298). Arguably, this understanding suggests the ultimate impossibility of substantiating the psychopathological status of psychosis.

Whereas Focal Setting Three has chiefly focussed on binary models and concepts for differentiating psychotic from psychospiritual experiences (punctuated by critical analysis challenging this view), Focal Setting Four explores the idea that these states of being are essentially indistinguishable. It is therefore prudent, in closing, to provide quotations from commentators that depict an apparent common source for psychotic and psychotic-like states of consciousness. These are presented in chronological order to demonstrate that such thinking has existed within various disciplines over time.

- "The shaman differs from an ordinary patient ... in possessing an extremely great power of mastering himself ... [and though often] on the verge of insanity ... the shaman never passes this verge" (Czaplicka, 1914, pp. 169, 172).
- "The power of understanding is exhibited not when madness is absent but when it is mastered" (Schelling, 1942, fn. 27, p. 148).
- "[T]he mentally ill patient proves to be an unsuccessful mystic or, better, the caricature of a mystic" (Eliade, 1964, p. 27).

- "Mystical experience always carries a potential risk of psychosis … Those sensitive enough to taste mysticism are often sensitive enough to fall into psychosis" (Clark, 1966, p. 79).
- "The entire mystic path may be understood to be a strengthening process whereby the mystic gradually develops the 'muscles' to withstand the experiences of this 'inner world' … The schizophrenic undergoes no such training or strengthening. His 'muscles' are undeveloped and when 'thrown' into this 'inner world' he is overwhelmed" (Wapnick, 1969, pp. 63, 64).
- "Mysticism is fusion without confusion; schizophrenia is fusion with confusion" (Wilber, 1975, p. 123).
- "The psychological basis of insanity is the same basis for enlightenment. It all depends on whether or not it is accepted and comprehended and ultimately worked with as the key to liberation" (Clifford, 1984, pp. 138–139).
- "Both the madman and the mystic have been cast upon the sea of the prepersonal unconscious" (Washburn, 1988, p. 184).
- "There may be a great deal of variation in the very nature or 'stuff' of consciousness within the human species itself. This would then explain why the mystic experiences the world in a different way as compared to others. Simultaneously, this view would also be able to account for the difference in consciousness of the psychotic" (Varma, 2005, p. 205).
- "In some sense, a psychotic is a failed mystic. Perhaps the same latent capabilities are activated in both psychosis and mysticism but, in the case of psychosis, a person is unable to psychologically integrate the experiences" (Barušs, 2007, p. 39).

Each of these authors arguably suggests a basic and common psychic or psychospiritual source in which, or from which, both psychospiritual and psychotic experiences may result.

Furthermore, in regard to "metaphysical delusions", Jaspers (1997 v1, p. 108) maintains that "religious experience remains what it is, whether it occurs in saint or psychotic or whether the person in whom it occurs is both at once". This arguably connotes the common nature and, conceivably, the common source of mystic and psychotic experiences. Indeed, Goretzki et al. (2009) conducted empirical research to ascertain whether or not there is a clear difference between psychotic experiences and spiritual emergencies. They found the two states chiefly differ in that spiritual emergencies "are 'managed'" via psychospiritual interventions that support their developmental trajectory, and subsequently concluded that "there is a strong relationship between self-report of experience of many psychotic symptoms, self-report of psychosis, and spiritual emergency, to an extent that suggests that they may be different aspects of the same thing" (ibid., pp. 91–92). Further research in this field may shed new light not only on the seeming possibility of psychotic and psychospiritual interconnectivity, but also on a deeper understanding of the nature of human consciousness.

10.8 Conclusion

This chapter has facilitated a conceptual transition from Focal Setting Three to Focal Setting Four. Whereas the former introduces and examines issues pertaining to discerning psychotic from psychospiritual experiences, the latter argues that such differentiation is seemingly impossible. The questionable validity of psychiatric diagnostic criteria illustrated throughout this Focal Setting Three intrinsically challenges differentiation practices, for how does one discern two poorly understood phenomena from each another? Additionally, the notion that psychosis may reflect innate human capacities, including non-psychopathological healing processes of renewal, further suggests that reductive diagnostic practices may best be superseded by deeper phenomenological investigation into the nature of psychotic-like occurrences.

FOCAL SETTING FOUR

UNDERSTANDING PSYCHOSIS: PSYCHOSPIRITUAL AND PSYCHOPATHOLOGICAL AS INDISTINGUISHABLE

Focal Setting Four argues that, in the absence of experientially attaining deep metaphysical knowledge, it is ultimately impossible to discern culturally normative psychotic-like experiences from psychotic instances, unless deep metaphysical understanding has been attained.

CHAPTER 11

Hearing voices and delusions

11.0 Introduction

In psychiatric diagnostics voice hearing and delusions are considered quintessential psychotic symptoms. In Focal Setting Three I demonstrate that psychotic and non-psychotic psychospiritual experiences often share seemingly identical characteristics and argue the subsequent impossibility of discerning psychopathological from psychospiritual instances. Extending from this, I undertake a critical appraisal here of the phenomena of voice hearing and delusions to demonstrate that they cannot be definitively substantiated as psychotic diagnostic criteria. Showing that these two core psychotic features commonly occur in non-psychopathological instances undermines their diagnostic veracity and represents a significant challenge to the psychiatric picture of psychosis. If voice hearing and delusional ideation are core defining features of psychosis, and it is not possible to absolutely discern psychotic from non-psychotic instances, then how can a diagnosis of psychosis be made with certitude? Does the psychiatric psychopathological model of reductionist diagnostics ultimately serve to impede, rather than advance, a better understanding of psychosis?

11.1 The psychopathology of hearing voices?

Is the experience of voice hearing essentially indicative of psychopathology? Generally, auditory hallucinations, or hearing voices, have been viewed as psychopathological within the psychiatric literature, and while the authors of the latest DSM manual acknowledge that "hallucinations may be a normal part of religious experience in certain cultural contexts" (APA, 2013, p. 88) the term 'hallucination' is primarily understood, and used throughout the text, as depicting psychopathology. However, there exists a growing body of evidence that challenges this assumption. For instance, in his book *Hearing Voices: A Common Human Experience* (1998), John Watkins provides a thoroughgoing appraisal of this issue with numerous examples of normal, non-psychopathological voice hearing. He notes that the term 'hallucination' generally infers psychopathology because, being "based on a strictly materialist view of the world it makes no allowance for the possibility that it might sometimes be quite normal for human beings to have vivid sensory experiences in the absence of an external physical stimulus" (ibid., p. 266). However, despite the fact that hearing voices is "often considered to be one of the classic hallmarks of severe mental disorder" (p. 5), his extensive research reveals that voice hearing frequently occurs within the normal population. Some famous voice hearers listed by Watkins (p. 30) are Freud, Jung, Gandhi, Socrates, William Blake, and Martin Luther King. In light of his overall findings, he draws the conclusion that:

> the tendency of mainstream psychiatry to focus almost exclusively on the biological aspects of schizophrenia ... has resulted in a neglect of the vitally important psychological, social and spiritual aspects of this condition ... The whole question of the personal meaning and significance of the voices of schizophrenia remains virtually unexplored. (p. 111)

Ironically, this suggests that medical psychiatry's reductive thinking works to discount or ignore pathways of inquiry that may reveal answers to the fundamental question it aims to resolve as a discipline. That is, what is the true nature of psychosis and its attendant symptoms? In light of the seeming fact that voice hearing can occur in both psychotic and normal circumstances, it appears the psychiatric belief that voice hearing is simply the errant effect of faulty brain-wiring is illogical. This infers that all voice hearing experiences are psychopathological, when it is clear that, in many instances, they are not.

11.1.1 Voice hearing in mainstream society

As stated above, it appears that voice hearing is a natural human experience that can occur in both normal and anomalous contexts. Indeed, non-psychopathological views of voice hearing are not new to psychiatric or scientific inquiry. For instance, in the mid-nineteenth century the French psychiatrist Alexandre De Boismont (1859, p. 70) noted that hallucinatory experiences, including voice hearing, were commonplace among sane people and that "the hallucination of the sound mind may be seen to glide into the hallucination of insanity, without its [sic] being possible always to point out the boundary which separates the one condition from the other". This paradoxically acknowledges the notion of 'sane hallucinatory experience', which, apart from a few cultural exceptions, is absent from contemporary psychiatry. That De Boismont perceived his investigation of hallucinations to be of a scientific nature is evident in his comment that "the intelligent reader ought now to recognize the scientific character of our opinion, and to perceive that it is based on a legitimate induction from a principle inherent in the nature of man" (ibid., p. 339). Additionally, his book's opening sentence clearly portrays his recognition of the fundamental psychospiritual context of hallucinatory experience: "At all epochs in the history of man, in every climate, under the most opposite forms of government, and with every variety of religion, we constantly find the same belief in spirits and apparitions" (p. 1). He subsequently maintained that the global ubiquity of hallucinations over millennia "renders their study of the highest importance" (p. 8). Rather than depicting hallucinations (including the auditory variety) as reified and meaningless diagnostic criteria to be used for discerning states of psychopathology, he described them as natural human phenomena that occur in both states of sanity and insanity. Furthermore, he held that it is difficult, if not impossible, to discern sane from insane voice hearing and that it is imperative that psychiatry strives to attain a deeper understanding of such experiences. Intriguingly, this view from nascent psychiatry is ostensibly closer to better understanding the nature of psychosis, and its attendant symptomatology, than is contemporary psychiatry with its strong biogenic focus.

De Boismont, however, has not been the only investigator to view voice hearing as being common to both normality and insanity. Later in the nineteenth century, two censuses were conducted by psychologists seeking to provide empirical data regarding the incidence of hallucinatory experiences among sane people. First, Gurney et al. (1886a, p. xxxi) undertook research in 1883, via the methodology of a census, which sought to ascertain the incidence of "transient hallucinations of the sane". They found that "of the 5705 persons who have been asked the question,[117] it appears that 96 have, within the last 12 years, when awake, experienced an auditory hallucination of a voice" (Gurney et al., 1886b, p. 12). This was about 1.7 per cent of respondents. Soon after, Sidgwick et al. (1894, p. 25) conducted a "statistical inquiry into the spontaneous hallucinations of the sane" with 17,000 people, via census, over a three-year period.[118] Their findings showed that 553 sane people (about 3.3 per cent) indicated that they had heard voices (ibid., pp. 40–41). The findings of these empirical studies contest the prevailing psychiatric practice of identifying auditory hallucinations as characteristically psychotic, for they substantiate the longstanding awareness that voice hearing is relatively common among the sane.

More recent empirical research corroborates this. For instance, Posey & Losch (1983) presented a questionnaire to 375 college students that asked for a 'yes' or 'no'

---

[117] The census question was:

> Since January 1, 1874, have you when in good health, free from anxiety, and completely awake had a vivid impression of seeing or being touched by a human being, or of hearing a voice or sound which suggested a human presence, when no one was there? Yes or no? (Gurney et al., 1886b, p. 7)

[118] The census question was:

> Have you ever, when believing yourself to be completely awake, had a vivid impression of seeing or being touched by a living being or inanimate object, or hearing a voice; which impression, so far as you could discover, was not due to any external physical cause? (Sidgwick et al., 1894, p. 33)

response to a list of fourteen different types of voice hearing experiences. In total, seventy-one per cent of students "reported some experience with brief, auditory hallucinations of the voice type in wakeful situations" (ibid., p. 99), none of which showed signs of psychosis according to clinical profiles conducted to assess possible psychopathology (p. 106). Furthermore, in his comparative appraisal of Sidgwick et al.'s findings and the NIMH Epidemiologic Catchment Area Program data,[119] Tien (1991, p. 292) concluded that there is an "incidence of 10–30 cases per 1000 people per year" for hallucinations within the general population. These results of a one to three per cent incidence reflect those of Gurney et al. and Sidgewick et al. one hundred years earlier. Finally, in their empirical research into the incidence of voice hearing in "normal child populations", Pearson et al. (2001, pp. 401, 406) propose the likelihood of "a continuum of non-pathological hallucinatory experiences from children to adults in the normal population", while in their appraisal of epidemiological literature Sommer et al. (2010, p. 633) conclude that "epidemiological studies suggest that auditory verbal hallucinations (AVH) occur in approximately 10%–15% of the general population, of whom only a small proportion has a clinically relevant psychotic disorder". Combined, these clinical views and studies, spanning a period of about 170 years, strongly suggest that the phenomenon of voice hearing is not *intrinsically* psychopathological.

11.1.2 Hearing Voices Network: coping and recovery

Psychiatry's view that voice hearing is a key diagnostic indicator of psychotic experience is further challenged by the advent and global proliferation of the Hearing Voices Network (HVN). This global movement emerged from a 1987 incident whereby Dutch psychiatrist, Marius Romme, was persuaded by his patient, Patsy Hage, to put aside his psychopathological beliefs regarding auditory hallucinations and consider the possibility that the voices she heard were real (Escher & Romme, 2012, p. 385). This led to him discovering Hage's feelings of being overwhelmed by the voices were alleviated when enabled to share her experiences with other voice hearers (ibid.). Subsequently, Romme and Hage appeared on a Dutch television program to invite other voice hearers to contact them, resulting in 450 responses, of which 300 people reported struggling to cope with their voices, and 150 people reported having developed ways of coping with them (Romme & Escher, 1989, p. 209). A questionnaire was then sent to each person in the latter group to ascertain the nature of their respective coping skills. From this, twenty respondents, who were particularly clear in elucidating their coping strategies, were selected as key presenters at a 1987 hearing voices congress held in the Netherlands (ibid., p. 210). At the congress, an organisation called Resonance was established to conduct further research into the presence or absence of coping skills in voice hearers, which, in turn, led to the formation of the

---

[119] According to the Interuniversity Consortium for Political and Social Research (2016) "the Epidemiologic Catchment Area (ECA) program of research was initiated ... to collect data on the prevalence and incidence of mental disorders and on the use of and need for services by the mentally ill".

first UK HVN group in 1988 (Escher & Romme, 2012, p. 386). Since then, the number of HVN groups has expanded exponentially with hundreds established throughout thirty-one countries (Intervoice, 2021a).

This development is of considerable consequence for it demonstrates that alternative understandings of, and remedial approaches to, voice hearing are possible. For instance, two key HVN tenets assert that "hearing voices is a normal though unusual and personal variation of human experience [and ...] the problem is not hearing voices but the difficulty to cope with the experience" (Intervoice, 2021b). Furthermore, the UK HVN *Position Statement on DSM 5 & Psychiatric Diagnoses* affirms that "rather than seeing voices, visions and extreme states as symptoms of an underlying illness, we believe it is helpful to view them as meaningful experiences", which subsequently calls for "seeing mental distress as human and, ultimately, understandable" (Hearing Voices Network, 2013). These views diverge from classic psychiatric assumptions regarding so-called hallucinatory experiences. They also represent a major conceptual challenge to psychiatry's depiction of voice hearing as an innately psychopathological key diagnostic criterion for identifying psychosis.

The therapeutic efficacy of HVN groups and approaches also challenges the validity of psychiatry's psychopathological understanding of voice hearing. Because psychiatry views voice hearing as unreal, the possibility that people can learn coping skills to mitigate and/or regulate them does not enter the field of clinical reckoning. It is evident, however, from the work of unconventional psychiatrists such as Romme, that a different approach to understanding voice hearing is both possible and efficacious. In their initial research, Romme & Escher (1989, p. 210) observed that learning to cope with voices involved three general phases:

1. The startling phase: the usually sudden onset, primarily as a frightening experience.
2. The phase of organization: the process of selection and communication with the voices.
3. The stabilization phase: the period in which a more continuous way of handling the voices is acquired.

Additionally, four broad coping strategies employed by voice hearers were identified as "distraction, ignoring the voices, selective listening to them, and setting limits on their influence" (Romme et al., 1992, p. 99). However, within these four coping approaches the types of strategies are idiosyncratic and manifold.[120] Furthermore, for practitioners who employ the HVN model it is essential to "make allowance for the fact that voice hearers actually do hear voices"; "accept the reality of the experience"; and "accept the possibility of hearing voices as nonpathologic" (Escher & Romme, 2012, p. 392). This is opposite from standard psychiatric practice where the assertion by persons that their voices are real is perceived by clinicians

---

[120] For example, see: Hearing Voices Network Australia, 2013; Hearing Voices Network, 2012.

as signifying a psychopathological lack of insight. However, Romme and company found that accepting the reality of voices is an essential precursor to enabling the teaching, learning, and application of coping skills.

A growing body of empirical research indicates that HVN groups, and the use of coping skills by voice hearers, have positive therapeutic outcomes. For instance, Wykes et al. (1999, p. 180) found that a group of people diagnosed with schizophrenia demonstrated increased control over voices, decreased distress levels, and increased effectiveness in applying coping strategies after only six sessions of cognitive-behavioural skills training within a twenty-four week period. In light of the application of coping strategies, Wykes (2004, p. 38) later concluded that "there is ample evidence that factors other than biology have an effect on the experience of auditory hallucinations". Meddings et al. (2004) conducted an evaluation of a UK HVN group two years after its formation, finding that participants experienced a decrease in their incidence and duration of hospitalisation, and an increase in empowerment, proficiency in skills application, self-esteem, and social or vocational functionality. Furthermore, in her doctoral research project, which examined adult voice hearing experiences in the New Zealand adult population, Beavan (2007, p. 141) found that on a seven-point Likert scale for rating the effectiveness of coping strategies, "the majority of strategies (68.4%) had an average rating of at least four, indicating that on the whole, participants found the strategies they used to be at least somewhat effective".[121] These are but a few examples, from a considerable body of research, that demonstrate beneficial outcomes of HVN groups and/or coping practices for voice hearers.[122]

There also exists a growing qualitative literature in which people provide personal accounts regarding the efficacy of using coping skills to contend with the distress and disruption of their voice hearing experiences. For example, an edited book by Romme et al. (2009) titled *Living with Voices: 50 Stories of Recovery* presents an exemplary collection of such instances. The authors assert that "this book demonstrates that it is entirely possible to overcome problems with hearing voices and take back control of one's life" (ibid., p. 1). They further claim that the first-person accounts throughout the book, many of which are related by long-term psychiatric patients, prove that people can "overcome the disabling social and psychiatric attitudes towards voice hearing" (p. 2). Indeed, it is their view that people who embark on such a recovery process learn that "their voices are not a sign of madness but a reaction to problems in their lives that they couldn't cope with" (ibid.). Hence, there appears to be substantial evidence suggesting that HVN and other skills training groups have therapeutic efficacy for diagnosed and undiagnosed voice hearers alike.

---

[121] In her measure, "1 indicated 'not effective at all' and 7 indicated 'very effective'" (Beavan, 2007, p. 140).

[122] For further examples see: Beavan et al., 2017; Longden et al., 2018; Dos Santos & Beavan, 2015; Oakland & Berry, 2015; Leff et al., 2014; van der Gaag et al., 2014; Dillon & Hornstein, 2013; Howard et al., 2013; Milligan et al., 2013; Corstens et al., 2012; Goldsmith, 2012; Casstevens et al., 2006; Coleman & Smith, 2006; Meddings et al., 2006; Haddock et al., 1996.

A final important point is the difference between how psychiatry and HVN understand recovery. For psychiatry, full recovery occurs only when voice hearing ceases and functionality is restored. However, a guiding principle of the hearing voices movement is that "'recovery' is not about getting rid of voices but about the person understanding their voices in relation to their life experiences, and the person changing their relationship with their voices so that the voices become harmless and/or helpful" (Dillon, 2010, p. 35). In other words, rather than being clinically construed as unreal and incomprehensible, voice hearing can be appreciated as real, comprehensible, manageable, and meaningful. Therefore, the effectiveness of the HVN approach calls to question the veracity of psychiatry's core belief that voice hearing is essentially psychopathological and characteristically psychotic.

11.2 The psychopathology of delusions?

As is the case with 'auditory hallucinations', the presence of delusional thoughts is also understood by psychiatry to be a key characteristic of psychotic disorders. In fact, in DSM-5 their presence is listed as the first of five domains of "abnormalities" that define "schizophrenia spectrum and other psychotic disorders" (APA, 2013, p. 87). Therefore, unlike voice hearing, which can occur in both normal and psychospiritual contexts, it evidently appears that delusional ideation is particular to psychotic states and is undeniably psychopathological. This is seemingly exemplified in Schreber's (1988) book *Memoirs of My Nervous Illness*[123] that abounds with autobiographical accounts of experiences and beliefs which, from the perspective of consensus reality and psychiatry, are utterly insane. For instance, he believed himself to be the victim of "soul murder" (ibid., p. 35) and that God had transformed him into a woman with breasts and female genitals (p. 181). His memoir is also replete with accounts of assorted "miracles" caused by "rays" of a psychospiritual nature that manifested in his body and the world around him. This included the belief that he was the last real living person and that "the few human shapes I saw apart from myself ... were only 'fleeting-improvised-men' created by miracle" (p. 85). Schreber maintained these beliefs with utter conviction for years.

A contemporary, yet equally bizarre example is provided by Chadwick (2010, p. 70) in recounting his reasoning immediately prior to stepping in front of a bus. Fortunately, he survived to tell the tale:

---

[123] At the time of his first episode of 'nervous illness' in 1884, Daniel Schreber was the Chief Justice of the Supreme Court of the state of Saxony, in Germany. His *Memoirs*, which was first published in 1903, is an account of his second episode of 'nervous illness' from 1893–1902 (Schreber, 1988, pp. xii, 2–4). This book subsequently influenced the thinking of luminaries such as Freud, Jung, Kraepelin, Bleuler, and Jaspers and had considerable impact upon the development of psychoanalytic and psychiatric theory. Indeed, in a 1910 letter to Jung, Freud affectionately referred to him as "the wonderful Schreber, who ought to have been made a professor of psychiatry and director of a mental hospital" (McGuire, 1974, p. 113).

New King's Road in Fulham obviously was the perfect location for my nemesis. Me, the Antichrist, must be destroyed on 'the road of the new king'. When I was dead, Satan, 'the old king' would be thrust out of my mind and Jesus, 'the new king' would come into the world to reign. As usual, it all fitted so well it surely had to be true! This was no delusion, this was *really happening*!

At face value, such beliefs and assertions certainly appear to be psychopathological. However, upon closer examination, it becomes evident that this view represents a very limited understanding of a phenomenon that is enigmatic and fascinating, though potentially lethal.

According to psychiatric diagnostics, there are three features which essentially characterise delusions as psychopathological. These are:

1. Incorrigibility—This refers to the unshakable conviction 'delusional' people have that their beliefs are real, despite all proffered evidence and argument to the contrary. In this context, the DSM-5 glossary defines "delusional conviction" as "a false belief based on incorrect inference about external reality that is firmly held despite what almost everyone else believes" (APA, 2013, p. 819). The manual also explains that "the distinction between a delusion and a strongly held idea is sometimes difficult to make and depends in part on the degree of conviction with which the belief is held despite clear or reasonable contradictory evidence regarding its veracity" (ibid., p. 87). While, 'conviction' and 'incorrigibility' represent two distinct nuances of delusional ideation, they are fundamentally interrelated and, therefore, examined below as a composite phenomenon.
2. Dysfunctionality—In psychiatry, a diagnostic corollary to delusional ideation is the degree to which the beliefs undermine a person's capacity to function normally. As stated in DSM-5, "when poor psychosocial functioning is present, delusional beliefs themselves often play a significant role" (p. 93). Indeed, an essential diagnostic criterion for schizophrenia is that the "level of functioning in one or more major areas, such as work, interpersonal relations, or self-care, is markedly below the level achieved prior to onset" (pp. 99–100).
3. Incomprehensibility—A commonly held psychiatric supposition about delusions is that their nature and content are bizarre, incomprehensible, and meaningless. As explained in DSM-5, "delusions are deemed *bizarre* if they are clearly implausible and not understandable to same-culture peers and do not derive from ordinary life experiences" (p. 87).

The critical appraisal below of each of these three key delusional features aims to challenge the veracity of 'delusions' as a psychotic diagnostic criterion. This correspondingly suggests that a better understanding of unusual beliefs (delusions) is impeded by the reductionist psychiatric approach of viewing them only in terms of psychopathology.

11.2.1 The incorrigibility of delusions?

In terms of incorrigibility, psychopathology has long been seen by psychiatry as evident when a person maintains a resolute belief that is at odds with consensus reality. Indeed, in 1838 the French psychiatrist Jean-Étienne Dominique Esquirol (1845, p. xi) noted the "tenacious" nature of delusions in that such psychopathological beliefs were held with utter conviction despite their apparent illusoriness. Zaehner (1961, pp. 89–90) also explains that, for the person experiencing delusional psychosis, "fantasy is fact: indeed it is a great deal more real than the majority of things that pass for fact in everyday life … For him they really are, and nothing can persuade him that they are not". The futility of trying to refute such beliefs is cleverly depicted by Torrey (2013, p. 25) in his analogy that "reasoning with people about their delusions is like trying to bail out the ocean with a bucket". However, as Jaspers (1997 v1, p. 105) explains, "*delusion proper* is incorrigible because of an *alteration of personality*, the nature of which we are so far unable to describe, let alone formulate into a concept, though we are driven to make some such supposition". In other words, psychiatry's depiction of delusional incorrigibility as typically psychotic is assumed, but ultimately not substantiated.

It appears, however, that the psychopathological status of so-called delusional incorrigibility is questionable because such conviction of belief is also common to psychospiritual contexts. For instance, as Podvoll (1979, p. 575) notes, "ecstatic states have always been greatly esteemed by both mystics and the insane … These experiences are frequently seen as ultimate and irrefutable, and ideas contained within them may reach the level of full conviction". Indeed, during his experiments with active imagination Jung (2009, p. 338) reported that, although his rational everyday mind regarded his experiences with suspicion, he was often swayed by their compelling veracity:

> Through uniting with the self we reach the God. I must say this, not with reference to the opinions of the ancients or this or that authority but because I have experienced it. It has happened thus in me … I wish I could say it was a deception and only too willingly would I disown this experience. But I cannot deny that it has seized me beyond all measure and steadily goes on working in me … I recognize the God by the unshakeableness of the experience.

There is a marked parallel here between Jung's reported experience of God-identification and the frequent occurrence of the same, or similar, during psychotic episodes. Hence, it seems that, rather than being an incomprehensible and quintessential marker of psychosis, the act of maintaining unusual beliefs with utter conviction may be a manifestation of a deep psychic function that is yet to be understood by Western psychiatry.

While the unshakable nature of seemingly psychotic beliefs appears beyond understanding within the conceptual framework of materialism, this phenomenon can be better understood from a psychospiritual perspective. Throughout his works, Merrell-Wolff describes intricacies of subjective psychic experience that provide possible insight into psychospiritual mechanisms underpinning the incorrigible conviction of beliefs common to both mystic and psychotic states. For example, he maintains that a "marked characteristic" of peak mystical states of consciousness is that the person who experiences them "is above doubt. He is not believing, but KNOWING … His knowledge carries an authority, or rather this knowledge, this consciousness, carries an authority that is more than ordinary" (Merrell-Wolff, 1938, p. 38). Here he alludes to a supramental state of human consciousness whereby an immediacy of 'knowing' is experienced that transcends the normal process of belief formation via incremental rational deduction. According to Merrell-Wolff (1995, pp. 188–189), the apperception of reality from this perspective "carries with it a superlative order of assurance—one knows without doubt that here is Truth … One has found a base upon which to stand against the opinion of the whole world, if necessary". Clearly, this view, if considered free of its mystical context, could well reflect incorrigible psychotic delusions.

Sri Aurobindo similarly discusses the human mystic capacity to directly experience knowledge, in contrast to the normal mode of reality perception and knowledge formation. He describes conventional "indirect knowledge" as an inferior mental act of "groping and seeking" that is facilitated by "logical processes of deduction, induction, all kinds of inference" (Sri Aurobindo, 1999, p. 482). In contradistinction, he refers to the "spontaneous certitude" and the "true and direct knowledge" of mystical experience that "begins with the opening of the psychical consciousness and the psychical faculties" (ibid., pp. 477, 893). Even though expressed using different terminology, this essentially mirrors Merrell-Wolff's contention, and while neither of these two psychospiritual authorities suggest there is a correlation between mystic certitude and the incorrigible delusions of psychosis, the similarities between the two states of consciousness, in terms of conviction of 'knowing', begs the question: Does psychotic delusional incorrigibility stem from the same psychic structures that facilitate the certitude of mystic 'knowing'? Although this is a speculative proposition, it proffers a potential line of investigation beyond the psychiatric view that bizarre beliefs held with unshakable conviction are inherently psychopathological. This aside, it appears that both mystic and delusional experiences share a similar incorrigibility of conviction, therefore, it is not diagnostically sound to claim that delusional incorrigibility is absolutely indicative of psychosis.

11.2.2 The dysfunctionality of delusions?

As with incorrigibility, presuming a fundamental correlation between delusions, dysfunctionality, and psychopathology is also questionable. Although it is well documented that delusional beliefs can often result in psychosocial dysfunction, this is not universal, as there are reported instances whereby people maintain highly functional lives while harbouring beliefs that, from a psychiatric perspective, would constitute classic psychotic delusions. Such is the case for Elyn Saks (2013), a law professor at the University of Southern California, and a diagnosed schizophrenic who continues to have "delusions crowding my mind" despite her high level of functionality and professionalism.[124] According to Saks (ibid.), "conventional psychiatric thinking and its diagnostic categories say that people like me don't exist", yet she participated in a research project evaluating the coping strategies of twenty people in Los Angeles who "were able to maintain a high level of daily responsibility despite active, ongoing symptoms of schizophrenia", particularly delusions.[125] This research found many instances of 'functional-psychopathology' in the Los Angeles area, which possibly reveals a relatively common but unrecognised phenomenon.

Indeed, such musing about the prevalence of undetected 'functional-psychopathology' is seemingly corroborated by other research into the presence of psychiatric-type delusions in the normal population. For instance, van Os et al. (2000, p. 16) found that "4.2% of the general population had psychiatrist-rated evidence of delusions or hallucinations". Similarly, in context of delusion and hallucination frequency among mainstream children and adolescent populations, Kelleher et al. (2012, p. 1861) conclude that "the relatively high prevalence of these symptoms would suggest a lack of specificity in terms of risk for psychosis". Also, in a meta-analysis of empirical studies of the prevalence of delusions in clinical and non-clinical populations, Freeman (2006, p. 191) found that "approximately 1% to 3% of the nonclinical population have delusions of a level of severity comparable to clinical cases of psychosis". Additionally, in their measure of "delusional ideation in the normal population", Peters et al. (1999, pp. 553, 562) found that about ten per cent of "healthy individuals" showed higher scores than deluded psychiatric patients. They subsequently proposed that there are "differences that enable the former to function adequately in society, while the latter suffered a severe breakdown and required hospitalization" (ibid., p. 562). Consequent to this finding, Peters (2001, p. 207) argued that "what makes people cross the psychotic 'threshold' is not necessarily the content but the consequences of their beliefs: it is not *what* you believe, it is *how* you believe it". Indeed, in considering the ambiguous nature of delusional beliefs, psychiatrist Joseph Pierre (2001, p. 170) proposes that the DSM definition for 'delusion' should include mention that "delusional thinking can span the continuum from normalcy to pathology, but is not alone indicative of mental illness or psychiatric disorder" and, therefore, should only be "an appropriate target for clinical attention" if it causes undue distress or dysfunction. Arguably, then, the existence of highly functional 'delusional' people suggests that delusional ideation is not psychopathological per se. Rather, as with voice hearers, it seems the difference between a person's capacity to

---

[124] Saks relates her personal journey from schizophrenia diagnosis to professorship in her autobiography *The Centre Cannot Hold* (2007).

[125] Saks (2013) describes the research group, which was conducted in Los Angeles, as consisting of "graduate students, managers, technicians and professionals, including a doctor, lawyer, psychologist and chief executive of a nonprofit group". (For more details about this project see—Glynn et al., 2010).

function, or not, is dependent on their ability to attain and apply skills for coping with bizarre beliefs.

Although groups teaching coping skills for delusional ideation are few in comparison to the Hearing Voices Network, there has been a nascent development in this area. The key initiator of this project is Tamasin Knight, a UK medical doctor who, inspired by the work of Romme and the Hearing Voices Network, considered the possibility of transposing the same support and training framework into the context of learning to cope with overwhelming delusions (Knight, 2010, p. 21). This enterprise first took the form of a research project conducted from 2001–2003 that aimed to "determine methods of helping people cope with beliefs that others may consider to be unusual", and which identified a raft of effective coping strategies used by such people (Knight, 2009, p. 12). From this emerged the establishment of a weekly "unusual beliefs" group in 2003 which, according to a 2005 follow-up qualitative evaluation, had effectively established a support forum with diverse benefits for participants (pp. 36–37). For instance, Knight (p. 7) notes that while "mainstream psychiatric treatment attempts to remove or reduce conviction in these beliefs", group members actually derived many benefits from sharing their unusual beliefs and experiences in a non-judgemental setting. Examples of such benefits are: not having their beliefs "dismissed as illness" and clinically labelled; feeling supported by members to disclose "issues they may be too afraid to discuss with psychiatric professionals for fear of the consequences"; "reduced anxiety"; "a sense of safety"; "able to speak freely"; a "sense of belonging and reducing isolation"; and having "a space where people who have had a crisis or breakdown could explore the factors that may have led up to it" (pp. 37–39). Although such groups remain few in number, and there appears to be no evidence-based evaluation as to their general efficacy, it is anecdotally evident that they enable therapeutic benefits.

While unusual beliefs groups are seemingly beneficial, can they provide coping skills that enable people to contend with overwhelming delusions and improve functionality? According to UK clinical psychologist, Rufus May (2007a, p. 30; 2007b, p. 124), they can. He observed in the unusual belief groups he facilitated that the support and coping skills provided enabled participants to develop enhanced levels of functionality. This suggests the efficacy of using coping skills to contend with disabling beliefs. Indeed, empirical research conducted by Turkington et al. (2015, pp. 56, 57) with a group of psychiatric patients demonstrates that the judicious use of cognitive behavioural therapy can decrease the overall level of belief conviction in patients, and improve their social functioning "to a marked degree". Hence, it arguably appears that psychopathological dysfunction is characterised more by the absence of coping skills than the presence of 'delusions' per se.

If so, then medical psychiatry's depiction of delusions as being essentially characteristic of psychosis is questionable. Although such unusual beliefs are often distressing or destructive and can lead to dysfunction, this is apparently not universal, but relative to the degree that psychosocial support and coping skills have been provided and acquired. It is subsequently plausible to suggest that, in the context of dysfunctionality, psychiatry's depiction of delusions as essentially psychopathological is more prescriptive supposition than clinical fact.

11.2.3 The incomprehensibility of delusions?

Are delusions as incomprehensible as psychiatry presumes and asserts them to be? It seems not, for the possibility of appreciating them beyond the limited purview of clinical diagnostics has already been demonstrated above. For instance, it appears:

1. There is a marked commonality between delusional and mystical incorrigibility, which may indicate they share a common psychic source.
2. Psychotic-like delusions occur, and are indistinguishable, within both psychiatric and normal populations.
3. It is possible to circumvent the social dysfunction that often stems from delusional beliefs via the acquisition and application of coping skills.

These three possibilities alone establish lines of potential investigation that move beyond the superficial psychiatric depiction of delusional ideation as a static diagnostic criterion. Additionally, other views expressed within the literature offer potential pathways for better understanding the nature of the phenomenon of harbouring unusual beliefs. For instance, can delusions be construed as serving a functional purpose?

While psychiatry sees a strong causal link between delusions and dysfunctionality, many commentators understand delusions to serve a functional purpose. This view was exemplified eighty years ago in Boisen's (1936, p. 29) appraisal of delusions as "attempts to organize our experience in such a way that we can go on living and functioning in the world of men". He also observed that, despite their unusual appearances in comparison to normal beliefs, delusions serve the function of preventing a person from "going to pieces" and to "maintain a certain degree of integration and poise" (ibid.). Others have similarly depicted delusions as a functional attempt to establish a semblance of existential stability in the face of the chaos and collapse of psychosis. For instance, Siegler et al. (1969, p. 956) see delusions as being pragmatic though "desperate attempts" to make sense of "thought changes" in psychotic states, while Brett (2002, p. 329) likewise suggests that, in psychosis, when "the previous frameworks of meaning have been eroded", there is a need for the "emergence of new patterns of meaning" in the form of delusions. From a slightly different perspective, Deikman (1971, p. 486) describes delusional formation as a default strategy for contending with the chaos of an unresolved spiritual emergency. He notes that, whereas the mystic resolves such crises through spiritual transformation, "the psychotic person … creates a delusion to achieve a partial ordering and control". Finally, some commentators view delusions as fulfilling an efficacious role. For example, from a psychodynamic and cognitive psychology perspective, delusions are seen as serving the unconscious function of circumventing irresolvable and painful psychic states and life events (Martindale, 2015, p. 61; Turkington et al., 2015, p. 51). Inasmuch, they are partially remedial in nature. Black (2008, p. 80), however, takes this idea a step further to propose that "the developed delusional system … should be considered as an attempt at recovery rather than the primary illness" because its chief purpose is to establish meaning in the midst of chaos.

These views on the functionality of delusions challenge psychiatry's depiction of them as being essentially incomprehensible. For instance, delusional formation can be understood as an unconscious attempt on behalf of the self or psyche to make sense of a chaotic and overwhelming psychotic or psychospiritual experience. Hence, in this light, the formation of delusions can be understood as an unconscious *act* that serves a functional purpose, a possibility lost to medical psychiatry's view that delusions are incomprehensible and psychopathological *things*. This poses the intriguing possibility that, while delusions appear to be psychopathological at face value, they may paradoxically represent a self-healing gesture at an unconscious or transpersonal level. This idea is supported by the ensuing examination of John Weir Perry's model for understanding so-called delusions.

11.3 John Weir Perry and better understanding delusions

As discussed in Chapter Ten, Section 10.6.4, Perry endorses the view that psychosis can be seen as a process of self-healing and transformative renewal. However, he also understands this process of renewal to be fundamentally driven by what psychiatry refers to as 'incomprehensible delusions'. Perry (1974, p. 2) eschews the "shackles of medical thinking with its special taste for signs and symptoms of pathology" in favour of an open-ended, phenomenological, investigative approach. From his training in Jungian psychotherapy, and his observations of, and interactions with, many 'psychotic'[126] people over many years, he came to understand 'delusions' as *archetypal* formations that reflect the "language of the unconscious, emotional psyche" (ibid., p. 11). Hence, he rejects the term 'delusions' with its psychopathological meaning and clinical assumptions. Instead, he has coined the term "affect-images" to signify the mythic-type ideation that is central to the renewal process (Perry, 1999, p. xv). As he explains: "When activated, an archetype manifests in the form of an emotion and an image and a pattern of behaviour; its charge of energy is intense. I have suggested the term *affect-image* to designate these forms" (ibid.). The idea of 'delusions' as affect-images invests the supposed incomprehensibility of such phenomena with evident and profound meaning. Whereas psychiatry sees a 'delusional' experience as being an inscrutable psychopathological symptom, Perry understands this to be an intrinsically functional dynamic that is native to the deeper human psyche.

---

[126] Again, as in Chapter Ten, throughout this section I adopt Perry's practice of placing inverted commas around psychiatric words such as 'psychosis' and 'delusions'.

Further to this, Perry (1974, p. 140) maintains that affect-images, or 'delusions', serve the purpose of facilitating "some very much needed changes in the organization of the self and the emotional life". He explains that,

> the image renders the meaning of the emotion, while the emotion lends the dyna-
> mism to its image. On this account the images lead to the lost affects. They are the
> means by which the affects become processed in nature's own way, unfamiliar as it
> is to us. (ibid., p. 141)

Here, Perry adds a further layer of meaning in terms of the general nature and functional dynamics of the phenomenon of 'psychotic delusions'. Far from being incomprehensible and psychopathological, he construes them as natural archetypal forms that play a principal role in a psychic process of attempted self-actuation and remediation. Although 'delusions' appear abnormal in context of mainstream normalcy, if Perry is correct, then they are not 'false' as psychiatry claims, nor even abnormal in an absolute sense, because they are real and normal within the context of archetypal psychic processes. Analogously speaking, then, rather than being seen as incomprehensible and illogical, 'delusions' may be likened to a 'foreign language' that clinicians ideally need to learn and understand if they are to respond with apposite therapeutic effectiveness.

In general, Perry's description of the 'psychotic' process is essentially psychospiritual in that it is orchestrated through archetypal dynamics of the transpersonal self. This principle applies also to affect-images. According to Perry (1999, p. 129) affect-images "have the function of implementing the processes of the spirit: of liberating and transforming its energies, which will then slip out of the old structures lingering on the recent past and into new ones geared to the near future". Significantly, however, he does not see this view as being incompatible with biomedical psychiatric thinking because he perceives a holistic and correlative relationship between psyche and soma (ibid., p. 145). He subsequently endorses a holistic aetiological view and believes that ascribing specific causal primacy to psyche or body is erroneous (ibid.). This is a maverick idea, for it infers a mixed aetiology in psychosis whereby physical and psychic-cum-psychospiritual causes are not separate, but co-causal. In other words, he suggests a matrix of causality wherein body, mind, and spirit are inextricably inter-active and cannot be isolated from each other.

It is evident, thus far, that Perry's depiction of a 'psychotic delusion' as an affect-image challenges its status as a key psychiatric diagnostic criterion. Indeed, if Perry is correct, then far from being psychopathological in nature, such 'delusions' or affect-images may conversely represent an intrinsic and poorly understood recovery process of psychic renewal. Indeed, after years of working with 'psychotic' people he came to believe that the apparent inscrutable chaos of the 'psychotic' process may in fact be following "some sort of order or groundplan" (Perry, 1974, p. 28). By analysing his case notes he elicited ten apparent thematic categories of 'psychotic' affect-images that he understood to represent "some form of drama or ritual performance" that unfurls in the form of a mythological psychic process (ibid., pp. 28–29, see Table 9, below).

Table 9. Perry's ten thematic categories of affect-images.

Category	Description
A. Center	A location is established at a world center or cosmic axis (point where sky world, regular world, and underworld meet; between opposing halves of the world; center of attention).
B. Death	Themes of dismemberment or sacrifice are scattered throughout and make themselves evident in drawings (crucifixion, pounding or chopping up, tortures, limbs or bones rearranged, poisoning). A predominant delusional statement is that of having died and of being in an afterlife state (people look like living dead; in hell or in heaven; or in prison as equivalent to death).
C. Return to Beginnings	A regression is expressed that takes the person back to the beginnings of time and the creation of the cosmos (Garden of Eden, waters of the abyss, early steps of evolution, primitive tribal society, creation of the planets). There is a parallel regression, of course, to emotions, behaviour, and associations of infancy (surrounded by parent figures; crawling, suckling; needs for touch and texture; oral needs).
D. Cosmic Conflict	There arises a world conflict of cosmic import between forces of good and evil, or light and darkness, or order and chaos (surprisingly often expressed nowadays as democracy and communism; Armageddon, or the triumph of the Antichrist; destruction or end of the world, or the Last Judgement; intrigues, plots, spying, poisoning—for all to gain world supremacy).
E. Threat of Opposite	There is a feeling of a threat from the opposite sex, a fear of being overcome by it, or turned into it (drugs to turn one into the opposite; identifications with figures of the other sex; supremacy of the other sex; moves to eradicate the other sex).
F. Apotheosis	The person experiences an apotheosis as royalty or divinity (as a king or a queen, deity or saint, hero or heroine, messiah).

(Continued)

Table 9. (Continued)

Category	Description
G. Sacred Marriage	The person enters upon a sacred marriage of ritual or mythological character (royal marriage, perhaps incestuous; marriage with God or Goddess; as Virgin Mother, who conceives by the spirit).
H. New Birth	A new birth takes place or is expected of a super-human child or of oneself (ideas of rebirth; Divine Child, Infant Savior, Prince, or Reconciler of the division of the world).
I. New Society	A new order of society is envisioned, of an ideal or sacred quality (a New Jerusalem, Last Paradise, Utopia, World Peace; a New Age, a New Heaven and New Earth).
J. Quadrated World	A fourfold structure of the world or cosmos is established, usually in the form of a quadrated circle (four continents or quarters; four political factions, governments, or nations; four races or religions; four persons of the godhead; four elements or states of being).

Source: Perry, 1974, pp. 29–30.

Perry explains that, although these themes are not present in all 'psychotic' instances, and do not occur as prescriptive and sequential patterns, they do seemingly unfold in a broad developmental trajectory whereby "the themes of the regression and cosmic conflict tend to come early, and those of new birth, new social order" generally occur later (p. 30). Furthermore, he warns against reifying these themes and stresses that they "must be understood to be purely arbitrary assignments and arrangements for purposes of descriptive study and formulation" (p. 28). Hence, he sees them as heuristic and provisional concepts that may be used to guide a progressive understanding of 'psychotic' experience and to correspondingly formulate psychiatric theories and practices that work with, rather than against, what may potentially be a renewal process.

Arguably, then, Perry's notion of 'psychosis' as representing a meaningful renewal process, in which 'delusions' play a functional role, proffers a viable alternative to psychiatry's psychopathological understanding of the same. Indeed, Perry's model invests so-called 'incomprehensible psychotic delusions' with profound meaning as to their form, content, and course. Hence, it is feasible that further research may yield an enhanced understanding about the nature and functional potentialities of such experiences.

11.4 Conclusion

It is evident voice hearing and delusions can occur in non-psychopathological forms identical to, yet indiscernible from, psychotic manifestations. This calls to question the veracity of their use as primary criteria for diagnosing psychosis and also challenges psychiatry's modus operandi of a reductive seeking for psychopathology. If voice hearing and delusional ideation are not definitively psychotic then how can psychosis be diagnosed? Perry's answer to this conundrum is to abandon psychiatry's diagnostic and psychopathology–seeking approach and, instead, investigate the possibility that 'psychosis' represents a meaningful renewal process. I further examine this diagnostic conundrum throughout Chapter Twelve in the context of cross-cultural and psychospiritual understandings of psychosis.

CHAPTER 12

Cross-cultural considerations

12.0 Introduction

Chapter Twelve continues Chapter Eleven's trajectory of inquiry by critically examining psychiatric diagnostics within a cross-cultural context. Here, the conundrum of squaring psychiatric materialism with metaphysical cultural relativity is explored: What substantiates the psychiatric view that an anomalous experience deemed psychotic in a Western context can be viewed as non-psychotic and normative in another cultural context? It is shown that psychotic-like experiences are commonly reported in relation to traditional healing, shamanic initiatory processes, and spirit possession. Cross-cultural conundrums resulting from Western materialism, rationality, and cognicentrism are also examined. The aim here is to further challenge the veracity of psychiatric diagnostic and psychopathology-seeking practices by demonstrating, though a cross-cultural lens, the seeming impossibility of discerning psychotic from psychospiritual experiences.

12.1 Psychiatry and the cross-cultural conundrum

It has become accepted practice within mainstream psychiatry to assert that psychospiritual beliefs or experiences deemed psychotic in one cultural setting may be normative in another. Upon closer investigation, however, it appears illogical to proclaim that a given experience is intrinsically psychotic in a mainstream Western cultural context but not psychotic in the context of other cultural psychosocial or psychospiritual norms. For instance, the proposal that hearing voices is psychotic for mainstream Westerners, but not for Indigenous healers, fails to explain the phenomenological nature of the voices in each instance. Is psychiatry suggesting that Western psychotic voice hearing is 'out of touch with reality', but Indigenous shamanic voice hearing is not? If so, what is the difference between non-real voices and real voices? Does culturally normative voice hearing constitute an experience whereby people are in communication with invisible disembodied entities? If spirits are real, then why are they only real in non-Western contexts, beyond which they are deemed imaginary or insane? What discerns the culturally valid hearing of spirit voices from psychotic voice hearing (i.e., what differentiates those who are really hearing the voices of spirits from those who are having psychotic auditory hallucinations)? Such critical questions are neither posed nor answered by psychiatry.

12.1.1 The epiphenomenal problem

At the core of this conundrum are epistemological assumptions about the nature of reality. As discussed in Chapter Two, Section 2.3, medical psychiatry is based on the materialist assumption that mind is epiphenomenal to physicality; hence, psychopathology is reflective of an anatomical malfunction, probably in the brain. In such a worldview, metaphysical realities do not actually exist, regardless of cultural context. This is seemingly evident in the DSM-5 authors' (2013, p. 758–759) suggestion that "connections between cultural concepts may help identify … underlying biological substrates". Although DSM-5 also explains that "cultural concepts are important to psychiatric diagnosis" because they enable clinicians to "avoid misdiagnosis … (e.g., unfamiliar spiritual explanations may be misunderstood as psychosis)" (ibid., p. 758), it appears that psychospiritual cultural explanations are ultimately deemed to be the epiphenomenal and presumably fanciful products of 'underlying biological substrates'. As such, psychiatry has seemingly anchored cultural relativity within the fabric of biological determinism, and diagnostic differentiation is achieved by observing degrees of distress or divergence from cultural norms. This, however, fails to phenomenologically explain what, exactly, differentiates psychotic from non-psychotic 'spiritual explanations'.

That these 'spiritual explanations' may be indicative of actual psychospiritual realities does not seem to feature in the medical psychiatric purview. As Sanderson (2003, p. 2) observes, "the established scientific view that consciousness is a by-product of brain activity has had the effect of imposing a selective blindness on our thinking". Indeed, from a quantum physics perspective it is understood that "looking for consciousness in the brain is like looking inside a radio for the announcer" (Haramein in Vacariu, 2016, p. 137). Hence, the axiomatic materialist assumptions upon which psychiatry is founded establish a limited scope of investigative inquiry that proscribe questions such as: Do the 'unfamiliar spiritual explanations' within other cultures signify something that is ontologically real? If so, can they also be real in mainstream Western contexts, and if so, what does this say of our core beliefs regarding psychopathology anchored in biological determinism? Rather than attempting to empirically categorise cross-cultural and psychospiritual explanations, an investigation of their phenomenology might better guide an understanding of psychosis within psychiatric research. To what degree, then, are the conundrums that cross-cultural considerations present to psychiatry the result of its failure to consider the possibility that the expression and experience of psychospiritual states of consciousness may be generically inherent to the human psyche and, therefore, can appear in all cultures? For example, if spirits do ontologically exist, then the notion that psychopathology is indicated by deviation from cultural norms becomes redundant because it is feasible to suppose that all people within all cultural settings can potentially be subject to influence by spirits. The same theoretical reasoning also pertains to other forms of psychospiritual experience.

12.1.2 The problem of cognicentrism

A related cross-cultural issue which arguably limits psychiatry's capacity to consider psychospiritual explanations of psychotic-like experiences is that it has adopted and operates by the Western cultural assumption that rationality is a superior faculty of perception and knowledge formation. This is known as 'cognicentrism', which Walsh (1993, p. 740) defines as "the tendency to assume that one's own usual state is optimal". Ackerknecht (1943, p. 55), however, refers to such assumptions as "faulty conclusions" in that they "spring from the supposition that a society is only able to function normally insofar as it is rational. History proves that this 'criterion of rationality' is but a delusion". Further to this, Waldram et al. (2006, p. 129) assert that "rationality must be understood to be a culture specific notion; one culture's rational thought is not necessarily the same as another's. Indeed, the rational thought that underlies scientific inquiry and biomedical practice is but one type of thought". In discussing the pros and cons of the rational function from a mystic perspective, Sri Aurobindo (2005, pp. 13, 66–67) acknowledges that "the rationalistic tendency of Materialism has done mankind this great service", but he also notes it is limited in that "rational action is incapable of knowing what is, it only knows what appears to be, it has no plummet by which it can sound the depths of being, it can only survey the field of becoming". It can hence be argued that while rationality is a valid and valuable form of cognition, it is limited in its scope of apprehension, and therefore, can be blind to aspects of reality that are accessible via other human cognitive capacities. However, it appears the limitations inherent to rationality are ironically compounded by cognicentrism because the belief in rational superiority eclipses awareness of its limitations. It also obviates the serious investigation of 'irrational' notions regarding psychospiritual realities and their possible influence in psychotic experiences.

This has significant implications for better understanding psychotic and psychotic-like experiences. For instance, a basic characteristic of rationality is to depict reality in terms of bifurcated opposites, a practice exemplified in psychiatric diagnostics. On this point, Noll (1983, p. 447) asserts that "the psychological states involved in shamanism and schizophrenia have been imprisoned in the limiting context of the abnormal/ normal or pathological/non-pathological dichotomy, the familiar either/or criterion of cognicentrist thought". It appears, then, that the rules of rationalism, combined with cognicentrism, limit the ways in which reality can be understood and construed, and consequently overlook dialectical considerations such as the idea that psychotic-like occurrences may be integral aspects of a larger transformation process. Therefore, despite the merits and validity of rationalism, when it is coupled with cognicentrism, the exploration of 'irrational' (i.e., metaphysical) domains of reality are generally deemed unworthy of consideration and overlooked by psychiatry. This translates into the formation of a binary diagnostic model (i.e., psychopathology versus non-psycho-pathology) and also essentially denies the consideration of possible psychospiritual determinants in psychosis.

12.1.3 Explicating the cross-cultural challenge

The idea that psychotic-like experiences may possibly reflect psychospiritual developmental processes raises the critical and challenging question: *To what degree does psychiatry inadvertently pathologise that which is potentially healing and transformative and consequently employ treatment approaches that may do more harm than good?* If a shamanic initiatory process, or transpersonal transformative process, is facilitated through psychic or 'psychotic' upheaval, and if this is a phenomenon native to the human psyche and common to all cultures, then pathologising this process, and attempting to curtail or reverse it via enforced hospitalisation and medication, may indeed result in iatrogenic harm.

In light of these considerations, the ensuing investigation further challenges the veracity of psychiatry's psychopathology-based diagnostic model of understanding by examining various psychotic-like psychospiritual phenomena and experiences within the cultural contexts of:

1. Psychospiritual experiences of traditional healers.
2. The shamanic initiatory process.
3. The phenomenon of spirit possession.

The aim here is to look deeply into these experiences in order to elicit a better understanding of their nature and ontological reality and to subsequently demonstrate the seeming impossibility of formulating differential diagnostic criteria in such instances. This, by no means, constitutes a full investigation of the innumerable forms of cross-cultural, psychotic-like, psychospiritual experiences. However, it demonstrates that such research is possible, and adds weight to the idea that better understanding psychosis requires better understanding the many psychospiritual realities that exist beyond the conceptual horizons of psychiatric materialism, biological determinism, cognicentrism, and psychopathology-seeking.

12.2 Psychospiritual experiences of traditional healers

An examination of various cross-cultural understandings regarding anomalous psychospiritual experiences proffers a further and considerable challenge to the diagnostic psychopathology model. Indeed, the anthropological and cross-cultural literature is replete with examples of culturally normative psychotic-like experiences among traditional healers that have seemingly occurred within all cultures throughout the history of humanity. Citing a few such examples suffices to demonstrate the conundrum they pose for psychiatry because, at face value, from a psychiatric perspective, they exemplify definitive signs and symptoms of psychotic disorders. It is apposite to keep in mind that the following reported observations and experiences are not only similar to those observed and reported in psychotic experiences, but are essentially indistinguishable from them. For instance, from an anthropological perspective, Benedict (1934, p. 60) observes that traditional healers exhibiting what appear, by psychiatric standards, to be psychotic "delusions of grandeur or of persecution", are able to "function at ease and with honor" within their own cultural settings. Similarly, Kroeber (1940, p. 204) explains that amongst northern Californian Native American societies, it is common for shamanic practitioners to experience seizures, and both auditory and visual hallucinations.

Indeed, first-person accounts from contemporary Native American traditional healers corroborate these anthropological observations. For example, in describing a healing ceremony she conducted for a person suffering from apparent spirit possession, the Karuk medicine woman, Tela Star Hawk Lake, states that "I could see the bad spirit in a psychic way ... a weird-looking creature that was half-human, with large bat like wings, terrible red eyes, and long claws" (Star Hawk Lake, 1996, p. 102). Her Karuk shaman husband, Medicine Grizzlybear Lake (1991, p. 139), likewise attests to the common occurrence of spiritual causes in "such psychopathological cases as autism [and] juvenile schizophrenia" and proffers the example of an autistic girl who "was locked in a spiritual dimension under the protective custody of the Little People". Both of these shamanic practitioners have achieved healing outcomes when working with such possession cases by utilising traditional psychospiritual skills and understandings. However, if they were to relate the same experiences to a psychiatrist in a clinical setting, independent of a culturally normative context, they would probably be diagnosed as exhibiting clear signs of hallucinatory or delusional behaviour. This begs the question: If their exorcism approaches have achieved healing outcomes with ostensible spirit possession cases, then, are the spirits real, and if so, how might a psychiatrist discern between psychotic and valid reports from patients about being tormented or possessed by spirits?

Another example of Native American shamanic reality, which would likely be considered as psychotic magical thinking by psychiatry, is the ability to engage in two-way communication with non-human creatures and other natural or spiritual forms and forces. For example, the Chippewa medicine man Sun Bear asserts that "we can talk to the trees, to the Earth, to the Creator ... We've been doing it for thousands of years. *It's not supernatural. It's perfectly natural*" (Sun Bear et al., 1983, p. 208). Similarly, the Lakota medicine man, Frank Fools Crow (in Mails, 1990, pp. 183, 184), maintains that a transformative experience he had during a vision quest ceremony resulted in:

> my ability to talk with animals, birds, and thunder beings ... I also have a special song that has been given to me to use when I want to talk to the winds, clouds, and thunder, to stop the rain, or to split the clouds.

Further to this, Fools Crow reports the 'magical' appearance of objects in his body that he uses in healing practices. He claims that after a visit to a sacred site "I now have seven small stones in my body ... One is in my back ... the rest are just under the skin of my left arm and hand" (ibid., p. 183). Although such experiences may sound bizarre by mainstream Western standards, and potentially psychotic by psychiatric standards, it is pertinent to note that the above-described capacities and experiences are not presented as symbolic or imaginative, but as real. These examples represent just some of the many phenomena reported by Indigenous healers (and religious mystics) worldwide that are actualised, either intentionally or spontaneously, when following prescribed traditional psychospiritual practices.

Traditional Australian Indigenous healers relate having similar experiences and powers. For instance, three traditional healers (*ngangkari*) from the Anangu Pitjantjatjara Yankuntjatjara lands of the Central Desert region in South Australia have recently shared their experiences to enlighten non-Indigenous Australians about their cultural and spiritual ways. As with their Native American counterparts this includes interactions and communications with the spirit world. For instance, Andy Tjilari explains that, at night "the ngangkaris' spirit bodies begin to fly around and to visit the sleeping spirits of other people to make sure all is well", while Naomi Kantjuriny states that "at night I see spirits. The kurunpa spirits talk to me" (Kantjuriny et al., 2013, p. 20). Intriguingly, like Fools Crow, these healers also speak of power objects entering their bodies. In discussing power objects called *mapanpa*;[127] Maringka Burton explains that:

> my mapanpa live in my body. I am a painter, and when I paint, my mapanpa move right up into my shoulder and sit up there, out of the way. If somebody comes

---

[127] Andy Tjilari describes *mapanpa* as follows:

> While all the ngangkari are gathered in the special camps, hundreds of mapanpa will come flying in. Mapanpa are special, powerful tools. They hit the ground with small explosions, "boom, boom, boom!" The ngangkari dash around collecting up the objects: kanti that look like sharp stone blades, kuuti that resemble black shiny round tektites, and tarka—slivers of bone. Each ngangkari gathers up the pieces he wants. These pieces become his own property. (Kantjuriny et al., 2013, p. 20)

References to the occurrence and use of flying stones also exist within a traditional Native American shamanic context (Albers, 2003; Standing Bear, 1978, pp. 215–216; Densmore, 1918, pp. 205–206).

to me, needing help, I would have to ease my mapanpa back into my hands again. Sometimes I would push them from one arm to the other. (ibid.)

Again, from the mindset of Western materialism these reported experiences may appear to be supernatural, superstitious, or psychopathological, yet, for these traditional healers, such reports reflect real experiences whereby access has been gained to psychospiritual domains of reality through their initiatory training processes.

While psychiatry's recent attention to, and acceptance of, culturally normative psychotic-like experiences is commendable, this falls short of addressing the conundrums posed by introducing cultural relativity into the epistemological bounds of a discipline governed by the tenets of medical materialism. However, while this is a challenging task, such an undertaking is possible. For instance, the successful collaboration between the Māori spiritual healer, Wiremu NiaNia, and psychiatrist, Allister Bush, demonstrates the viability and efficacy of psychiatry and Indigenous healers working together in mental health practice. Their book *Collaborative and Indigenous Mental Health Therapy* offers an exemplary portrayal of how "bicultural partnership frameworks can augment mental health treatment by balancing local imperatives with sound and careful psychiatric care" (NiaNia et al., 2017, back cover). Throughout this book, NiaNia and Bush relate their respective stories about working together with people undergoing psychotic-like experiences. In each instance, NiaNia offers a traditional spiritual perspective, and Bush a psychiatric perspective, about the nature of each person's experience and the effective outcomes resulting from working collaboratively. As NiaNia explains:

> The key for me is understanding. If Allister is able to develop that understanding of wairua and consider that alongside his other knowledge as a psychiatrist, then he is capable of looking outside the box of Western thinking. He'll never be a Māori, but he can be a healer in the broad sense of the word, because having that awareness that a problem could be spiritual may have a healing effect for a young person. (ibid., p. 163)

The Māori word 'wairua' roughly translates as 'spiritual' and, in light of his own 'supernatural' capacities for perceiving things invisible to others, NiaNia further asserts the importance for psychiatry to understand that psychotic-like experiences may have wairua origins (p. 2). He explains that from a Western psychiatric viewpoint:

> I would be in danger of being misdiagnosed. I could have been labelled as having hallucinations or being psychotic. And I strongly believe this has been a problem for many of our people … I'm not suggesting mental illness doesn't exist. But far too often the wairua side, the spiritual side, has gone unrecognised, which has had very negative outcomes for us as Māori. (ibid.)

Therefore, the conceptual tension created by bringing these two worldviews together arguably represents an opportunity for psychiatry to consider the validity of metaphysical realities and to reconsider its traditional understanding of psychosis as a form of psychopathology whereby people are 'out of touch with reality'. Ironically, psychiatry is seemingly out of touch with psychospiritual realities existing beyond the borders of its materialist purview, and consequently identifies these as psychopathological.

12.3 Psychosis and the shamanic initiatory process

The shamanic initiatory process[128] refers to the developmental and transformative training process through which a person becomes a shaman. In a general sense, Krippner (2007, p. 20) describes shamans as practitioners who "attempt to modify dysfunctional attitudes, behaviors, and experiences" within their sociocultural environments. However, he further notes that they are healers who attend to a community's "spiritual needs" and who "deliberately shift their phenomenological pattern of attention, perception, cognition, and awareness in order to obtain information not ordinarily available to members of the social group" (ibid., p. 16). In other words, integral to their healing practice is the ability to use technologies of consciousness to glean psychospiritual insight and guidance about the nature of and therapeutic responses to a problematic situation. According to Winkelman (2004, p. 152), the shamanic initiatory process is essential to providing a shaman-to-be with the requisite training and skills for adroitly navigating psychospiritual domains of reality. This often entails a lengthy period of upheaval that may appear classically psychotic from a psychiatric perspective.

The idea that psychotic-like occurrences are natural and integral features of shamanic initiatory processes is endorsed by both Indigenous and Western commentators. For example, in her doctoral dissertation which explores "Māori ways of understanding extra-ordinary experiences and schizophrenia", Taitimu (2007, p. 34) explains that, in psychiatry, a person experiencing psychotic-like symptoms is diagnosed as having "that thing [schizophrenia], but we would say he was a divine healer. If I ask if a person has these things, what would you call them? We would say a healer. But they say sickness and diagnose". Similarly, the African shaman, Odi Oquosa (in May, 2007b, p. 123), maintains that "madness is an initiation of a healing process; an awakening of the unconscious mind. For this healing to be enabled it is important not to suppress these experiences as western psychiatry has tended to do". In terms of Western commentators, Eliade (1958, pp. 89, 102) observes that, while the shaman "sometimes borders on madness … he has succeeded in integrating into consciousness a considerable number of experiences that, for the profane world, are reserved for … madness". Hence, for the shaman, madness is circumvented by understanding

---

[128] While I have already discussed similarities between the shamanic initiatory process and Western notions of the psychotic process, particularly in light of differentiating shamanic experience from psychopathology (for instance, see the Grofs' notion of 'shamanic crisis' in Table 5, Chapter Eight, Section 8.2), my focus here is to elucidate the seemingly indiscernible and interconnected nature of the two.

that psychotic-like occurrences signify a calling to learn how to withstand and navigate metaphysical realities. As Winkelman (2004, p. 152) notes, rather than seeing psychotic-like occurrences as psychopathological "the shamanic paradigm provides a useful framework for addressing these experiences as natural manifestations of human consciousness, and as developmental opportunities" whereby the skilled shamanic practitioner "re-interprets symptoms of acute psychosis, emotional disturbance, hallucinations, ASC [altered states of consciousness], and interaction with spirits as symbolic communications for personal development". Likewise, in his appraisal of shamanic initiatory processes, Robbins (2011, p. 110) maintains that psychiatry's understanding of psychosis could be advanced by pondering the question: "Might psychosis be thought of as personal disharmony with the cosmos requiring spiritual healing"? In this context, the presence of psychotic-like phenomena is not a call to identify psychopathology, or to differentiate psychotic from psychospiritual instances, but signifies the need to provide a person with support and guidance so that integration and transformation can occur.

It is important to clarify, however, that the term 'shamanic initiatory process' does not only infer instances that occur within cultures where shamanism is practised. It is my contention that such psychotic-like processes may be intrinsic to human nature and can possibly occur within Western society independently of an established shamanic context. For example, African shaman Malidoma Somé (in Marohn, 2003, p. 170), recollects the affront and dismay he experienced when he first visited America and was exposed to the treatment of 'psychotic' patients in a psychiatric ward:

> I was so shocked. That was the first time I was brought face to face with what is done here to people exhibiting the same symptoms I've seen in my village ... 'So this is how the healers who are attempting to be born are treated in this culture. What a loss! What a loss that a person who is finally being aligned with a power from the other world is just being wasted'.

Here, Somé clearly suggests that psychotic-like shamanic experiences are intrinsic to being human and can occur within all cultural settings. This is an idea that extends beyond psychiatry's limited definition of "cultural syndromes" as "clusters of symptoms and attributions that tend to co-occur among individuals in specific cultural groups" (APA, 2013, p. 758), with the general inference being in non-Western contexts. Somé (in Russell, 2014, p. 265) subsequently maintains that "the easy labelling of clinical psychotics ... is a reflection of a profound misunderstanding, because the structure of the world afforded by people like this has not been studied sufficiently". In other words, a better understanding of the nature of so-called 'psychosis' may be gleaned through the heuristic investigation of psychospiritual phenomenology, which concomitantly eschews psychiatry's primary focus of seeking to identify and name forms of psychopathology.

The feasibility of such an approach is personified by New Zealand clinical psychologist and shaman, Ingo Lambrecht, who draws on both shamanic and traditional

Western approaches in his therapeutic practice.[129] He argues that "our science of consciousness is so poor we just have no idea" about shamanic altered states of consciousness, and from his own experience proposes that "the psychological process of voluntary culturally determined trance states may be similar to the involuntary dissociative or psychotic trance states" (Lambrecht, 2017). Further to this he explains that when "shamans have an initiation illness … it could be viewed as a spiritual crisis … a strange entanglement of madness and the transformation, finding its expression in the *ukutwasa* of South African *sangomas*" (Lambrecht, 2015, p. 7).[130] In terms of challenging Western cognicentrism, Lambrecht (2017) describes the shaman as "the first psychologist or psychiatrist". Indeed, he explains that "it is the shaman who is waiting for modern Western discourse to wake up and catch up with what has always been known in other cultures and for modern Western discourse to bring with it its own unique and valuable contributions" (Lambrecht, 2009, p. 15). This suggests that, contrary to Western science's cognicentric stance, it is largely ignorant of knowledge pertaining to psychospiritual domains of reality that shamans have long mastered.

Lambrecht, however, appears to have bridged this epistemological gap. As a healer who has trained in both shamanic and Western clinical therapeutic modalities, he demonstrates the possibility of reconciling scientific materialism with cross-cultural metaphysical worldviews and, from this dialectical position, forging new ways of understanding psychotic-like human experiences beyond the psychiatric approach of psychopathology-seeking. This, of course, raises questions as to what essentially defines the shamanic initiatory process. Are psychic upheavals that occur in shamanic cultures fundamentally the same as those occurring in Western psychotic instances, in the sense of their transformative potential? Is it this potential that defines them as 'shamanic' or is it the facilitative guidance of a shaman that makes them so? Does this suggest that all apparent psychoses are actually shamanic initiatory processes in potential? In this sense, does 'psychosis', as psychiatry understands it, actually exist? Can psychiatric efficacy be advanced by practitioners learning how to utilise technologies of consciousness, navigate metaphysical domains of reality, and train 'psychotic' patients to do likewise? These are questions that cannot be answered here. However, they characterise the type of speculations and investigations that may arise from extending scientific and psychiatric epistemic parameters to include the consideration of metaphysical views of reality.

---

[129] Lambrecht (2017) describes himself as "privileged to undergo an intense shamanic training as a sangoma, a South African traditional healer" and notes that his field of expertise and research interests include "the relationships between culture, psychosis, and spirituality".

[130] Lambrecht (2015, p. 4) explains that the term *ukutwasa* (or *ukuthwasa*) refers to a shamanic apprenticeship that:

> allows you to take on your new identity, but this process is feared, as it entails madness, insane pain, and acts of wild behavior; the more you resist the call, the more severe this process is. Death through madness is a real danger in this rebirth needed to become a *sangoma*.

In light of the above, my ensuing investigation aims to support the idea that psychotic-like experiences may represent potentially transformative and healing processes that are natural to the human psyche. In this sense, 'psychotic' instances seemingly call for a therapeutic response of psychospiritual tutelage and not the diagnostic identification of psychopathological symptoms. Indeed, from this perspective, the notion of 'psychopathology' becomes highly ambiguous because it is impossible to isolate any symptom that is definitively psychopathological. This task is undertaken in two contexts:

1. Challenging the veracity of key psychiatric symptoms for diagnosing psychosis by demonstrating their prevalence in shamanic contexts.
2. Challenging the veracity of the notion that the duration of psychotic-like episodes differentiates psychopathological from shamanic instances.

Such investigation also supports my proposal that it is ultimately not possible to distinguish between shamanic initiatory and psychotic occurrences.

12.3.1 Psychotic indicators: the veracity of symptoms?

Contrary to assertions that shamanic and psychotic experiences are discrete, the descriptions in Table 10 of experiences occurring during shamanic initiatory processes appear identical to those identified by psychiatry as being characteristically psychotic.

Table 10. Descriptions of shamanic initiatory psychotic-like symptoms.

Cultural context	Description
Native American shaman (Chukchee)	Thus a Chukchee female shaman, Telpina, according to her own statement, had been violently insane … during which time her household had taken precautions that she should do no harm to the people or to herself. (Czaplicka, 1914, p. 172)
Zulu shaman	He habitually sheds tears, at first slight, then at last he weeps aloud … a man becoming a diviner causes great trouble, for he does not sleep, but works constantly with his brain; his sleep is merely in snatches, and he wakes up singing many songs … And then he leaps about the house like a frog; and the house becomes too small for him, and he goes out leaping and singing. (Benedict, 1934, p. 63)
Native American shaman	All through native northern California the onset of shamanistic power is marked by a seizure in which the candidate experiences an hallucination—always auditory and usually visual also. (Kroeber, 1940, p. 204)

(Continued)

Table 10. (Continued)

Cultural context	Description
Siberian shaman	He who is to become a shaman begins to rage like a raving madman. He suddenly utters incoherent words, falls unconscious, runs through the forests, lives on the bark of trees, throws himself into fire and water, lays hold on weapons and wounds himself, in such that his family is obliged to keep watch on him. By these signs it is recognised that he will become a shaman. (Ackerknecht, 1943, p. 42)
Native American shaman	Inspirational medicine men who communicate directly with the spirits … exhibit the most blatant forms of psychotic-like behaviors. These include grossly non-reality-oriented ideation, abnormal perceptual experiences, profound emotional upheavals, and bizarre mannerisms … One sees strange meanings in everything about one, and one will soon be sure of only one thing—that events, people, and places are not what they seem … Causal relationships are perceived against a background of magic and animism. Everything is now capable of being related to everything else in terms of a mental orientation that is grossly subjective. New ideas crowded in upon the anxious individual, are experienced as real things. Reality becomes something else. Chaos prevails. (Silverman, 1967, pp. 22, 27)
Shaman (generic)	During the initial crisis … shamans-to-be may experience themselves as tormented and controlled by spirits. They may exhibit considerable confusion, emotional turmoil, withdrawal from society, and a range of unusual and even bizarre behavior such as going naked, refusing food, and biting themselves. (Walsh, 1997, p. 111)
Balinese balian	When the balian's life histories are examined in detail, it becomes evident that the pattern of disturbance described is in fact far closer to chronic psychosis, or schizophrenia … The superficial resemblance to the course of schizophrenia is of the greatest importance since … from the perspective of Western diagnostic categories, the balian described in this article prior to their taking up the vocation could be identified as schizophrenic, meeting all the major criteria of delusions, hallucinations and disturbed behavior. (Stephen & Suryani, 2000, p. 21)
South African sangoma	A sangoma … would understandably from a Western psychiatric standpoint be considered to have psychotic symptoms, dominated by auditory hallucinations and social withdrawal, i.e. positive and negative symptoms of schizophrenia … In South African shamanism … during the *ukuthwasa* or initiation illness, the voices are experienced as persecutory and are experienced as fragmenting the ego. (Lambrecht, 2009, pp. 6, 11)

These descriptions evidently reflect classic psychiatric symptoms of psychosis such as: auditory and visual hallucinations; persecutory voices; bizarre beliefs and delusions; distortions of reality; bizarre and socially deviant behaviour; interpersonal and vocational social dysfunction; social isolation; extreme affective states; harm to self, others, or property; disrupted sleep; high levels of anxiety, confusion, and distress; garbled speech; catatonia; ego fragmentation; hyperreflectivity; and experiencing an intensity of meaning and interconnectivity between things and events. However, these 'symptoms' not only resemble psychiatric indicators of psychosis, but have also been identified by differential diagnosis proponents as indicating a psychotic rather than a shamanic experience. For instance, authors in my content analysis variously suggested that psychotic rather than psychospiritual instances are signified by the presence of: social isolation or dysfunction; ego anomalies; auditory hallucinations; persecutory voices; risk of harm to self or others; bizarre delusions, behaviour, and speech; aggressive outbursts; and so on.

Hence, it appears that psychiatry's entire framework of psychotic diagnostic and descriptive features can occur within the context of a shamanic initiatory process, as can all proposed criteria for discerning psychotic from psychospiritual experiences. If so, then it is plausible to propose that psychotic and psychotic-like psychospiritual experiences are ultimately indistinguishable and that there is no solid hook on which to hang the hat of psychopathology in either. If psychopathology cannot be discerned from normative cultural anomalies, or from natural transformative psychotic-like experiences, then psychosis cannot be substantiated. This is not to deny the existence of distressing and anomalous experiences called 'psychoses', but suggests that the practices of psychopathology-seeking and psychopathology-labelling seem to eclipse rather than illuminate the nature of such experiences. In light of the fact that the full gamut of psychotic-like behaviours and experiences can occur within shamanic and other transformative psychospiritual contexts, the validity of psychiatry's model of diagnostic psychopathology-seeking is rendered dubious, as is the respective construal of psychosis. Such an approach seemingly finds only that which it is looking for and overlooks the expertise and knowledge of Indigenous healing systems that demonstrate a sophisticated understanding of the human psyche and its myriad psychospiritual dynamics and capacities.

12.3.2 Psychotic indicators: the veracity of duration?

The ambiguity of the issue of 'duration of experience' as a differentiation marker has already been touched upon in Chapter Nine, Section 9.3.4. However, it warrants further examination within a shamanic context because initiatory training and transformation processes can entail lengthy periods of psychotic-like experiences. For instance, Czaplicka (1914, p. 172) reports a Native American Chukchee shaman who underwent three years of psychotic-like disturbances throughout her initiatory process. Similarly, Benedict (1934, p. 62) observes that the Siberian shamanic initiatory crisis can last for several years, and Stephen & Suryani (2000, p. 21) note the same in a

Balinese shamanic context. In a Christian context, the Franciscan mystic Brother John of La Verna experienced a protracted state of psychotic-like ecstatic trance in which "his heart was kindled with the fire of love divine, and this flame lasted in him for full three years, in the which time he received marvellous consolations and visitations divine, and oftentimes was rapt in God" (Rhys, 1912, p. 89). Such instances clearly challenge the idea that the duration of an anomalous experience is a criterion for discerning psychotic from psychospiritual experiences. They also challenge the veracity of the DSM-5 assertion that schizophrenia can be diagnosed if "continuous signs of the disturbance persist for at least 6 months" (APA, 2013, p. 99). Although the DSM includes culturally sensitive considerations to circumvent such diagnostic problems, this is based on the presumption that genuine psychopathology is distinct from normative psychotic-like cultural experiences. There is no consideration of the possibility that spontaneous, psychotic-like upheavals of transformative potential and long duration are native to the human psyche and can therefore occur within both Western and non-Western cultural settings.

For contemporary medical psychiatry, a significant dilemma is posed by the notion that a psychotic-like psychospiritual upheaval, of long duration, can represent an intrinsic developmental function of the human psyche. If true, then many people within Western psychiatric settings may likely be diagnosed as schizophrenic or psychotic when they are actually exhibiting features of a natural and protracted psychospiritual transformative process. A brief examination of three cases elucidates and supports this theoretical view.

First, is the example of Egan Bidois (in Robbins, 2011, pp. 99–110), a Māori man who was diagnosed as psychotic when overwhelmed by an array of metaphysical experiences. These consisted of hearing voices, seeing spirits, and a psychic sensitivity that swamped him with unbidden intuitive 'feelings' and insights into other people's subjective lives: "their attachments, their histories, their pains" (ibid., p. 102). From a Māori perspective, such experiences would generally be understood as incipient signs of a calling to the vocation of seer or healer. However, circumstances led Egan to a psychiatrist where the same experiences were seen as the hallucinations, delusions, distress, and dysfunction of psychosis (p. 103). He was subsequently hospitalised and recalls that: "What followed was many years of involvement with the mental health system. No amount of anti-psychotics or western intervention helped. Finally I was discharged as being 'treatment resistant'" (ibid.). Upon discharge, he returned to his community where he received initiatory training from traditional healers, which gradually enabled him to control the overwhelming influx of metaphysical content and to become a healer himself. Ten years later, during which time he had no further contact with the mental health system, he reported that "I see, hear and feel at levels beyond anything I ever have before; well beyond even those that pushed me into unwellness" (p. 104). Hence, experiences that had once rendered him dysfunctional and 'psychotic' had become, with appropriate training, experiences and capacities that enabled him to operate effectively as a healer.

A second example is that of Alex, an American teenager who, after four years of ineffective medical treatment for severe psychotic and depressive symptoms, was taken by the African shaman, Malidoma Somé, to a West African village. According to Somé (in Marohn, 2003, pp. 173–174), after residing eight months in the village, Alex "became quite normal" and subsequently stayed in Africa for four years, training with local healers before returning to America where he completed a psychology degree at Harvard University and became a healer in his own right. In regards to Alex's apparent 'psychosis', Somé explains that "he was reaching out. It was an emergency call. His job and his purpose was to be a healer … no one was paying attention to that" (ibid., p. 174). Arguably, had Alex not undergone shamanic training in Africa then he would likely have continued to be a patient in the American psychiatric system.

Similarly, from her personal experience as an American psychiatric patient, Ekhaya Esima (2017)[131] reports that, "I started having experiences that some would say are characteristics of psychosis or mental illness. My experiences included disturbing visions, voices, and confusion". However, after years of being in the mental health system she met, and become apprenticed to, an African American sangoma who told her she was "gifted" and described her experiences as the "Ancestors waking her up" to her vocation as a healer (Borges & Tomlinson, 2017). Within two years of her initiation she had parted ways with the mental health system, and though still experiencing visions and voices, these now served her in her capacity as a healer (ibid.). As with Egan, both Alex and Ekhaya also experienced a protracted period of psychotic-like symptoms that were deemed psychopathological by psychiatry and unsuccessfully treated accordingly. However, in all instances, when these psychiatric patients were introduced to a shamanic setting where the potential for a psychic transition was recognised and supported, the outcome was integrative and positive.

Such instances demonstrate that the duration of psychotic-like experiences is not a reliable diagnostic indicator of psychopathology. They also lend credence to the idea that apparent shamanic initiatory processes can spontaneously occur within Western populations. In sum, it is clear that protracted, psychotic-like episodes are a common feature of shamanic initiatory processes and, presumably, other psychospiritual transformative processes. Hence, 'duration of symptomatology' is not a failsafe criterion for discerning psychotic from psychospiritual experiences, or for diagnosing chronic psychotic disorders such as schizophrenia. From a shamanic perspective, instances of so-called 'psychosis' are not generally seen as indicative of severe psychopathology but as a natural and potentially beneficent process of developmental transformation that requires skilled support and can be thwarted by well-intentioned but misinformed diagnostic labelling and pharmacological interventions.

---

[131] Ekhaya is one of the two people whose stories are documented in the film *CRAZYWISE* that explores the question: "What can we learn from those who have turned their psychological crisis into a positive transformative experience?" (Borges & Tomlinson, 2017).

12.4 Spirits and spirit possession

Throughout the history of humanity, the belief in spirits and spirit possession has been ubiquitous. Yet, with the advent of scientific materialism in modern Western societies, belief in a psychospiritual domain and spiritual entities is commonly deemed superstitious, irrational, unempirical, and, in the case of psychiatry, indicative of possible psychopathology. As observed by Gutberlet (1913, p. 43) in his description of 'Materialism' in the *Catholic Encyclopedia*, "absorption in the study of material nature is apt to blind one to the spiritual". However, it was the conviction of the eighteenth-century Swiss scientist and mystic Emanuel Swedenborg (2009 [1758], p. 499) that "the spiritual world cannot be separated from the natural, nor the natural world from the spiritual". Indeed, Swedenborg stated this not as a conceptual conviction, but in light of his own metaphysical explorations and experiences. He explained later in his life that "it has been granted to me now for many years to speak with spirits and to be with them as one of them, even in full wakefulness of the body" (Swedenborg, 1905 [1758], p. 379). This is not an isolated instance, for research conducted in the late 1960s by the American anthropologist Erika Bourguignon (1973, pp. 10–11, 16–17) regarding the spiritual beliefs and practices of 488 global societies, found that ninety per cent had "institutionalized forms of altered states of consciousness" and seventy-four per cent maintained a "belief in possession by spirits". Therefore, despite the relatively recent dismissal of spiritual realities by mainstream scientific, psychiatric, and psychoanalytic disciplines, it appears the belief in spiritual beings and spirit domains still prevails globally.

What, then, might these spirits be, and how do they relate to the phenomenon of psychosis? Both of these questions point to a deeper understanding of spirits and so-called 'psychosis' in terms of psychospiritual phenomenology. While psychiatry's acknowledgement of culturally normative and non-psychopathological beliefs in spirit possession is a progressive step, it fails to take the logical further step of inquiring into the nature of these spirits. This failure is arguably due to the conceptual framework of bifurcating rationalism which governs and limits the psychiatric worldview. For instance, Huskinson & Schmidt (2010, p. 12) maintain that a better understanding of spirit possession is curtailed by "the blind endorsement of unwarranted dichotomies", while Samuel (2010, pp. 35, 37) argues that "spirit possession and trance seem to fit particularly badly into a conceptual framework built around a rigid mind-body distinction" and that "reducing of everything to cognitive categories … excludes other questions … (e.g. what in fact is spirit possession and how does it operate?)". It therefore appears that understanding spirit possession, and its relation to psychosis, is eclipsed by psychiatric rationalism and materialism.

12.4.1 DSM on spirits and spirit possession

Psychiatry assumes and asserts that spirit possession, outside of normative cultural beliefs, is psychopathological. As Sanderson (2003, p. 1) points out, this may be because "spirit possession, according to contemporary science, is impossible".

Generally, psychiatry understands so-called 'spirit possession' to be a dissociative disorder involving "the splitting off of clusters of mental contents from conscious awareness" that may occur as "possession-form presentations" with intrusive symptomatology such as "voices; dissociated actions and speech; intrusive thoughts, emotions, and impulses" (APA, 2013, pp. 820, 292). Indeed, this view has prevailed within psychiatric epistemology since the late nineteenth century when the French psychiatrist Pierre Janet introduced the notion of dissociation into the clinical lexicon in reference to "the existence of double personality and double consciousness as hysteric phenomena", including reported instances of spirit possession (Avdibegović, 2012, p. 368). Hence, in mainstream Western psychiatric settings, people who claim to be possessed by spirits, or attribute their anomalous experiences to spirit influences, are likely to be diagnosed as psychopathologically out of touch with reality.

While notions of spirits and spirit possession were absent in DSM I-to-III, they entered the sphere of diagnostic considerations in both DSM-IV and DSM-5. Intriguingly, despite the psychotic-like appearance of beliefs in spirit possession, the DSM chiefly provides instruction about this phenomenon in terms of cross-cultural considerations and dissociative disorders, and not in the context of psychotic disorders. This diagnostic separation of psychotic and dissociative disorders creates ambiguity in DSM references to spirit or trance possession. For instance, while DSM-IV infers a psychotic dimension in stating that Dissociative Trance Disorder cannot be diagnosed if an ostensible trance possession occurs "exclusively during the course of a Psychotic Disorder" (APA, 1994, p. 729), the difference between psychotic and dissociative trance possession is not explained. Such ambiguity is also reflected in the updated DSM-5 manual, which emphasises that "dissociative identity disorder may be confused with schizophrenia or other psychotic disorders" (APA, 2013, p. 296), but further instruction as to why and how this is so is not provided. Overall, then, the DSM makes only tenuous diagnostic links between psychotic disorders and spirit possession.

However, despite the ambiguity of references to spirits and spirit possession in the DSM, the broader literature indicates that such experiences can often be perceived as psychotic. For example, Pfeifer (1994, p. 252) observes that "belief in demonic influence has repeatedly been described as a delusion in schizophrenic patients" while Teoh & Dass (1973, p. 62) also note that unless cross-cultural considerations are taken into account "one may diagnose spirit possession as schizophrenia or other forms of psychosis". Beyond acknowledging the validity of spirit possession in the context of culturally accepted norms, psychiatry seems disinterested in considering the nature of reported 'spirits'. However, as is evidenced below, such investigation is not only possible, it can glean deeper insights into understanding the seemingly conjoint psychotic and psychospiritual dynamics of the human psyche.

12.4.2 Beyond psychiatry: what might these spirits be?

Outside the purview of medical psychiatry, there exists a significant body of literature that proffers both psychosocial and metaphysical explanations as to the nature of 'spirits' and their play in psychotic experiences. Those who have engaged this subject appear to fall into two conceptual camps: one, that spirits are ultimately of a psychological nature; and two, that spirits exist as actual metaphysical beings. It is pertinent to note that, in both instances, spirit possession is seen as effectively 'real' in that a person's mind or being is influenced or controlled by an autonomous, subliminal, or supernatural 'something'.

From a mainstream psychological perspective, purported experiences of spirit possession are not seen as real, but generally understood to represent a case of self-protective mental dissociation and projection. For example, from a psychodynamic viewpoint, Ward & Beaubrun (1980, p. 206) describe possession as a form of dissociation that offers a person "escape from unpleasant reality, and diminution of guilt by projecting blame onto an intruding agent", while Huskinson (2010, p. 85) equates "spirit possessions" to "dissociative ego-states". Similarly, from a sociological and anthropological perspective, instances of dissociative 'spirit possession' are generally understood to represent an unconscious reactive coping mechanism against oppressive social mores, such as forced marriage or gender inequity (Child, 2010; Samuel, 2010). Such views essentially reflect the understanding of psychoanalytic psychiatry that the existence of spirits is scientifically impossible and, therefore, reported instances can be explained as psychopathological forms of unconscious dissociation whereby aspects of the psyche become autonomous (i.e., spirits).

Other authors in this field of research consider spirits to be ontologically real. For instance, from an anthropological perspective, Bourguignon (1973, p. 22) observes that spirits "may be ancestors, foreigners, or other humans, animals, or spirits that never had been embodied in human or animal form". This clearly depicts spirits as extant entities. Betty (2005, p. 13) describes spirits as "more or less intelligent beings, insensible to us, with a will of their own who seem to bother or oppress us or, in rare cases, possess our bodies outright, and with whom we can relate in a variety of ways". She subsequently maintains that psychiatry should heed the "growing evidence for demonic possession" (ibid., p. 14). Here, Betty seems to call on psychiatry to step beyond simply recognising the belief in spirits and spirit possession as culturally idiosyncratic, and to acknowledge that these may be metaphysical realities that can impact upon the mental health of all people. Further to this, Caygill & Culbertson (2010, p. 44) note that Indigenous Pacific Islanders "complain that western psychiatrists … Do not understand how thin is the veil that separates human beings from the 'invisible'". Indeed, Azaunce (1995, p. 255) questions whether the phenomenon of spirit possession should be understood as "a major symptom of a mental disorder, such as schizophrenia, and … treated with psychotropic medication and psychotherapy", or, instead, should "such alternative curative interventions as spiritual healing be more seriously examined as viable ways of defining and treating mental illness"? Interestingly, Jaspers (1997 v1, pp. 107–108) also counselled clinicians to give serious consideration to patients' reports of metaphysical experiences:

> Patients may display their delusions in some supra-natural mode and such experiences cannot be adjudged true or untrue, correct or false … We have to regard this

experience as such and not merely as some perverted psychological or psycho-pathological phenomenon if we really want to understand it.

It seems, however, that psychiatry has not adopted this proposal, for it generally dismisses the veracity of psychospiritual occurrences, including the possible reality of spirits and spirit possession.[132]

As Jaspers observes above, it is common for psychiatric patients to attribute their experiences to psychospiritual influences. Indeed, a significant degree of voice hearers understand their experiences in such terms. For example, in a national survey of participants in American Hearing Voices groups, Jones et al. (2016, pp. 110–111) found that 84.5 per cent of discussion relates to the perceived "religious/spiritual connections" of voices, while 68.8 per cent pertains to "paranormal phenomena". Similarly, in terms of voice-hearing aetiology, Romme & Escher (1989, p. 214) found that about forty-five per cent of a sample of twenty voice hearers identified their voices as deriving from "gods or spirits"; Jones et al. (2003, p.203) found that many mental health service clients believed "people may hear voices when a spirit possesses their body"; and 45.5 per cent of respondents interviewed by Beavan (2007, p. 91) maintained that the voices they heard "belong to other types of beings, e.g., God(s), spirits, guides". Research also indicates that patients have identified the influence of spirits as being a general causal factor in psychotic or psychotic-like experiences. For instance, Pfeifer (1994, pp. 247, 250) found that of the 343 religiously-oriented out-patients interviewed at a Swiss psychiatric clinic, 37.6 per cent believed in "the possible causation of their problems through the influence of evil spirits", particularly for those diagnosed with psychotic disorders. Additionally, Esterberg & Compton (2006, p. 223) found that, of the family members of hospitalised urban African American schizophrenia patients they interviewed, 26.2 per cent believed that the cause of schizophrenia was "very likely" to be "possession by evil spirits". It therefore appears spirit possession, or the influence of spirits, is a commonly held explanatory belief for people having psychotic-like experiences.

Although such widespread belief does not prove the existence of spirits, nor does clinical disbelief prove their non-existence. Arguably, then, the ubiquitous belief in spirits across cultures constitutes grounds for psychiatry to at least consider the possibility that such spirits exist. In fact, Bourguignon (1973, pp. 11, 12) concludes that, in light of the prevalence of trance induction in societies throughout the world, the human ability to experience altered states of consciousness is "a psychobiological capacity of the species, and thus universal". If the capacity for trance induction is

---

[132] There are rare exceptions to this general trend. For instance, a one-day conference titled 'Spirit possession and mental health' was held in London in 2013 and promoted as being "relevant to all professionals in the field of Mental Health and Social Care", including psychiatrists. The conference considered "the critical themes and debates on spirit possession from an anthropological, social, psychological, medical and religious perspective using a range of illustrative case study, clinical practice and research" (Ethnic Health Initiative, 2013). Though an exception to the traditional psychiatric rule, this demonstrates the feasibility of Western clinicians learning about metaphysical realities.

universal then it is logical to suggest that the spirits people report communicating with in altered states of consciousness, including psychosis, may represent a real and universal phenomenon. The ensuing sections investigate further views on the nature of spirits and their play in psychosis, in the context of Carl Jung's psychoanalytic understanding, and psychologist Wilson van Dusen's unique phenomenological research. Both share in common the explication of a psychospiritual theory of mind in relation to spirits and psychosis, though each differs in its nuanced understanding of the nature of spirits. Also, their respective works demonstrate the feasibility of conducting robust research into the prospect that humans have the universal capacity to access psychospiritual domains and, concomitantly, into investigating the possibility that the altered state of consciousness called 'psychosis' may, in part, or full, reflect the influence of spirits or psychospiritual determinants.

This line of investigation ostensibly proffers a plausible solution to the conundrum of how, exactly, does deviance from cultural norms constitute psychopathology? Arguably, this conundrum results from psychiatry's attempt to force fit cross-cultural considerations into a bifurcating model of diagnostics, while failing to provide a cogent explanation as to how a particular experience and behaviour can be deemed normal in one cultural setting, yet psychotic in another. However, if materialist assumptions about the nature of reality are set aside and the possible generic existence of spirits and psychospiritual realities is accepted, then such conceptual dilemmas are circumvented. Furthermore, acknowledging the prospect that spirits may exist and that spirit possession may, therefore, be universal, raises new investigative questions: If spirits exist, what might they be, what roles might they play in psychosis, and how might a better understanding of this impact upon psychiatric thinking and practice?

12.4.3 Jung on spirits and spirit possession

As discussed above,[133] Jung sees the collective unconscious as a fundamental psychic structure common to all of humanity. To him, this is the realm of "primordial images which have always been the basis of man's thinking" and also the source of the mythic imagery that abounds in psychotic experiences (Jung, 1969, pp. 310–311). Accordingly, the study of spirit possession was very much an aspect of his investigations into the mechanisms of the unconscious self. Indeed, he makes frequent references to spirits and spirit possession throughout his writings. For example, in the following excerpt from his *Memories, Dreams, Reflections*, Jung (1965, pp. 190–191) proffers an intriguing account of a poltergeist-like phenomenon he experienced:

> Around five o'clock in the afternoon on Sunday the front doorbell began ringing frantically. It was a bright summer day; the two maids were in the kitchen, from which the open square outside the front door could be seen. Everyone immediately looked to see who was there, but there was no one in sight. I was sitting near

---

[133] See Chapter Ten, Section 10.6.5.

the doorbell, and not only heard it but saw it moving. We all simply stared at one another. The atmosphere was thick, believe me! Then I knew that something had to happen. The whole house was filled as if there were a crowd present, crammed full of spirits. They were packed deep right up to the door, and the air was so thick it was scarcely possible to breathe. As for myself, I was all a-quiver with the question: "For God's sake, what in the world is this?" Then they cried out in chorus, "We have come back from Jerusalem where we found not what we sought". That is the beginning of the *Septem Sermones* [the title of a subsequent book written by Jung, also known as *The Seven Sermons to the Dead*]. Then it began to flow out of me, and in the course of three evenings the thing was written. As soon as I took up the pen, the whole ghostly assemblage evaporated. The room quieted and the atmosphere cleared. The haunting was over.

Had he been a psychiatric patient reporting this experience to a resident clinician he probably would have been considered mad, yet this depicts an actual event in his life.

Although the belief in spirits is traditionally dismissed within scientific circles as being fanciful and irrational, if not psychotically delusional, Jung was adamant that his study of this subject represented the scientific investigation of extant psychic phenomena. This is evident in his 1920 paper, titled 'The psychological foundations of belief in spirits', in which he affirms that spirits are "psychic facts of which our academic wisdom refuses to take cognizance" (Jung, 1969, p. 316).[134] Hence, it appears he paradoxically views the general refusal within scientific circles to investigate the 'psychic fact' of spirits as an unscientific stance. Yet, conversely, while Jung's unique views on spirits and spirit possession may appear 'unscientific' from a conventional perspective, they potentially proffer new pathways for better understanding issues pertaining to psychiatry, metaphysics, cultural relativism, psychopathology in general, and psychosis in particular.

In stating that spirits are 'psychic facts', Jung does not mean that they are actual discarnate entities. Rather, he sees them as autonomous manifestations of the deeper psyche that influence human experience. Although he understands the psyche to be a composite of various interconnected parts, he also views these parts as being "relatively independent" phenomena that can manifest as "autonomous complexes", or 'spirits' (Jung, 1969, p. 307). Accordingly, he defines spirits as "unconscious autonomous complexes which appear as projections", and asserts that "dreams, visions, pathological hallucinations, and delusional ideas" are examples of such 'spirits' (ibid., pp. 308–309). He further explains that spirits are artefacts of the collective unconscious that manifest when "a complex of the collective unconscious becomes associated with the ego" (p. 311). In other words, a spirit 'comes into being' when a collective unconscious complex enters the ego-conscious sphere. Jung maintains that people often experience these complexes, or spirits, (in both malevolent and benevolent forms), as foreign and alien to the self and he suggests that such instances may represent a

[134] Jung's 1920 paper is reprinted in the 1969 edition of his *Collected Works (Volume 8)*.

"characteristic symptom marking the onset of many mental illnesses" (p. 312). Indeed, in terms of psychopathology, he makes the somewhat sweeping assertion that "the insane person has always enjoyed the prerogative of being the one possessed by a demon, which is, by the way, a correct rendering of his psychical condition, for he is invaded by autonomous figures and thought-forms" (Jung, 1939, p. 1007). At this level of explication, his construal of spirits is essentially congruent with the aforementioned DSM-5 notion of the 'splitting off of clusters of mental contents from conscious aware-ness' in dissociative disorders. His understanding, however, goes deeper than this to postulate generic psychic structures that are native to, and encompass, the entire cross-cultural gamut of humanity.

Like contemporary psychiatry, Jung also views cultural relativity as an important factor in discerning between healthy and psychopathological expressions of spirit possession. For instance, he explains that when such experiences are mediated within a supportive framework of cultural beliefs and practices, curative outcomes may occur whereby "the driving forces locked up in the unconscious are canalized into consciousness and form a new source of power" (Jung, 1969, p. 315). In the absence of such supportive cultural frameworks, however, he holds that the forces remain unintegrated and the situation can become psychopathological because "the collec-tive unconscious may take the place of reality" (ibid.). Jung's reference here to cultural relativity is similar to views espoused by psychiatry regarding cross-cultural diagnos-tic considerations, however, his essential understanding is markedly different from the psychiatric view. For instance, while psychiatry does not apply culture-related considerations when diagnosing mainstream Western patients, Jung's culture-related considerations apply in all instances, regardless of ethnicity. Accordingly, he under-stands spirit influence, or possession, to be a generic cross-cultural phenomenon: "I am convinced that if a European had to go through the same exercises and ceremonies which the medicine-man performs in order to make the spirits visible, he would have the same experiences" (p. 303). For Jung, then, the phenomenon of 'spirits' is univer-sal, and whether a spirit's influence has a beneficial or psychopathological outcome depends on the presence or absence of a supportive framework of cultural beliefs and practices. If an apposite support framework exists, then the spirit may be integrated into ego-consciousness. If not, then a regression into psychopathology may occur.[135]

Overall, it appears that Jung's theory on spirits and spirit possession has much to say about the possible nature of psychosis and proffers an alternative way to con-tend with the vexing issue of how to differentiate culturally normative spirit posses-sion from psychopathology. For example, building on Jung's work, Huskinson (2010, pp. 71, 85) endorses "a non-pathological diagnosis of spirit possession" approach

---

[135] Intriguingly, while Jung endorses a psychodynamic understanding of spirits, it seems he was also ambiv-alent regarding their ultimate nature. For instance, in a footnote appended to his definition of spirits as "unconscious autonomous complexes" he clarifies that "the question of whether spirits exist *within them-selves* is far from having been settled. Psychology is not concerned with things as they are 'in themselves', but only what people think about them" (Jung, 1969, p. 309, fn. 5). This statement suggests that spirits *might* exist beyond his psychological rendition of them.

whereby "spirit possession should not be evaluated according to the intensity of its presentations, but according to one's capacity to endure it". Such an approach could apply equally to understanding spirits as dissociated psychological complexes or as actual metaphysical entities. If spirits are psychic facts, as Jung proposes, then it ironically seems psychiatry is 'out of touch with reality' in failing to recognise them as such. If spirits are universal and can influence all people then it is erroneous and futile to adopt a binary diagnostic model of understanding that acknowledges the validity of non-Western cross-cultural instances of spirit possession while deeming the same to be psychopathological in a Western context. Arguably, the latter situation does not reflect the presence of mental disorder, but the lack or absence of a framework of knowledge and skills to assist people to contend and cope with psychospiritual crises. In light of this possibility, it can be hypothesised that in failing to accept the ostensible reality of spirits and to provide the requisite framework of beliefs and practices to cope with instances of spirit possession, the medical psychiatric approach may inadvertently precipitate the 'mental illness' outcomes it aims to prevent.

12.4.4 van Dusen on spirits and spirit possession

Research conducted by American clinical psychologist Wilson van Dusen during the 1960s proffers another view regarding the nature of psychosis in relation to spirits and spirit possession. Although his work reflects Jung's in some ways, it is otherwise unique and radically different. For instance, he explains that "the first step is to see that spirits and affections are the same thing", which mirrors Jung's notion of spirits as affective archetypal complexes (van Dusen, 1974, p. 112). He further adds that "it is more accurate to see them as inner ruling tendencies than to view them in their individual identities as Joe or Mary", which, like Jung, portrays spirits as unconscious aspects of the metaphysical self (ibid.). Indeed, van Dusen (p. 115) explicitly states that the view "of mind as based on the presence of spirits is not observably different from the modern dynamic theories of the nature of mind". Be this as it may, his theory of mind and spirits was formulated in researching the works of Emanuel Swedenborg,[136] whose theory of mind and views on the nature of spirits significantly differ from Jung's.

---

[136] Swedenborg (1688–1772) was an eminent scientist who dedicated his earlier life to becoming an authority in the major sciences of the day. He is described by Bucke (1901, p. 285) as "one of the great men of all time—a great thinker, a great writer, a great scientist, a great engineer". Similarly, van Dusen (1970, p. 60) notes that Swedenborg was "fluent in nine languages, wrote 150 works in 17 sciences, was an expert in at least seven crafts, was a musician, member of parliament, and a mining engineer". In his later life, he turned to the study of psychology and religion for answers to the nature of reality and it was here that he "broke through into the spiritual world" (ibid.). This entailed daily communications with spirits of many types (Jones & Fernyhough, 2008, p. 6). Appendix Seven presents an overview of Swedenborg's theory of mind. This provides an elucidation of his views regarding the interconnection between humans and spirits, which informed van Dusen's work with 'psychotic' voice hearing and spirit possession.

Swedenborg's theory of mind was adopted by van Dusen to help him better comprehend the possible nature of psychotic experiences. Taking Swedenborg's explication on the interrelationship between spirits and humans, he suggests that:

> *there is no real way of distinguishing our own potentialities and the potentialities of spirits with us* ... there is a correspondence between the spiritual worlds and the mind of man. The specific line of correspondence in the individual is through the affective spirits with him, into his affects and thence into all other levels of the mind. (p. 14)

In other words, from this perspective, while spirits have an independent existence, they are also intrinsically connected to human beings through the commonly shared medium of affective states of being, which, in turn, can interact with and influence the cognitive function of everyday human consciousness.[137] However, Swedenborg (1905 [1758], p. 230) further maintains that "these spirits have no knowledge whatever that they are with man; but when they are with him they believe that all things of his memory and thought are their own". Hence, extending this thinking in context of psychopathology, van Dusen (1974, p. 117) proposes that "man's life involves an interaction with a hierarchy of spirits. This interaction is normally not conscious, but perhaps in some cases of mental illness it has become conscious". Here, he diverges from Jung's thinking. Whereas Jung sees psychosis as the irruption of unconscious 'spirit' complexes into the conscious mind, van Dusen suggests that, in some instances, psychosis results in a 'lifting of the veil' that ordinarily conceals the connection between spirits and humans. Hence, some psychotic people can become aware of the spirits that are naturally with us, but which normally remain hidden from personal consciousness.

If this idea is given credence, it opens new lines of investigative consideration. For one, it offers another way of understanding 'spirit possession' beyond the standard view of spirits possessing humans, for it appears that spirit possession can be construed as a universal and natural phenomenon whereby humans and their spirit counterparts coexist in a perpetual and unconscious state of mutual 'possession'. Additionally, this view depicts the workings of the mind as intimately wedded with, and influenced by, psychospiritual forces and beings. Therefore, counter to the prevailing psychiatric practice of relegating psychospiritual matters to the fringes of clinical inquiry, it is possible that a better understanding of mental health and psychopathology requires an advanced knowledge about the larger psychospiritual realities of being human.

---

[137] Although van Dusen generally discusses spirits as if they are actual beings, there are instances where he speculates on this issue. For instance, he muses, "I wonder whether hallucinations, often thought of as detached pieces of the unconscious, and hallucinations as spiritual possession might not simply be two ways of describing the same process. Are they really spirits or pieces of one's own unconscious?" (van Dusen, 1970, p. 69).

12.4.4.1 van Dusen's research on spirits and psychosis

In terms of psychosis research, van Dusen used Swedenborg's theory of mind to guide a unique investigative experiment he conducted with patients regarding their 'hallucinatory' experiences. His research represents an investigative shift from a reductive psychopathology-based approach to a phenomenological approach, and his subsequent findings demonstrate the potential efficacy of the latter approach in gleaning better insights into the enigmatic nature of psychosis.

In 1964, after sixteen years in practice as a clinical psychologist with psychotic patients, van Dusen (1974, pp. 117–118) inadvertently discovered a marked correlation between patients' reported symptomatology, especially voice hearing, and Swedenborg's descriptions of spirit-human coexistence. One day, when working with "a young woman who was distressed about her love affair with an unseen lover", he decided, "just for the heck of it", to directly converse with the invisible lover via the patient, and was surprised when a response was forthcoming (van Dusen, 1981, p. 136). Over the ensuing years, he chose patients "who could distinguish between their own thoughts and the things heard and seen" (van Dusen, 1974, p. 118) as subjects for his further phenomenological research into the nature of the voices that people reported. He explains that during sessions with these people he would "hold long dialogues with a patient's hallucinations and record both my questions and their answers" (van Dusen, 1970, p. 61). This patently runs counter to standard psychiatric practice of dismissing the content of so-called hallucinations as unreal, meaningless, and incomprehensible. On this point, van Dusen (ibid.) explains that "I treat the hallucinations as realities because that is what they are to the patient". He further notes that "in no case did patients accept the term hallucinations for these experiences. The term was offensive. It implied they were not real" (van Dusen, 1981, p. 140). As discussed below, the subsequent findings of his research demonstrate the feasibility of investigating so-called psychotic symptoms to ascertain whether or not they represent psychospiritual phenomena unknown to psychiatry.

Far from being meaningless and illusory, the 'hallucinatory' voices interviewed by van Dusen demonstrated degrees of apparent cogency and agency independent from the person who was hearing them. From his documented communications with these voices he was able to produce a "roughly accurate phenomenological map" (ibid., p. 152) of a realm of spiritual entities. However, his analysis of these communications is not merely limited to what was said by the voices. If this were so, then his comparison of them with the symptoms of psychosis could rightly be dismissed as pure conjecture. In addition to the voices' content, he also noted patterns of behaviour and personality that suggested manifest types of being. Indeed, he reports that he was able to "give the Rorschach inkblot test to a patient's voices separately from the patient's own responses" (van Dusen, 1974, p. 129). The types of beings he discerned fell into two broad categories. As he explains, "in my dialogues with patients I learned of the two orders of experience, borrowing from the voices themselves, called the higher and the lower order" (van Dusen, 1970, p. 62). The key differentiating characteristics of each are listed in Table 11 below.[138]

Of particular significance for van Dusen was the marked correlation between the nature and content of the voices he recorded and the near identical appearance of the same in Swedenborg's writings. Hence, counter to psychiatry's view that spirit possession represents a cultural belief or superstition, van Dusen maintains it may possibly be a generic, pervasive, and natural psychospiritual reality.

A related and pertinent finding was that this potentially rich source of phenomenological material was not only ignored by psychiatry, but ironically, also rendered invisible by its disbelief in psychospiritual realities. It was van Dusen's (1981, p. 138) discovery that many patients consequently hid the content of their voice-hearing experiences from clinicians for fear of being diagnosed and stigmatised with a psychiatric label. However, in gaining the trust of his patients by being open-minded and dropping the usual pathologising clinical mindset, van Dusen was afforded the opportunity to make some novel observations about the possible nature of voices in

Table 11. Typology of van Dusen's higher order and lower order voices.

Higher order voices	Lower order voices
Less prevalent (about twenty per cent of cases)	Most prevalent (about eighty per cent of cases)
Benevolent, helpful, and supportive	Malevolent, wilfully destructive, and hypercritical
Respectful of a person's autonomy	Strive to control a person's will
Rarely speak	Talk endlessly
Intrinsically religious or spiritual	Highly irreligious and adverse to spiritual matters
Vocabulary and knowledge often transcendent to a person's own	Vocabulary and knowledge limited— "they cannot report more than the patient sees, hears, or remembers"
"Thinks in something like universal ideas"	Incapable of sequential reasoning
Communications possess "an almost inexpressible ring of truth"	Communications are deceitful

Source: van Dusen, 1970, pp. 62–63.

---

[138] For van Dusen's full description of the characteristics of higher and the lower order spirits, see Appendix Eight. I have placed this important material in an appendix, rather than in the main body, because it is several pages in length and is quoted verbatim. This constitutes a unique body of writing in terms of its phenomenological description of different types of spirits that may possibly explain the occurrence of various "psychotic symptoms"; especially voice hearing. The fact that this research was conducted by an experienced clinical psychologist within a mainstream mental health setting adds to its importance in that it sets potential precedence for further such investigation into possible psychospiritual determinants in voice hearing and other "psychotic" symptoms.

psychosis, an opportunity that is largely lost to mainstream psychiatry due to people hiding the phenomenological details of their experiences from disbelieving clinicians. In communicating with people's 'hallucinatory' voices he made discoveries that may be pivotal to better understanding not only the nature of 'psychotic' experiences, but also innate psychospiritual human experiences.

12.4.4.2 van Dusen on spirits and causes of psychosis

If coexistence with spirits is intrinsic to being human, then under what circumstances does such natural 'spirit possession' become psychopathological, or psychotic? This question was addressed by van Dusen in two ways. First, at a symptomatic level, he highlighted parallels between his own findings, Swedenborg's descriptions, and the descriptive material in psychiatric texts about psychotic auditory hallucinations and other reported anomalous experiences. Second, at a conceptual level, he mused on the possible psychospiritual machinations of psychosis.

In terms of the symptomatic focus, he found that lower order voices mirror typical descriptions in mainstream psychiatric literature regarding the pernicious nature of auditory hallucinations. From his dialogues with patients' voices, he noted a predominant presence of spirits that exercised a "persistent will to destroy" a person (van Dusen, 1970, p. 62). Such voices:

> tease and torment just for the fun of it ... find a weak point of conscience and work on it interminably ... call the patient every conceivable name, suggest every lewd act ... threaten death ... suggest foolish acts ... invade every nook and cranny of privacy, work on every weakness and credibility ... [and] undermine the patient's will. (ibid.)

This reflects Swedenborg's (1905 [1758], p. 185) report, from his personal experience with spirits, that a fundamental objective of malevolent spirits is to seek to break a person, for they "are such that they hold man in deadly hatred, and desire nothing so much as to destroy him both soul and body". Another commonly reported psychotic symptom is the belief that 'something' is attempting to take control of a part of a person's body. On this issue, van Dusen (1970, p. 62) observes that "the lower order can work for a long time to possess some part of the patient's body", while Swedenborg (2010a [1747–1765]) likewise describes the wish of spirits "to possess ... wherefore they also inflow with man, from the head as far as to the mouth, and to the breast—others from the feet as far as to the genitals", and that people in such states of possession sometimes "behaved like insane persons" (2010b [1749–1756]). Additionally, van Dusen (1981, p. 148) holds that spirit-induced hallucinations "were very clearly the basis for delusional ideas", an idea seemingly corroborated by Swedenborg's (2010c [1749–1756]) observation that "if spirits were to flow into man from the exterior memory, he could not think from his own memory, but only from that of the spirit". These are but a few of many examples in both van Dusen's research findings and Swedenborg's texts that closely correlate with symptoms of psychosis as identified by mainstream psychiatry. This is not to say that the works of van Dusen and Swedenborg irrevocably prove the role of spirit possession or influences in psychosis. However, they do present plausible and intriguing phenomenological possibilities that warrant further investigation.

Additionally, van Dusen considers the effect that the presence or absence of psychospiritual skills can have on psychotic outcomes. He proposes that, in contrast to the mystic's conscious and voluntary entry into psychospiritual domains, the unwitting and unprepared person can become psychotic when exposed to the same. For instance, he suggests that Swedenborg's entry into the realm of spirits was voluntary, as opposed to the involuntary experience of psychosis: "My guess is that Swedenborg systematically explored the same worlds that psychotic patients find themselves thrust into … the worlds beyond this one, inside this one" (van Dusen, 1974, pp. 135, 137). He also notes that Swedenborg warned of the considerable dangers of dabbling into these realms and strongly counselled against doing so (van Dusen, 1970, p. 65; 1974, p. 137; 1981, p. 152). From this perspective it appears that psychosis results from involuntarily breaching the barrier separating worlds where unskilled or unprepared people find themselves at sea and subject to spirit attack. Elsewhere, he compares Swedenborg's active use of yogic breathing techniques with the schizophrenic withdrawal into fantasy (van Dusen, 1970, p. 65). This suggests that Swedenborg was able to avoid insanity through the acquisition and skilled application of technologies of consciousness, in contrast to van Dusen's patients who somehow found themselves in other realms of being that they were ill-equipped to navigate. This arguably supports the idea that advanced conceptual and experiential knowledge about psychospiritual realities may help to better understand and navigate through distressing states of consciousness, be they spirit possession, spiritual emergencies, or other psychotic-like experiences.

Overall, van Dusen's research represents a landmark in psychosis research for it seems his approach has not previously been attempted by other clinicians, nor has it been replicated since. His reported findings challenge present-day psychiatry's portrayal of issues of spirit possession as a peculiar cultural-religious factor that is incidental to the bigger endeavour of identifying mainstream forms of psychopathology. Like Jung, Swedenborg saw 'spirit possession' as a natural and universal phenomenon and van Dusen's dialogues with his patients' voices appear to support this idea. *His work also suggests that psychotic experiences of spirit influences cannot be psychopathologically differentiated from culturally normative experiences of the same.* Indeed, this calls into question the veracity of psychiatry's prevailing practice of equating 'noncultural' psychospiritual experiences with psychopathology. *If psychopathology cannot be accurately delineated, then it seems prudent and justifiable to refrain from insisting on its validity and, instead, adopt a phenomenological approach to investigating and better understanding anomalous states of being and consciousness.*

12.5 Conclusion

Psychiatry fails to explain how experiences deemed intrinsically psychotic in mainstream Western contexts are deemed normative and non-psychotic in 'other' cultural contexts. How can it be, for example, that reports of spirit possession by Western patients are considered unreal and psychotic, yet are viewed as normative and non-psychotic in patients from 'other' cultures? Indeed, my investigation throughout this chapter suggests that experiencing psychospiritual realities is a natural and pancultural human capacity. This arguably calls upon psychiatry to transcend its limited materialist and cognicentric worldview to incorporate metaphysical considerations within its epistemic scope. My ensuing exploration of Tibetan Buddhist psychiatry in Chapter Thirteen exemplifies the efficacy of using a phenomenological approach to open-endedly investigate both physical and metaphysical phenomena in order to better understand psychopathology, psychosis, and the mysteries of being human.

CHAPTER 13

Tibetan Buddhist psychiatry: spirit possession and psychosis in practice

13.0 Introduction

This chapter deepens my exploration of psychosis and spirit possession within the context of Tibetan Buddhist psychiatric epistemology and practice. As a culminating challenge to Western materialist psychiatry, this provides a concrete example of a holistic model of psychiatry that understands psychosis to be essentially psychospiritual in nature and aetiology. Examining the texts of three expert commentators on Tibetan Buddhist psychiatry demonstrates the metaphysical depths to which psychosis can be understood and the therapeutic efficacy that such an understanding enables. Doing so anchors this book's driving argument that psychospiritual considerations are essential to better understanding psychotic and psychotic-like experiences.

13.1 Tibetan Buddhist psychiatry and psychopathology

Tibetan Buddhist psychiatry appears to have a deeper understanding of the nature of psychopathology than Western psychiatry. Indeed, a core focus throughout this book has been to systematically challenge the validity of Western psychiatry's psychopathology-seeking approach to understanding psychosis. I have argued and aimed to demonstrate that the proposed constellation of diagnostic criteria that constitute 'psychosis' is a tenuous construct shaped by materialist supposition and limited phenomenological observation. This does not infer that psychopathology is non-existent. Rather, I argue that the materialist approach adopted by Western psychiatry enables only a limited understanding of psychopathology due to its superficial scope of investigation. Likewise, for researchers who aim to discern psychotic from psychospiritual instances through rational and physical sense-based approaches alone. Indeed, it seems that identifying and understanding the deeper nature of psychopathology requires that clinicians and researchers have the capacity to explore metaphysical domains of reality via the use of technologies of consciousness. Indeed, it appears that while psychopathology-seeking and diagnostic differentiation are ineffectual in a *materialist model* of psychiatric practice and investigation, the effective diagnosing of psychopathology is often enabled in holistic approaches where practitioners are adept in using technologies of consciousness to explore psychospiritual domains.

As demonstrated below, throughout Section 13.3, the Tibetan Buddhist psychiatric approach exemplifies how a profound understanding of psychopathology may be gleaned through a deep phenomenological investigation of physical, psychological, and metaphysical realities. Within such a framework of understanding and practice, where psychospiritual knowledge is fundamental, practitioners are enabled to directly perceive and identify the causal roots of psychosis, and discern psychopathology from developmental psychospiritual experiences. Subsequently, Tibetan Buddhist psychiatry has a high rate of reported therapeutic efficacy. For example, Clifford (1984, p. 199) observes that "Tibetan psychiatric remedies ... are held in wide esteem by the Tibetans for their effectiveness", while Begley (1994, p. 323) similarly notes that for centuries throughout Asia the discipline "has been highly respected for its effectiveness". It is therefore feasible to suggest that Western psychiatry might gain a better understanding of psychosis, psychopathology, and human developmental potential through investigating cross-cultural psychospiritual bodies of knowledge.

13.2 Tibetan Buddhist theory of mind

Before investigating the nature of spirit possession and psychosis within Tibetan Buddhist psychiatry, it is first apposite to provide a brief overview of the theory of mind upon which the discipline is based. This provides an epistemological backdrop for my later examination of three texts concerning how Tibetan Buddhist psychiatry understands mental health and illness, and the dynamics of spirit possession in psychosis.

The Tibetan Buddhist theory of mind is vast, complex, and largely foreign to the worldview of Western materialism. Hence, it is necessary to restrict the scope of description here to key understandings. Although modern psychiatry and psychology share common ground with Buddhist psychiatry in that they are all primarily concerned with issues pertaining to mental health and dysfunction, Buddhism differs markedly in its understanding of the nature of mind. In simple terms, the Tibetan Buddhist teacher Lama Yeshe (2003, p. 75) explains that, from a Buddhist perspective, mind is understood to be composed of two interrelated aspects, "the relative and the absolute". At face value, this appears similar to the psychoanalytic view of the conscious and unconscious mind. However, the Buddhist understanding of absolute mind goes far beyond Freud's introjected unconscious material, and Jung's autonomous archetypal domain, to encompass a meaning of cosmological proportions.

Lama Yeshe (ibid.) describes the relative mind as the "dualistic" mind that "perceives and functions in the sense world". However, from a Buddhist perspective, relative mind is but the microcosmic expression of macrocosmic mind or "the absolute true nature of the mind, which is totally beyond the duality" (ibid.). Similarly, Evans-Wentz (1968, pp. 6, 12) refers to macrocosmic mind as "One Mind" or "Cosmic Consciousness", in comparison to ego mind, which is seen as the existential province of the "unenlightened man" and "illusion-based belief". One Mind is also the omnipresent source of all creation that "illuminates the innumerable myriads of finite minds" and "contains all things" (ibid., p. 10). Clifford (1984, pp. 5, 66) further maintains that the macrocosmic Mind is "the basis of all phenomena", hence, in Tibetan Buddhist psychiatry, the "entire universe is seen to be within the individual" and all illness, both physical and mental, is the product of failing to understand and mediate this mystic dimension of self. From this viewpoint, physical reality is epiphenomenal to One Mind, which is inverse to the Western psychiatric understanding that mind is epiphenomenal to physicality.

Tibetan Buddhist psychiatry, then, is fundamentally informed by the understanding that all things are interconnected within the cosmological matrix of One Mind. Further to this, Clifford (ibid., p. 151) explains that Buddhism understands the universe to be "like an immense field of electromagnetic energy" in which all things are interconnected, impermanent, in flux and, despite appearances, not solid. Rather, the entirety of existence, both physical and metaphysical, "consists of radiations of energy vibrations emitted as rays or as fields of force and at varying rates of speed and thus solidity" (ibid.). What appears to be a solid and discrete object is in fact "a dynamic manifestation of vibrations" and, correspondingly, each person is seen as "a bundle of perceptions" that are in constant flux (ibid.). Western quantum physics poses a similar theory. For instance, American physicist Harold Puthoff (2001, p. 41) contends that:

> all of us are immersed, both as living and physical beings, in an overall interpenetrating and interdependent field in ecological balance with the cosmos as a whole, and even the boundary lines between physical and 'metaphysical' would dissolve into a unitary viewpoint of the universe as a fluid, changing, energetic/informational cosmological unity.

Hence, the universal matrix of vibrational interconnectedness encompasses and contains everything from stars, to geographical landforms, to trees, to human beings, to mental states, to metaphysical beings such as spirits.

A related core concept is that of *prana*, which denotes the form and nature of the One Mind matrix of universal interconnectivity. Sri Aurobindo (2005, p. 283) describes *prana* as "the life-stuff, the substantial will and energy in the cosmos working out into determined form and action and conscious dynamis of being", and Lama Govinda (1969, p. 137) further explains that "all forces of the universe, like those of the human mind, from the highest consciousness to the depths of the subconscious, are modifications of 'prana'". According to Epstein & Topgay (1982, p. 67), while *prana* acts as a "vital force or energy that pervades the human organism", demons are also manifestations of *prana*. Hence, the human mind and demons are different manifestations of the same *pranic* energy that permeates and constitutes all phenomena.[139] As such, they are immutably interconnected. Overall, Tibetan Buddhist psychiatry sees all aspects of physical and psychospiritual reality as integrated, and integral to self, with One Mind as the omnipresent source of all creation that contains all things.

Finally, while Tibetan Buddhism understands all things to be interconnected within One Mind, it paradoxically also understands that the perception of 'self' and 'things' within corporeal reality is ultimately illusory. As Clifford (1984, p. 17) explains, the notion of "no self" is fundamental to Buddhist epistemology and reflects the ultimate understanding that "there is no independent self-entity, no self either in ourselves or in the phenomenal world around us. There is only contained experience". Indeed, she maintains that a person "strays into delusion" when perceiving his or her 'self' as being concrete and individuated (ibid.). Hence, according to this philosophical view, the idea of self as a unique 'I' is ultimately illusory. This applies not only to the idea of an individuated 'self' but also to the entirety of corporeal reality. For instance, Goddard (1938, pp. 102–103) notes that in Buddhist cosmology "all the mind's arbitrary conceptions of matter, phenomena, and of all conditioning factors and all conceptions and ideas relating thereto are like a dream, a phantasm … the phenomena of the physical appearance is wholly illusion". It therefore follows that normal ego function, which Western psychiatry understands to be 'mental health', is ultimately seen as a delusory form of 'mental illness' from a Tibetan Buddhist psychiatric perspective.

On this point, Lama Yeshe (2003, p. 38) holds that because "our mistaken perception processes the information supplied by our five senses and transmits incorrect information to our mind" the consequent outcome is that "most of the time we are hallucinating, not seeing the true nature of things". He understands this to be a form of mental illness and further explains:

> By mental illness I mean the kind of mind that does not see reality … In the West, you wouldn't consider this to be mental illness, but Western psychology's interpretation is too narrow. If someone is obviously emotionally disturbed, you consider that to be a problem, but if someone has a fundamental inability to see reality, to understand his or her own true nature, you don't. Not knowing your own basic mental attitude is a huge problem.

According to Evans-Wentz (1968, p. 11), the ultimate state of reality-based mental health is achieved when "the microcosmic becomes one with the macrocosmic" within a person. In other words, "realization of the One Mind, through introspectively attaining understanding of the nature of its macroscopic aspect innate in man, is equivalent to the attainment of the … Full Awakening of Buddhahood" (ibid., p. 12). Therefore, optimal mental health is achieved with mystical Enlightenment, part of which

---

[139] The notion of *prana* is further discussed in Section 13.3.1 in the context of spirit possession and psychosis.

includes becoming aware that the seeming separateness of things, and the experience of the individuated 'I', (which are both born of dualistic thinking), are illusory and out of touch with ultimate One Mind reality.

This has major ramifications for Western psychiatry's practice of diagnostically discerning 'mental illness' from 'mental health' because both are delusional from a Tibetan psychiatric framework of understanding. Such an idea essentially undermines the Western notion of 'psychopathology', for what differentiates the delusional nature of ego normality from psychotic delusional states? The depiction of corporeal reality as being ultimately 'unreal' is a repeated theme throughout mystic literature and fundamentally challenges conventional psychiatric thinking about psychopathology. The ensuing investigation of Tibetan Buddhist psychiatry and spirit possession demonstrates how a deep psychospiritual understanding of the nature of reality enables greater insight into the nature of the human condition as a whole.

13.3 Tibetan Buddhist psychiatry and spirit possession

The Tibetan Buddhist understanding of spirit possession is complex and comprises a sophisticated body of knowledge regarding the nature of spirits, or demons, and their deleterious effects on the human condition. The scope of their influence in human life extends far beyond the Western psychiatric depiction of them as idiosyncratic cultural norms and beliefs. For instance, Clifford (1984, p. 148) explains that, from a Tibetan psychiatric perspective, demons:

- "represent a wide range of forces and emotions which are normally beyond our conscious control";
- "prevent well-being and spiritual development";
- "are outer and inner factors";
- "can include such 'demons' as laziness, lust, bad companions, dualistic thinking, hypersensitivity, increased emotionality, attachment to wealth, sectarianism, spiritual pride, and clinging to tranquillity".

Hence, unlike Western psychiatry which refutes the existence of spirits, Tibetan Buddhist psychiatry sees spirits as having a pervasive impact on human life personally, interpersonally, socially, and globally. This includes matters common and normal to Western secular society, such as attachment to wealth, indulging ego desires and appetites, and sectarianism. Intriguingly, Tibetan Buddhist psychiatry also views 'dualistic thinking' as a form of demon, presumably because it is a function of relative mind that is inherently prone to misconstruing the nature of reality due to its limited scope of cognition and perception. From this perspective, Western medical psychiatry, which is grounded in dualistic thinking, might be seen as the product of demon or spirit influence.

What, then, is the nature of these demons? There are differing views amongst commentators about whether the 'demons' of Tibetan Buddhist psychiatry are actual entities or symbolic psychological projections. According to Deane (2014, p. 448), translators have generally represented the Tibetan psychiatric worldview in Western psychological terms to establish mutual grounds of understanding. For instance, Clifford (1984, p. 149) maintains that the notion of 'demon' symbolically represents that which is "primarily a psychological phenomenon associated with the multitude of mental and emotional obscurations", while, in psychoanalytical terms, she holds that "these demons are in the role of the id trying to obstruct the super-ego's higher promptings". In regards to psychopathology, she further explains that "in the pre-Freudian terms of Tibet, 'demons' and 'devils' are appropriate names for the forces of life and emotion that can drive the mind insane" (ibid., p. 150). However, Deane (2014, p. 448) questions the veracity of this psychological interpretation for, in her view, it misrepresents the belief by many Tibetan Buddhist practitioners that demons are "entities in their own right ... who had the ability to cause harm in the form of psychiatric or other illnesses". She sees Clifford's psychological translation of 'demon' as a compromise, as most Western professionals would be unable to accept them as actual beings. However, according to Clifford (1984, p. 129), her extensive experience with Tibetan Buddhist psychiatrists reveals that, while the general Tibetan population believe spirits to be real, "learned Tibetans" understand the term 'demons' to symbolically represent the deeper psychospiritual dynamics of human existence. From another perspective, Plakun (2008, p. 422) takes the middle ground in suggesting "there may ultimately be little difference between the views". This seems to infer that unconscious psychological projections and demons may be essentially the same.

My investigation throughout the remainder of this chapter delves deeper into the nature of demons and of spirit possession in psychosis by examining the views of three leading commentators on Tibetan Buddhist psychiatry epistemology. This provides an explication of key concepts and terms in Tibetan Buddhist psychiatry that are integral to understanding psychotic experience and spirit possession. These authors and their works are:

1. Epstein & Topgay's (1982) description of the interplay between *prana* and *rlung*;
2. Burang's (1974) consideration of the impact of *skandhas*; and
3. Clifford's (1984) description of *gdon* (demons) and their relation to madness.

It is beyond the scope of this investigation, however, to elaborate on the complex array of related factors within the multidimensional matrix of Tibetan medicine. Still, my limited undertaking here demonstrates how a sophisticated phenomenological knowledge of psychospiritual matters can lead to better understanding psychosis and to informing effective psychiatric therapeutic practices, beyond that which is possible within the Western materialist model of psychiatry.

13.3.1 Tibetan Buddhist psychiatry and spirit possession in psychosis (Epstein & Topgay, 1982)

Epstein & Topgay (1982) provide an explication of the causal role of spirit possession in madness across a spectrum of dynamics ranging from specific to universal. Their views are drawn from analysing a key fourth-century Tibetan medical text titled *rGyud-nShi*, which includes a section on "nervous and mental disease" (ibid., p. 69). Central to this explication is Tibetan Buddhist psychiatry's concept of '*rlung*'. According to Epstein & Topgay (p. 71), "in order to understand mental illness from the Tibetan point of view, an understanding of the nature, properties, and functions of *rlung* is essential". Fundamentally, the term '*rlung*' denotes the movement and flux of *prana* (p. 69). In other words, *rlung* is to *prana* what currents are to the ocean. At a macrocosmic level, *rlung*-action operates throughout the entire universe. However, it also operates microcosmically within the body-psyche complex of each person. In terms of the latter, consciousness "is carried by the currents of *rlung* as it changes its object moment to moment" (p. 71), hence, the faculties of human cognition are essentially dependent on the underlying presence of this psychospiritual force. Indeed, Tibetan Buddhist psychiatry sees the human mind as "inseparably linked to the body through the medium of *rlung*", and mental disorder or illness is the result of distortion or disturbance of *rlung* (p. 72). Finally, *rlung* manifests in five interconnected currents of varying solidity, ranging from physical to ethereal (p. 71). Of these five currents, the life-sustaining or life-bearing current, known as sok-*rlung*, operates "as the basis of conceptual consciousness" and is chiefly related to mental disorders and spirit possession (pp. 72, 76–77). Hence, it appears that through the application of technologies of consciousness that are little understood by Western psychiatry, Tibetan Buddhist practitioners have been able to identify subtle psychospiritual dynamics that can cause mental disorders.

Furthermore, Tibetan Buddhist psychiatry understands that mental disorders resulting from sok-*rlung* disturbances are ultimately precipitated by the detrimental influence of spirits (p. 76). As Epstein & Topgay (p. 77) explain, "Tibetan conceptions of psychopathology see spirit possession as an activating condition of psychosis". However, harmful spirit incursion is itself enabled by "predisposing causes" such as negative mental states and poor lifestyle choices (p. 76). More specifically, "psychosis is said to result when the space or channel containing the subtle life-bearing *prana* is forcefully entered by another energy, usually a spirit … disturbing the relationship between *pranic* flow and mind" (ibid.). Upon entry into the *pranic* body the invading spirit is understood to form a blockage, therefore "occluding or reversing the current of *prana* upon which the mind rests. Thus, control over the functioning of mental process is lost, with loss of memory and hysterical behavior proceeding to full-fledged psychosis" (p. 77). The authors further explain that "the spirit forcefully enters the site of the life-bearing current, dis-localizing it and functioning itself in that space", which consequently initiates an internal power struggle:

> This is akin to 'two people forcefully living together in the one room'; when one becomes more powerful, the other loses control and struggle becomes commonplace. No longer does the affected person's mind bear its original nature, but that individual has not totally lost his mind either. (ibid.)

Interestingly, the struggle described here mirrors reports by psychotic individuals in Western society who claim they are under attack by invisible alien forces that seek to control their minds and bodies. It is also markedly similar to Bleuler's (1950, p. 9) portrayal of schizophrenia as a "clear-cut splitting of the psychic functions" and Jung's (1939, p. 1004) picture of psychosis as "a psyche at war with itself". In the Tibetan instance, however, the identified cause is a subtle psychospiritual agent in the form of a possessing spirit.

Arguably, then, the understanding that psychosis results from the seat of consciousness being disrupted, blocked, or controlled by attacking spirits, suggests that the 'delusional' belief of many psychotic people about being possessed by spirits may, in fact, reflect reality. Indeed, Epstein & Topgay (1982, p. 77) claim that "those spirits that cause psychosis come primarily from the realm of hungry ghosts",[140] which are driven by malevolent and negative inclinations and are "sometimes attracted to humans predisposed to their influence". While the standard Western psychiatric response to such instances is to attempt to quell the 'delusional' beliefs with medication, the Tibetan psychiatric response is to use a holistic array of remedial methods to restore balance and to remove the possessing entity (ibid., p. 76). In Tibetan Buddhist psychiatry, then, the clinical scope for identifying psychosis is not limited to simply noting physically observable signs and symptoms, but extends into metaphysical domains that are ostensibly the causal source of such disruptions. This raises the following questions. If spirit possession (however it is understood), is a primary causal agent in psychotic episodes, are biological treatments, such as antipsychotic medications, the optimal therapeutic approach? If psychospiritual dynamics are the basic causal determinants in psychosis, do such medications have any curative effect at all?

13.3.2 Tibetan Buddhist psychiatry and spirit possession in psychosis (Burang, 1974)

Examining the work of Burang (1974) offers further insight into psychosis and spirit possession within a Tibetan Buddhist framework of understanding. After spending many years learning the Tibetan language and studying Tibetan medicine and psychiatry,[141] Burang (1974, p. ix) concludes that "in contrast to the standpoint of Western research, it acquaints us with unusual spiritual foundations ... and often displays a masterful observation of nature". As such, he depicts Tibetan Buddhist psychiatry as a therapeutic discipline based on robust phenomenological observation and a subsequent deep psychospiritual understanding of the nature of human mental health and disturbances. Burang's examination of the ancient Indian notion of *skandhas*, which Tibetan psychiatry has adopted, offers further elucidation on the role of spirit possession in psychosis.

---

[140] According to Epstein & Topgay, (1982, p. 77), hungry ghosts represent one of the six realms of Tibetan cosmology. Groves (2014, p. 987) explains that "the hungry ghost realm is described as a state of intense and unsatisfied craving".

[141] Clifford (1984, p. 10) claims that, to her knowledge, Burang is the "only Westerner to have examined the whole range of Tibetan psychiatric treatment first-hand in Tibet".

As explained above in Section 13.2, Tibetan Buddhist philosophy understands the seemingly real sense of self to actually be a composite "bundle of perceptions" (Clifford, 1984, p. 151). Further to this, Burang (1974, p. 89) explains that, within Indian and Tibetan cosmology, "man is considered to be an aggregate of 'vehicles' (*skandhas* in ancient Indian philosophy and *pung-po* in the Tibetan)". In other words, he depicts *skandhas* as 'vehicles', or modalities of life-stuff, that coalesce to form the corporeal experience of being human. He notes that Tibetan physicians "devote detailed description and speculation to the various vehicles of the aggregate", and that "after death, these vehicles or component parts of man are dismantled by varying degrees according to set laws" (ibid., pp. 89–90). Descriptions by other authors help to elucidate the notion of *skandhas*. For example, Clifford (1984, p. 17) explains that there are five *skandhas*, each of which represents a composite part of a person's whole "conditioned experience". She describes these as:

> the five aggregates or psycho-physical groupings ... [which are] form, feeling, perception, concept, and consciousness. The first three are instinctual processes; the last two are volitional. It is the dynamic interplay of these five rather than a permanent ontological self that describes the ego-sense. (ibid.)

Furthermore, in a broad context, Lama Govinda (1969, p. 70) describes *skandhas* as a composite of "the individual's active and reactive functions of consciousness in the sequence of their increasing density or 'materiality' and in proportion to their increasing subtlety, de-materialization, mobility, and spiritualization". Hence, that which a person experiences as an individuated 'I-self' is actually a no-self aggregate of *skandhas*.

Burang also discusses the notion of *skandhas* in the context of psychotic experience. For example, he explains that psychosis can occur when the influence of "interfering vehicles" results in "a discordant interaction of vehicles in the vehicle aggregate of man", which, in turn, can precipitate "a displacement of layers of personality of which the integrated self is normally composed", and consequently lead to "changes of consciousness" for the afflicted person (Burang, 1974, p. 90). More specifically, he maintains that such disruption and dysfunction within the body of *skandhas* can lead to "the kind of split in consciousness which the Western psychiatrist encounters in schizophrenia" (ibid.). Such instances, then, whereby interfering vehicles detrimentally affect the integrity of *skandhas*, constitute the precipitation of psychosis by spirit possession.

Burang's exposition on spirit possession is similar to Epstein & Topgay's, though couched in different terminology. While Epstein & Topgay (1982, p. 73) refer to spirits as "external forces", Burang depicts them as 'vehicles'. For instance, he explains that spirit possession occurs as "the occupation of component parts of the personality by vehicles from the outside" (Burang, 1974, p. 91). These occupying 'vehicles' are the demons of Tibetan cosmology, which he intriguingly describes as "psychic fields of force, either natural or contrived" (ibid., p. 92). It appears, here, that he understands possessing spirits may be both ontological (natural) or psychological (contrived) in nature. Indeed, his other descriptions support this idea. For example, he describes spirit-vehicles stemming from "the decaying vehicle aggregate of dead people", which seems to suggest that, after death, the aggregate of *skandhas* that comprise an embodied person disintegrate into separate 'vehicles' or independent post-mortem spirits. However, he also depicts spirit-vehicles in a psychological context in that they "owe their origin either to an act of will exercised by a malicious person, or to consciously or unconsciously transmitted thought forms" (ibid.). Therefore, in terms of the question regarding whether spirits are psychological or ontological, it appears from Burang's understanding that they can manifest in both forms.

Overall, Burang's introduction to the Tibetan Buddhist domain of psychiatric knowledge and practice is illuminating. He provides insight into a highly complex field of psychiatry that is informed by deep psychospiritual knowledge and which, in turn, enables effective therapeutic interventions for people afflicted by psychosis and spirit possession. Indeed, according to Burang (p. 89), "the success rate of Tibetan methods in the treatment of mental illness is remarkable". Such therapeutic efficacy seems to give credence to the understanding within Tibetan Buddhist psychiatry that psychosis largely reflects the presence of possessing spirits.

13.3.3 Tibetan Buddhist psychiatry and spirit possession in psychosis (Clifford, 1984)

An examination of Clifford's appraisal of Tibetan Buddhist psychiatry demonstrates that it is possible for the discipline to operate via a model of understanding that incorporates physical, psychosocial, and metaphysical considerations into its epistemology. However, in contrast to the materialist medical approach of Western psychiatry, which is fundamentally concerned with understanding, identifying, and treating reified forms of psychopathology, the initial concern within Tibetan Buddhist psychiatry is to understand the ultimate psychospiritual nature of mental health, for in its purview all forms of mental illness stem from a failure to do so. Within this epistemological framework, psychospiritual factors are understood to have causal primacy in mental illness. For instance, Clifford (1984, p. 170) notes that when "we no longer act and think in a manner which is harmonious with our deepest coherence of being … we become insane, self-destructive, not really ourselves" and consequently open to spirit attack. Similarly, she argues that "we think we can hide from our spiritual deformity, since it is not immediately visible, but we can't. It eats away at us and creates mental and physical disease" (ibid., p. 156). In other words, mental illness is present to the degree a person is experientially estranged from his or her ultimate spiritual nature.

Another intriguing and related idea inherent to the Tibetan Buddhist psychiatric worldview is that mental health and illness are states of being that stem from the same psychospiritual source, whereby the former epitomises the ability to realise the reality of one's ultimate nature, and the latter represents varying degrees of the inability to do so. This is evident in Clifford's (p. 251) observation that, from the perspective of

Tibetan psychiatry, "insanity and spiritual advancement are the two possibilities that follow from insight into reality". Further to this she affirms:

> Herein lies the crucial point. The psychological basis of insanity is the same basis for enlightenment. It all depends on whether or not it is accepted and comprehended and ultimately worked with as the key to liberation. If it is not, it becomes … the cause of denial, repression, and, ultimately, mental illness. (pp. 138–139)

This reflects the idea I previously discussed,[142] whereby an outcome of madness or enhanced psychospiritual development is dependent on whether or not a person has acquired the requisite knowledge and skills to navigate the stormy seas of metaphysical realities. Psychosis, from this perspective, is fundamentally a psychospiritual problem by nature.

Clifford also provides an appraisal of the human psyche and psychosis in relation to the phenomenon of sok-*r*lung. To reiterate, Epstein & Topgay (1982, p. 74) refer to sok-*r*lung as the "life-bearing current". Clifford (1984, p. 132), however, refers to "sok-lung" as "life-wind", which is "the main support of consciousness" and, therefore, is intrinsic to mental function in both its healthy and psychopathological manifestations. She further notes that this "very subtle life-force" is subliminally seated in the heart region and that "disturbed consciousness, neurosis and psychosis" may result if it is disrupted (ibid., pp. 132, 138). (See Figure 5 for a Tibetan diagram showing the 'madness' location in the heart.)

Indeed, other commentators have also identified the heart as the subliminal seat of madness. For instance, Epstein & Topgay (1982, p. 76) note that the seat of the life-bearing current is in the heart region and that mental disturbances and psychosis originate in this area. In the context of kundalini research, Louchakova & Warner (2003, p. 139) explain that "the left side of the chest, which houses the anatomical heart, also is said to contain the center of cosmic, supramental consciousness". In her subsequent research of "spiritual systems such as Hesychasm, Vedanta, Shakta–Vedanta and Sufism", Louchakova (2005, pp. 87, 100, 105) reports that meditating participants were warned to not focus on the left side of the chest "to avoid the rapid opening of subconscious material" and the possible precipitation of psychotic-like instances of spiritual emergency.

In terms of causal factors in psychosis, Clifford (1984, p. 135) explains that the original disruption "is bought on by" any one, or combination, of a variety of psychosocial stressors, and she proffers several descriptions of consequent experiences that are very similar to Western psychiatric descriptions of psychotic symptoms. For example, when this subtle seat of consciousness is destabilised:

- "The mind power of the individual begins to disintegrate and hallucinations and all sorts of distortions in perception of reality arise" (p. 133);

---

[142] For example, see Chapter Nine, Section 9.3.6, and Chapter Twelve, Section 12.3.

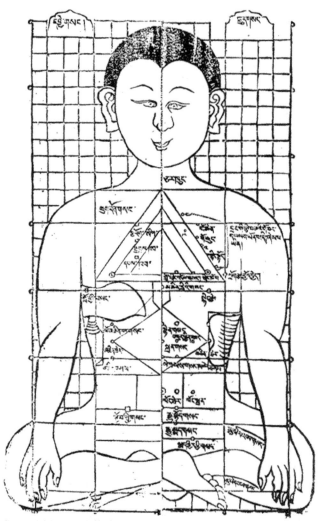

Figure 22 The front half of a medical chart from *An Illustrated Tibeto-Mongolian Materia Medica* (it is actually two folios aligned together). It shows the location of the "secret" points used to treat various diseases through moxibustion, acupuncture, etc. The triangle in the chest describes the heart center where the control of consciousness is said to reside. Just above the corner of the triangle on the viewer's right is the point for "madness made by the life-vein."

Figure 5. Tibetan illustration showing 'madness' centre in the heart.
Source: Clifford, 1984, p. 134.

- "There is a constant cycle between elation and depression, continuous changes back and forth in mood. If left untreated, it can develop into psychosis" (p. 135);
- "When the very subtle life-force supporting consciousness is out of place, then the consciousness which the person experiences feels 'wrong' or 'alien', which could give rise to the sense of being possessed by an outside force" (ibid.).

Further to this last point, she explains that such disruption can also create a gateway for possessing spirits which "are said to enter through various channels and make their way to the heart where they take over consciousness" (ibid.). This offers potential insight into the nature of psychotic hallucinations, delusions, depression, manic states, and beliefs regarding spirit possession, which Western psychiatry has generally construed as being essentially incomprehensible.

Clifford also explains that In Tibetan Buddhist psychiatry there are five chief causes of insanity. These are: "karma; grief-worry; humoral (organic) imbalance; poison (organic); and 'evil spirits'" (p. 137). Demons, or spirits, that are specific to causing mental illness are known as "*gdon*" (p. 148), which etymologically infers "to cause to come forth, to drive forth" (p. 150). Thus, in the context of causing mental illness, *gdon* generically refers to "those beings and forces that radiate negative effects" (p. 151). In sum, the Tibetan psychiatric system recognises 1,080 different types of *gdon*, which are divided into various subcategories (pp. 154–155).[143] Within this psychiatric framework of understanding there are also eighteen types of "elemental spirits" (known as *'byung-po'i gdon*) which represent "eighteen varieties of psychoses" (p. 176). These *'byung-po'i gdon* are derivative counterparts of the "five great elements"; namely, "earth, fire, water, air, and space", which are the "sub-atomic cosmic-physical principals" that operate collectively to form all corporeal reality (pp. 17, 251). Clifford (p. 195) notes the marked similarity between symptoms resulting from *'byung-po'i gdon* possession and classic symptoms of DSM-II psychoses, and maintains that such spirit possession results in "the sudden onset of behavior of a consistently alien nature … [which] suggest schizophrenia and manic depressive psychosis". Examples of such symptoms are: pronounced religious ideation; "unpredictable giggling, silly and regressive behavior and mannerisms"; manic speech and behaviour; garbled speech; beliefs in external forces of control; and difficulty in discerning one's own thoughts from alien thoughts (pp. 195–196). Hence, while Tibetan Buddhist and Western psychiatry share common ground in regards to psychotic symptomatology, they very much differ in their respective views as to the ultimate cause of such anomalies.

Clifford also addresses the question as to whether spirits are psychological or ontological by nature. For instance, she states that spirits "span a large range from the purely psychological—our own demons so to speak—to the cosmic forces which attack us in accordance with larger laws of karma" (p. 170). Thus, they are manifold, multivariate, and may manifest as both psycho-personal and cosmic-transpersonal forms and forces. She further explains that while spirits can be seen in the psychological sense as "ego-alien unconscious material and impulses that are projected as destructive forces that are perceived as an outer form which then possess us" (p. 152), she clarifies that they cannot be "regarded simply as projections of an unhealthy

---

[143] The descriptive material pertaining to these subcategories of *gdon* is detailed and complex and goes beyond the general focus of the investigation here. It does, however, provide further insight into the sophisticated intricacy of the Tibetan Buddhist model of psychiatric understanding. (See Clifford, 1984, pp. 154–195.)

mind" (p. 159). By this she means that "although they arose from projections, they are said to be real in a relative sense. That is, they have to be dealt with" (ibid.). Indeed, she emphasises that Tibetan lamas "refuse to relate to demons only as psychological phenomena in the Western sense", for they see such simplistic interpretations as lacking a deeper understanding of the ultimate paradoxical nature of reality, and as "typical of the materialist habits of modern man" (p. 162). Regardless of their actual nature, in the relative world spirits still represent "invisible negative forces and ... their negative effects are very much to be reckoned with" (ibid.). In this sense, they are seen as having autonomous ontology, even if psychological projections. It is therefore possible that spirits are neither psychological nor ontological, but psycho-ontological.

On the other hand, Tibetan Buddhist psychiatry paradoxically maintains that spirits ultimately do not exist at all. As Clifford (p. 161) notes, ultimately, within a Buddhist cosmological perspective, spirits "do not exist. Like everything else they have no self-nature. They are in fact empty". In order to help clarify this seeming contradiction, Clifford (ibid.) likens the belief in spirits (and all seemingly 'real' manifestations born of subject-object perception), to the experience of dreaming: "The dreams are not true, but they feel true when we are in them. All samsara ... is like this; ghosts are the same" (p. 159).[144] From this viewpoint, Tibetan lamas and spiritual practitioners understand that in "approaching ghosts and spirits from the level of absolute truth, we realize the nature of emptiness, theirs and ours, so nothing can harm us ... all sickness and negativity is subdued or dissolved. These distinctions simply do not exist" (p. 161). In this sense, while spirits exist in a relative sense, they do not in an absolute sense. The same applies to all physical and metaphysical phenomena.

This broad framework of understanding seemingly enables Tibetan Buddhist psychiatry to transcend the epistemological parameters of materialism and dualism that limit the thinking and practice of Western medical psychiatry. Whereas Western

---

[144] Clifford (1984, p. 19) does not directly define the term 'samsara', but infers its meaning in stating that "the source of all painful, conditioned phenomenal existence, samsara, is our acting in a state of not-seeing". Capriles (1990) also proffers an insightful elucidation on this Tibetan philosophical understanding:

> Tibetan spiritual systems regard as delusive, *both* the every day experience of human beings *and* the «supernatural» experience to which practitioners gain access by yogic and shamanistic means. This is not to say that both realms of experience are considered to be merely hallucinatory. Tibetan Teachings acknowledge that there is a *given* that, upon being processed by our mental processes, is experienced as the world in which we live, with its countless entities. Delusion arises when we are unable to see that entities do not have inherent, absolute existence, but depend both on the existence of other entities and on the functioning of our mental process in order to exist in the way they exist for us. Thus, delusion is a confusion about the mode of existence of entities, including the human subject: when we believe that ourselves and other entities exist inherently and substantially (in the sense of being self-existent and not needing anything other to itself in order to exist), that the relative is absolute, we are under delusion.

Thus, it appears the term 'samsara' infers the ultimately 'delusory' nature of normal human cognition, perception and existence.

psychiatry largely endorses a biomedical understanding of psychosis that splits mind from body and proscribes the consideration of possible psychospiritual determinants, Tibetan Buddhist psychiatry has a holistic understanding of psychosis that enables the dialectical integration of metaphysical and materialist factors. For instance, Clifford (p. 251) explains that when the 'byung-po'i gdon (i.e., elemental spirits) are excessively disrupted by mental-emotional stressors "then this can be interpreted as a disturbance of the basic biochemical ground that subsequently gives rise to eighteen basic divisions of perceptual distortions and disturbed consciousness". In other words, this portrays psychosis as the product of a disruptive interplay between mental-emotional states, spirits, and biochemistry. Hence, whereas a Western psychiatrist may see psychosis as caused by a biochemical brain imbalance, a Tibetan psychiatrist may see imbalanced brain biochemistry in psychosis as the product of elemental spirits being overly disrupted by mental-emotional stressors. While the former represents a materialist view stripped of psychological and psychospiritual determinants, the latter represents the holistic consideration of physical, psychological, and psychospiritual determinants. As such, Tibetan psychiatry demonstrates the possibility of better understanding psychosis via a holistic epistemological framework in which medical science and metaphysics, biochemistry and spirit possession, are seen as complementary aspects of a dynamic psychiatric whole.

Finally, while I have challenged the validity of Western psychiatry's practice of psychopathology-seeking throughout this book, the example set by Tibetan psychiatry suggests that it is not psychopathology-seeking per se that is problematic, but the way in which it is approached. For instance, the Tibetan psychiatric approach to psychopathology-seeking is holistic, heuristic, phenomenological, fundamentally inclusive of psychospiritual matters, and orchestrated by practitioners who are adept in using technologies of consciousness. Arguably, this investigative approach enables a profound understanding of the nature and multidimensional causes of psychopathology and correspondingly enables a practitioner to discern accurately between psychotic and psychotic-like psychospiritual developmental processes. Such open-ended investigation evidently leads to an advanced understanding of psychopathology. In contrast, Western psychiatric psychopathology-seeking is orchestrated through materialist, reductive, and cognicentric approaches that proscribe the investigation of psychospiritual matters that are seemingly essential to understanding the holistic nature of psychopathology. In addition, a lack of skills and knowledge regarding technologies of consciousness seemingly makes it impossible for Western practitioners to discern the characteristic diagnostic features of psychosis from identical features occurring in healthy cross-cultural and psychospiritual developmental contexts. This psychopathology-seeking approach arguably produces a narrow and ambiguous understanding of psychopathology and creates the many conundrums examined throughout this book. Indeed, it ultimately seems that the degree to which a therapeutic discipline can understand psychopathology and psychosis is proportionate to the degree that psychospiritual knowledge and skills are incorporated.

13.4 Conclusion

As a holistic discipline, Tibetan Buddhist psychiatry demonstrates the therapeutic efficacy of incorporating physical, psychosocial, and psychospiritual considerations into clinical thinking and practice. The integral influence of spirits in human health and wellbeing underpins the Tibetan understanding of psychopathology, and psychosis is essentially understood to be a disorder of psychospiritual aetiology. Intriguingly, despite my systematic challenge to Western psychiatry's psychopathology-seeking approach throughout this book, Tibetan Buddhist psychiatry exemplifies the ultimate clinical capacity to discern psychotic from psychospiritual experiences, but only when a deep and open-ended investigation of phenomena across the physical-metaphysical spectrum has been undertaken via the use of technologies of consciousness.

CHAPTER 14

Bringing it all together

14.0 Reiteration of core process and objectives

In response to psychiatry's limited and limiting depiction of psychosis as a fundamentally incomprehensible and biogenic form of psychopathology, this book has posed and engaged the research question: Can, and how can, psychosis be better understood by employing a phenomenological approach that includes psychospiritual considerations within its investigative ambit? As such, it has undertaken the joint task of drawing on psychospiritual considerations to glean a better understanding of psychosis, while challenging the materialist-based limitations of medical psychiatry. Accordingly, I have not aimed to definitively identify what psychosis is, but have embarked upon a heuristic investigative process to elicit a better understanding of psychosis than that proffered by mainstream psychiatry. This has entailed using four focal settings to systematically step beyond the epistemological borders of materialism and examine possible psychospiritual determinants in psychotic experience, which are customarily eschewed by psychiatry. Each of these focal settings represents a different conceptual framework of investigation for better understanding psychosis in light of psychopathological and psychospiritual matters. Hence, my scope of investigation has ranged across materialist and metaphysical domains of understanding with the aim to make more comprehensible that which has been deemed fundamentally incomprehensible. While traditional psychiatry has reductively construed psychosis as a discrete mental disorder (i.e., psychosis as a psychopathological entity that is clinically identifiable by characteristic symptoms), my open-ended approach has progressively opened new potential

247

investigative pathways for better understanding this enigmatic phenomenon, especially in the context of psychospiritual considerations.

Throughout this book I have aimed to demonstrate that a heuristic and phenomenological research approach can work to:

1. Challenge some fundamental psychiatric assumptions that underpin and limit the conceptualisation of psychosis.
2. Extend the parameters of perceived reality and knowledge formulation beyond the restrictive bounds of medical materialism to include psychospiritual reality.
3. Show that this broadened conceptualisation of reality, if adopted by psychiatry, can result in better understanding the nature of psychosis.
4. Set the stage for establishing new possible psychosis research pathways that fundamentally include psychospiritual considerations.

This book's content upholds my contention that the materialist-based and prescriptive model of psychiatric diagnostics limits the epistemological scope for understanding psychosis and essentially bars the inclusion of psychospiritual matters within clinical research and practice. Accordingly, I have demonstrated how a phenomenological investigative approach can reveal new possible ways for better understanding both psychotic and transpersonal states of human consciousness. Indeed, psychiatry's claim that psychosis is essentially incomprehensible seems, ironically, to say more about its own limited materialist outlook than it says about the nature of psychosis per se.

14.1 Key findings in better understanding psychosis

The systematic process of critical investigation throughout this book shows that the psychiatric term 'psychosis' has been imbued with a purely psychopathological meaning that represents a narrow understanding of this enigmatic phenomenon. Yet, even this narrow depiction is questionable, because the psychopathological nature and concrete existence of psychosis have not been scientifically or conceptually substantiated. Indeed, I have shown that, upon close examination, none of the key psychiatric criteria for defining and diagnosing psychosis are definitive. It therefore appears that psychosis is not indubitably psychopathological, as asserted by psychiatry, but is a term that represents a provisional and ambiguous construct of assumed psychopathology.

This critical view allows increased scope for better understanding psychosis, beyond the rigid conceptual strictures inherent to psychiatry's construal of the term. My use of the phrase 'better understanding psychosis' does not connote doing so in absolute terms, but in the relative sense of establishing a broader investigative scope through which many previously obscured dynamics and meanings of psychotic experience are revealed. As summarised below, my overall research process elicits and reveals several significant ways in which so-called 'psychosis' may be better understood beyond psychiatry's limited and materialist epistemic horizons.

14.1.1 Psychosis as comprehensible

The purported incomprehensibility of psychosis largely appears to reflect limitations set by psychiatry as to what is and is not primary reality. If psychological and cultural considerations in psychosis research are deemed epiphenomenal to physical causes, and metaphysical matters are deemed non-existent, then the ultimate scope of understanding is restricted to that which can be scientifically observed, measured, and explained. From this perspective, psychosis is largely incomprehensible. However, as is clearly demonstrated throughout this book, extending the scope of investigation to include psychospiritual and cross-cultural considerations reveals many ways of understanding psychosis and psychotic symptoms previously eclipsed by a biogenic research focus. Ultimately, psychosis is far more comprehensible when examined holistically.

14.1.2 Psychosis as having psychospiritual determinants

This book demonstrates that the consideration of psychospiritual matters appears to have significant relevance in better understanding the nature of psychosis. Indeed, the findings throughout indicate that such research is highly warranted. For instance, further investigation into Laing's theoretical phenomenon of ontological insecurity may lead to better comprehending unknown domains and dynamics of the deeper human psyche, from which psychotic and psychospiritual experiences ostensibly emerge. Likewise, a better understanding of psychospiritual determinants in psychosis may result from exploring Jung's idea of the transcendent function, Laing's metanoia, and the Grofs' transpersonal notion of spiritual emergence and emergencies. Psychiatry may also benefit from a close investigation of the multifarious global mix of cultural knowledge systems. For example, commentators on both the Zen Buddhist notion of 'nen' and the Tibetan Buddhist notion of 'sok-*r*lung' proffer sophisticated phenomenological explications as to how psychospiritual factors and forces operate to constitute psychotic behaviour and experience. Similarly, my detailed examination of the phenomenon of spirit possession reveals ways in which reality can be understood beyond materialism and how these may work to precipitate or influence psychotic experiences.

14.1.3 Psychosis as not necessarily psychopathological

An implicit aim of my employing a heuristic research approach has been to challenge the reductive psychiatric construal of psychosis as a psychopathological entity. There is considerable evidence to support this undertaking. My research indicates that *all* of the key diagnostic markers which define psychosis as a psychopathological disorder may also occur in culturally normative and non-psychopathological psychospiritual instances. This seriously undermines psychiatry's assumption that psychosis is fundamentally a form of mental illness. Efforts to differentiate psychotic from non-psychotic psychospiritual experiences have seemingly also failed. Indeed, the two types of experience may be coexistent and ultimately indistinguishable. There-fore, it appears the psychiatric practice of psychopathology-seeking represents and perpetuates a poor understanding of psychosis and does not reliably enable clinicians to identify psychotic-like experiences as psychopathological. Superseding this with a heuristic approach whereby psychotic-like phenomena are investigated openly and neutrally may foster a better understanding of psychosis and other mysterious depths of being human.

14.1.4 Psychosis as the absence of psychospiritual instruction

While psychosis is traditionally understood to signify the *presence* of medical psy-chopathology, my research shows that it can alternatively be seen as signifying the *absence* of the requisite skills, or technologies of consciousness, for competently navi-gating psychospiritual domains of reality. Campbell analogously portrays this as the psychotic person drowning in the same metaphysical waters in which the shamanic adept swims, thus depicting psychosis as the product of undeveloped psychospiri-tual functionality rather than of psychopathological dysfunctionality. While this view acknowledges the reality of distressing and debilitating occurrences, it sees psychotic-like experience as a state of imbalance more than a case of medical morbidity. Indeed, the results of my literature content analysis show that the 'absence of psychospiritual skills and/or teachers' is identified by authors as the fifth highest criterion for discern-ing psychotic from psychospiritual experiences. This raises the question: Might the provision of psychospiritual skills and knowledge be more beneficial than medica-tion and hospitalisation for certain people flailing in the stormy seas of transpersonal 'psychotic' upheavals?

14.1.5 Psychosis as a developmental and beneficial process

Considerable evidence exists to suggest that psychotic-like experiences may be inte-gral to natural processes of human self-healing and psychospiritual development. This idea is exemplified in Washburn's and Nelson's phrase 'regression in the service of transcendence' (RIST). However, while Washburn and Nelson differentiate psy-chotic from psychotic-like RIST processes, others such as Laing and Perry understand *all* instances of so-called 'psychosis' to represent a healing gesture on behalf of the deeper psyche. From this perspective, it is understood that if the 'psychotic' process is appropriately supported, rather than medically thwarted, it may culminate in a state of self-renewal. In terms of psychotic symptoms, the perception of metaphysi-cal realities (e.g., seeing visions, hearing voices, communicating with spirits) are also reportedly common for spiritual adherents as they advance along their path towards mystical illumination. Likewise, shamanic initiatory processes are typically marked by long periods of seemingly 'psychotic' experiences and behaviour. Indeed, a deep understanding of human psychospiritual realities is foundational to the practice of

Tibetan Buddhist psychiatry. These are fields of knowledge and expertise from which Western psychiatry may learn much, for they recognise both the beneficial and detrimental potential of psychotic-like experiences.

14.1.6 Psychosis as a holistic phenomenon

Although this idea has been forwarded by others, and particularly by Meyer in his psychobiological theory, it is evident that psychiatry's prevailing attempts to substantiate the biogenic theory of psychosis overlook many aspects of the holistic complex that constitutes psychotic experience. As is evidenced in Chapter Thirteen, Tibetan Buddhist psychiatry exemplifies the feasibility and efficacy of a holistic psychiatric model whereby therapy includes psychospiritual, psychosocial, and physical assessments.

14.2 Ramifications for psychiatric practice

This book's psychospiritual challenge to medical psychiatry has significant ramifications in terms of prospective change to its epistemology, research scope, understanding of psychopathology, and clinical training. Such 'change' does not simply entail swapping one psychiatric model for another. Rather, it involves a process of investigation and transition, whereby a deeper understanding of psychospiritual matters may gradually be integrated into the psychiatric corpus of knowledge, while avoiding the present materialist inclination toward reductive conceptualisation and categorisation.

14.2.1 Epistemology

As established in Chapter Two, Section 2.3, psychiatric epistemology has generally reflected a medical materialist purview that limits the investigative scope for understanding the nature of reality and psychosis to biogenic parameters. However, the incorporation of psychospiritual considerations into psychiatric thinking and practice necessitates establishing a new epistemological base and framework of understanding, whereby medical materialism is superseded by medical holism. Instigating such a change requires that psychiatry relinquish its present and predominant biological focus in exchange for a holistic focus that embraces the full metaphysical-materialist gamut of reality within its investigative remit. Doing so would enable the formation of a radically new model of psychiatry with radically new ways, and scope, for understanding the multidimensional nature and causes of apparent psychopathology.

Such an enterprise also necessitates considering ways to bridge the epistemological chasm between materialist and metaphysical worldviews. Although quantum physics and new disciplines such as neurotheology have already made advances in this direction, psychiatry remains predominantly entrenched in a modality whereby the axioms of medical materialism have been transposed into the domain of human psychopathology. As Powell (2001, p. 319) observes, the discipline of psychiatry "has largely focused on the biology of mental disorder" and that "the view taken by many is to regard mind as epiphenomenal, on the basis that the brain itself is somehow generating consciousness". However, from a Tibetan Buddhist psychiatric perspective, physical reality is epiphenomenal to universal consciousness, hence, the human brain is epiphenomenal to individual consciousness, hence, the aetiology of psychosis is psychospiritual. This is inverse to Western psychiatry's biogenic view of psychosis. Furthermore, while the Western materialist model eschews psychospiritual considerations in preference for biomedical research, the Tibetan holistic model investigates physical and psychosocial factors within its broader understanding that psychosis is essentially psychospiritual in nature. Arguably, this latter approach provides greater scope for better understanding the nature of reality, psychosis, and the human condition in their many interconnected forms. It also entails pursuing lines of investigation that naturally lead to bridging the seeming gap between materialist and metaphysical worldviews.

14.2.2 Research

Throughout the course of this book, I have investigated many psychospiritual views in order to demonstrate their research value in terms of better understanding psychosis. Doing so intrinsically constitutes a challenge to medical psychiatry to undertake similar research. Although my investigative process unveils prospective new psychosis research pathways, each of these warrants further investigation because they open fields of knowledge beyond medical psychiatry's present materialist scope and proffer potential ways of better understanding psychosis and other human states of consciousness and being.

In terms of psychosis research, then, a significant ramification for psychiatry is to inquire more deeply into psychospiritual matters. For example, throughout this book the phenomenon of kundalini and its potential to precipitate psychotic or psychotic-like experiences is touched upon several times. Kundalini experiences feature in the Grofs' spiritual emergency typology and have also been researched by the Royal College of Psychiatrists Spirituality and Psychiatry Special Interest Group (SPSIG). Indeed, Regner (1998, p. i) avers that "some nonordinary states of consciousness, viewed as aberrant by conventional psychiatry, may reflect the workings of a healing mechanism known as kundalini awakening". Rather than abjuring the investigation of such metaphysical realities, psychiatry may advance its knowledge about psychosis and other anomalous states of consciousness by following the lead already set by SPSIG in kundalini research. There exists an extensive body of literature pertaining to kundalini and the dangers it can pose to mental health. This is an untapped source of potentially rich knowledge in psychosis research.

My literature research process also reveals frequent references to the seemingly dreamlike nature of psychotic experience. For instance, Dean views both dreams and psychosis as metapsychiatry interest areas, while Robbins contends that they are both forms of primordial mental activity. Jung also notes parallels between dream and psychotic experiences and pointedly asserts that:

to say that insanity is a dream which has become real is no metaphor. The phenomenology of the dream and of schizophrenia is almost identical, with a certain difference of course; for the one state occurs normally under the condition of sleep, while the other upsets the waking or conscious state. (Jung, 1939, p. 1005)

Arguably, psychiatric research in this area may foster further insights into the nature of psychosis, dreaming, and the deeper unconscious self.

Furthermore, references to psychosis in the context of meditation are manifold within literature across many disciplines. For instance, commentators variously note that meditative practices can include psychotic-like experiences, induce psychosis, or, conversely, help to remediate psychosis. Dean identifies meditation as a prospective metapsychiatry research area while Jung warns how meditative practices, like active imagination, can lead the unskilled explorer into madness. Also, the diverse gamut of technologies of consciousness used by shamans and mystics are essentially meditative practices that may help 'psychotic' people integrate overwhelming subconscious content and experiences. Indeed, the profound depth of understanding of psychosis in Tibetan Buddhist psychiatry is the direct product of exploring psychospiritual domains of reality via meditative practices. Clearly, further research into meditation may likely advance psychiatric knowledge about the nature and causes of psychosis.

A final and fascinating area of prospective psychosis research is the mystic view that normal human faculties of perception and cognition allow only a limited and distorted apprehension of reality. From this perspective, the physical world that most people accept as solid and real is only so in a relative sense. However, from the mystic perspective of spiritual enlightenment, the world experienced through corporeal consciousness is ultimately illusory. This has profound ramifications in terms of better understanding psychosis for it poses the question: What differentiates the delusional nature of normal sense perception from psychotic delusional experience when both appear to be out of touch with ultimate reality? Indeed, despite its often distressing and disruptive nature, is psychosis a state of consciousness more in touch with deeper reality than is secular normality? Such questions call psychiatry to investigate psychospiritual knowledge systems in order to better understand the nature of reality, psychosis, and other mysterious vicissitudes of being human.

14.2.3 Understanding psychopathology

As suggested in my Chapter Thirteen investigation of Tibetan Buddhist psychiatry, it is seemingly not possible to truly identify instances of psychopathology until the nature of psychopathology is deeply and holistically understood. Hence, the transition from a biogenic model of psychiatry to a holistic model would entail major changes to the traditional practice of reductive psychopathology-seeking, which arguably represents an approach that prematurely diagnoses instances of psychopathology that are scarcely understood. Indeed, it appears that psychiatry inadvertently veils and perpetuates this lack of understanding via the assumption that psychotic-like happenings are intrinsically incomprehensible. However, as is shown throughout this book, such phenomena can be understood as deeply meaningful and non-psychopathological, especially when considered in light of cross-cultural and psychospiritual contexts.

A significant task and challenge for psychiatry-in-transition, then, is to abandon its standard and reductive practice of psychopathology-seeking in preference for a heuristic and phenomenological investigative approach whereby the discovery of new knowledge perpetually opens the way for further discovery. This approach would incorporate physical, psychological, and metaphysical considerations in its open-ended investigative scope. Arguably, only when a deep holistic understanding of the complex interplay of phenomenological factors within the metaphysical-physical nexus has been attained, is it then possible to identify psychopathology, and discern it from non-psychopathology, with a degree of comprehensive expertise.

14.2.4 Clinical training

Finally, my psychospiritual challenge to medical psychiatry also has profound ramifications for psychiatric training as it requires psychiatrists to become conceptually and experientially conversant with the nature of psychospiritual realities. In other words, rather than ignoring or giving secondary consideration to psychospiritual matters, psychiatrists would be required to develop a deep understanding of metaphysical realities within many cultural contexts. This may include considering the idea that physical reality is epiphenomenal to psychospiritual reality and, subsequently, that understanding the roots of psychopathology requires a deep understanding of the multifaceted nature of reality in its interrelated physical and non-physical forms. However, such conceptual knowledge would not be sufficient alone. As is evidenced by Tibetan Buddhist psychiatrists and shamanic healers, the most effective practitioners are adept in employing technologies of consciousness to perceive and directly work within metaphysical domains of reality. Ostensibly, psychiatrists may become 'soul doctors', who, through their advanced holistic understanding and psychospiritual expertise, can exhibit greater therapeutic efficacy when working with psychotic-like experiences and other manifestations of the body-mind-spirit complex.

APPENDICES

APPENDIX 1

A historical overview of uses of the term 'psychospiritual'

My challenge to medical psychiatry throughout this book is a *psychospiritual* one. Hence, elucidating the meaning of this core concept is important. While the definition provided in Chapter Two, Section 2.1 sufficiently fulfils this task in terms of articulating its essential scope and meaning, the historical overview here further fleshes out its significance and substance within the domain of metaphysical epistemology. Of particular pertinence are historical uses of the word 'psychospiritual' in reference to non-ordinary experiences and states of consciousness that may appear to be psychotic-like from a psychiatric perspective.

The word 'psychospiritual' was ostensibly first used as a scriptural idiom in 1879 by the American pastor Israel Warren, in his book *The Parousia* (1879).[145] Here, he referred to human nature as being "strictly psycho-spiritual", by which he meant that the essential spiritual self is wedded with the psychic self when embodied in human form (Warren, 1879, p. 280). Since Warren, the word psychospiritual has been used by commentators from various fields. However, two prominent metaphysical commentators who have used the term frequently in their respective works are the theosophist Helena Blavatsky (more commonly known as Madam Blavatsky), and the Indian scholar-mystic Sri Aurobindo.

Blavatsky first used the term 'psycho-spiritual' in her 1888 book *The Secret Doctrine*. Here, she refers to "psycho-spiritual man" as an existential conjunct to the "physical man" of scientific materialism (Blavatsky, 1888a, p. 528). She further argues that "the methods used by our scholars and students of the psycho-spiritual sciences do not

---

[145] After conducting an exhaustive search, this is the earliest use of the term 'psychospiritual' that I was able to find.

differ from those of students of the natural and physical sciences. Only our fields of research are on two different planes" (Blavatsky, 1889, pp. 1, 49). Hence, she sees the study of psychospiritual matters as a scientific endeavour. She also understands the term 'psychospiritual' to designate an extrasensory aptitude and challenged psychiatry's construal of such aptitude as mental illness. For instance, she muses:

> We ask: Do you know the nature of hallucination, and can you define its psychic process? How can you tell that all such visions are due merely to physical hallucinations? What makes you feel so sure that mental and nervous diseases, while drawing a veil over our *normal* senses (so-called) *do not* reveal at the same time vistas unknown to the healthy man, by throwing open doors usually closed against your scientific perceptions (?): or that a psycho-spiritual faculty *does not* forthwith replace the loss, or the temporary atrophy, of a purely physical sense? (Blavatsky, 1888b, p. 332)

Here, she questions the veracity of accepted materialist theory and strongly suggests that a psychospiritual perspective proffers further ways to consider, understand, and explain phenomena that might otherwise be deemed psychotic. This inclusion of psychospiritual knowledge within the ambit of scientific inquiry challenges medical psychiatry's biological-based view and has significant ramifications for understanding and diagnosing psychosis.

The Indian scholar and sage, Sri Aurobindo, also used the term 'psychospiritual' frequently in his writings throughout the first half of the twentieth century, whereby he emphasised and validated aspects and vistas of life which are generally absent from the materialist worldview. For instance, in an evolutionary context, he refers to "the psycho-spiritual plane" as an intermediary domain of human existence between secular life and "the spiritual consciousness proper", where a process of "psycho-spiritual change" is both pursued and experienced by the spiritual adherent (Sri Aurobindo, 1972). He sees this process of spiritual development as constituting "a complete psycho-spiritual and psycho-physical science of Yoga" that entails the use of "Yoga-systems of psycho-spiritual discipline and self-finding" and "inner mental and psycho-spiritual methods" (Sri Aurobindo, 1997, pp. 376, 190, 211). Additionally, he maintains that "psychospiritual means" can be actively harnessed for healing and therapeutic uses (2006, p. 375), and that "a psycho-spiritual transformation of this kind would be already a vast change of our mental human nature" (2005, p. 943). Hence, from an Aurobindoian perspective, the term 'psychospiritual' denotes many things, including a plane of existence, a scientific process in disciplinary practice of personal development and transformation, and the methods, experiences, and capacities therein.

Sri Aurobindo also describes normal psychospiritual experiences and powers that, from a psychiatric perspective, would be perceived as abnormal and probably diagnosed as symptomatic of psychosis. For instance, he explains that a notable and common feature of spiritual development is the occurrence of extrasensory "psychospiritual experiences" whereby the adherent's consciousness "opens to all kinds of things and to suggestions, and messages from all sorts of planes and worlds and forces and beings" (Sri Aurobindo, 2006, p. 371). In psychiatric practice such experiences are generally understood (or misunderstood) to be diagnostic indicators of a psychotic episode.

Although psychologists and psychiatrists have not used the term 'psychospiritual' as prolifically as metaphysical commentators such as Blavatsky and Sri Aurobindo, there is evidence of the term's use within their respective bodies of literature. For instance, an online keyword search for 'psychospiritual' or 'psycho-spiritual' in the American Psychological Association's PsychINFO database results in a total of 489 items, ranging from 1930–2013, with most appearing after 1990.[146] A similar search of psychiatric literature reveals that the terms 'psychospiritual' and 'psycho-spiritual' have been used in 108 articles between 1930–2013.[147] These findings demonstrate its significant use within psychological literature, and a lesser, though growing use in psychiatric literature. Therefore, it is clear that the term is not completely foreign to psychiatry and it is apposite to suggest that incorporating psychospiritual considerations into psychiatric epistemology does not require the integration of an alien concept. Rather, it requires the willingness by psychiatry to extend its parameters of thinking to encompass psychospiritual considerations that already exist, in latent and rudimentary form, within its epistemological body.

---

[146] Source: PsychINFO at http://www.apa.org/pubs/databases/psycinfo/index.aspx. This search was conducted on 27 October 2013 and restricted to books (n = 122), dissertations (n = 165), and journal articles (n = 202).

[147] There is no comprehensive psychiatric equivalent of PsychINFO. Therefore, I conducted an online keyword search for 'psychospiritual' or 'psycho-spiritual' in Psychiatry Online, PubMed and Google Scholar. The total results were then collated after omitting repeat articles. This search was conducted on 27 October 2013 and included journal articles only, as there were no instances of the terms being used in psychiatric books or dissertations.

APPENDIX 2

Key factors shaping the DSM-III revision process

A2.0 Introduction

The review process for transiting from DSM-II to DSM-III marked a radical shift from a psychodynamic model back to a medical model for psychiatry and understanding psychosis. It appears, however, that the DSM-III medical model is a provisional construct, the formation of which was influenced by a flux of non-scientific factors such as professional embarrassment, shifting psychosocial circumstances, ideological preferences, economic expediency, political wrangling, in-house voting processes, and the survival imperative for psychiatry to demarcate its operational territory as a profession. Despite the predominance of these factors, and the absence of any scientifically validated proof as to the biological roots of psychopathology, the reconfiguration of DSM-III set the stage for a subsequent biogenic revival. As noted by Stein (1991, p. 412) the DSM-III authors "narrowed diagnostic syndromes so that biological homogeneity is assured, and so fore-grounded biological explanations". In this multifaceted manner, the DSM-III task force, and other biologically oriented psychiatrists, successfully reconstituted a biomedical model within American psychiatry.

My ensuing appraisal of these factors provides a backdrop for better grasping the dynamics at play in shaping modern psychiatric thinking and practice, and the subsequent setting of the epistemological parameters for understanding psychosis. It is important to bear in mind the inextricable relationship between these dimensions of DSM-III formation. Although examined separately, these seemingly different factors worked together in a dynamic interchange of mutual influence.

A2.1 The DSM-III task force remit

The DSM-III review process formally began in 1974 when Robert Spitzer was nominated by the APA as Chair of the task force on Nomenclature and Statistics (APA, 1980, p. 2). Although the task force was initially formed to develop a manual that was useful to clinicians and researchers of various "theoretical orientations" (ibid.), it subsequently adopted a predominantly medical focus in keeping with Spitzer's intention and declaration that DSM-III would be a "defense of the medical model as applied to psychiatric problems" (Spitzer in Wilson, 1993, p. 405). This venture to establish, or re-establish, American psychiatry as a medical speciality was viewed as "a Kraepelinian revival" and earned the task force the appellation of "the neo-Kraepelinians" (Klerman, 1978, p. 106). As discussed below, various factors precipitated this endeavour to re-constitute American psychiatry as a medical discipline.

A2.2 The crisis in diagnostic reliability and validity

The credibility of psychiatry as a discipline depends on demonstrating diagnostic reliability and validity. Simply put, reliability is defined as "diagnostic agreement ... among practitioners" (Allardyce et al., 2010, p. 1), and validity as "the extent to which something represents or measures what it purports to represent or measure" (Schaler, 1995). During the 1960s and early 1970s, four concurrent incidents challenged the reliability and validity of American psychiatric diagnostics, and played a pivotal role in shaping DSM-III. First, the reliability of the DSM-II schizophrenia category was challenged by the results of a cross-national study of US and UK trial patient groups from 1965 to 1972, which showed that there "was a dramatic preponderance of schizophrenia in the New York samples as opposed to the London samples" (Professional Staff of the United States-United Kingdom Cross-National Project, 1974, p. 85). In other words, when presented with the same clinical data, American psychiatrists diagnosed schizophrenia far more frequently than British psychiatrists. Indeed, Spitzer (1989, p. 21) later acknowledged "the sorry state of psychiatric diagnosis" in America during the 1960s and early 1970s, whereby "clinicians and researchers consistently were unable to agree on the psychiatric diagnoses that they assigned to patients". The crisis this created for psychiatry as a discipline cannot be understated, for as DSM-IV Chair, Allen Frances, explains: "without reliability the system is completely random, and the diagnoses mean almost nothing — maybe worse than nothing, because they're falsely labelling. You're better off not having a diagnostic system" (Spiegel, 2005). The findings of the United States-United Kingdom Cross-National Project raised considerable concerns about diagnostic reliability in American psychiatric practice.

Concurrently, there was a threefold attack on psychiatric diagnostic validity. First, during the 1960s and 1970s, anti-psychiatrists disputed the veracity of psychiatric diagnoses because they were, in their view:

1. arbitrary, and hence, mythical constructs;
2. used as a hegemonic tool for fabricating professional legitimacy; and
3. used to exercise power and social control via labelling patients (Decker, 2007, pp. 343–344).

Second, in 1973, gay activists successfully lobbied the APA to revoke homosexuality from DSM-II as a mental disorder. This cast a pall of doubt over the validity of psychiatric diagnoses, for it inferred they "were strongly influenced not solely by scientific criteria, but by public opinion, social constructions of deviance, and political pressure" (Mayes & Horwitz, 2005, p. 258). Indeed, the final decision to revoke the psychopathological status of homosexuality was not the product of medical re-evaluation, but of a voting process whereby 5,854 APA members voted for, and 3,810 against, removing homosexuality from DSM-II (Butler, 1999, p. 22). This incident suggested the dubious validity of psychiatric mental disorder categories, because it seemed they were formulated more via subjective opinion than objective medical fact.

The third incident, which also occurred in 1973, was in the form of an experiment conducted by psychologist David Rosenhan (1973, p. 251), whereby several sane pseudo-patients approached different psychiatric hospitals and informed resident psychiatrists that they heard a voice saying "empty", "hollow", or "thud". Most were diagnosed as 'schizophrenic' and treated as such by staff, despite acting normally immediately upon admission, and were eventually released with the updated diagnosis of schizophrenia "in remission" (ibid., p. 252). As a result, Rosenhan (p. 257) scathingly concluded that "it is clear that we cannot distinguish the sane from the insane in psychiatric hospitals". These combined events highlighted "the absence of evidence about validity and causation" (Klerman, 1984, p. 541), and constituted a major public embarrassment for psychiatry. In response to this array of disconcerting occurrences, the DSM-III task force decided to implement innovative strategies to first improve diagnostic reliability and then to attempt to substantiate the validity of DSM-III mental disorders.

A2.3 Diagnostic innovations in DSM-III

The principal and galvanising objective of the DSM-III task force was to create a superior medical diagnostic instrument that redressed issues pertaining to reliability and validity. Samuel Guze (1982, p. 7), a task force consultant and key player in the review process, described diagnosis as "the keystone of medical practice and clinical research", while Feighner et al. (1972, p. 57), whose proposed diagnostic criteria model formed the basis of the DSM-III framework, also underscored the fundamental role of diagnosis in medical psychiatry. Consequently, between 1974 and 1980, the DSM-III task force sought to rectify the reliability and validity problem through several innovative developments, namely, the formation of:

1. A so-called 'atheoretical' model.
2. A generic definition for 'mental disorder'.

3. A set of operational diagnostic categories and criteria.
4. A multiaxial evaluation system.

A2.3.1 Positing an atheoretical model

The DSM-III task force maintained that the psychodynamic approach to psychiatric practice in America, heralded by DSM-I and DSM-II, was driven by unsubstantiated theories pertaining to aetiology. According to Tsuang et al. (2000, p. 1045), "a key innovation of DSM-III was its explicit separation of diagnostic criteria from speculation about etiology. At the time DSM-III was developed, this separation was essential because theories of etiology had not yet been subjected to empirical tests". Klerman (1984, p. 540) hailed DSM-III's ostensible scientific approach as remedying the unverified psychodynamic aetiological theories. Spitzer (1985, p. 522) referred to this DSM-III development as an "atheoretical" approach, by which he inferred:

> [a] descriptive approach [that] emphasizes classification on the basis of shared descriptive clinical features rather than on presumed etiology, and emphasizes the importance of specified diagnostic criteria for improving diagnostic reliability rather than the use of highly inferential clinical concepts for making a diagnosis.

According to the DSM-III authors, this "atheoretical approach" represented a nonpartisan framework that practitioners from "varying theoretical orientations" could adapt to suit their respective clinical approaches (APA, 1980, p. 7). At face value, this depicted the DSM-III upgrade as an egalitarian development that supported the views and approaches of both psychodynamic and medical disciplines. However, closer investigation reveals flaws in the task force's atheoretical claim.

Numerous commentators have disputed the veracity of DSM-III's supposed 'atheoretical' nature. These broadly constitute two different, though related, points of contention. The first is that, despite its purported atheoretical stance, DSM-III was itself a fundamentally theoretical document (Butler, 1999, p. 27; Wilson, 1993, p. 408; Carson, 1991, p. 305; Blashfield, 1984, p. 133). As McLaren (2007, p. xi) succinctly puts it:

> Psychiatrists can't have it both ways. They can't claim on the one hand to be functioning within a scientific framework yet, on the other, also claim that their diagnostic system is atheoretical. There is no such thing as a non-theoretical science as a science is necessarily committed to a theory; science just is the process of explicating and testing a theory.

Indeed, Faust & Miner (1986, pp. 962, 963) argued that DSM-III was modelled on Baconian empiricism, and hence, "replete with presuppositions and theoretical assumptions". This view was not only expressed by detractors, but also acknowledged by medical model proponents. For instance, Millon (1983, p. 808), a task force member, asserted that "it should be said that the categorical syndromes of the DSM-III are …

in the main, only theoretical constructs", while Klerman (1978, p. 107), an ardent supporter of the DSM-III project, alluded to the manual's theoretical nature in acknowledging that "mental illness and the medical model are social constructs; they are inventions of modern society". In fact, Spitzer (1984a, p. 546), as task force Chair, also declared that "all diagnostic categories are actually hypotheses; that is how we regard the diagnostic categories of DSM-III". This admission by Spitzer is surprising, for, on the one hand, he emphasises that the DSM-III atheoretical approach essentially differentiates it from the psychodynamic conjecture of DSM-II, yet on the other hand, he acknowledges the ultimate theoretical nature of DSM-III.

A further point of contention by commentators was that, despite the egalitarian assurances regarding the DSM-III atheoretical approach, the project, in fact, aimed to supplant psychoanalytic and psychotherapeutic approaches (Butler, 1999, p. 21; Rogler, 1997, p. 11; Wilson, 1993, p. 404; Gaines, 1992, p. 9; Blashfield, 1984, p. 21). For instance, Skodal (2000, p. 442) maintains that "Spitzer and other members of the DSM-III task force were blatantly antianalytic, not simply atheoretical". Spitzer (2001, p. 354) contested such criticisms, asserting that a number of DSM-III categories "were proposed by clinicians with a psychoanalytic perspective". However, one of the few psychoanalytically oriented DSM-III task force members resigned his position because "he felt that his suggestions for shaping the manual in a more psychodynamic direction had been dismissed out of hand" (Frosch in Wilson, 1993, p. 405). Additionally, Houts (2000, p. 947) concludes that, whether or not a biomedical agenda drove the DSM-III project, "the fundamental concepts of psychoanalytic theory were expunged from the official psychiatric nomenclature". Overall, it therefore appears that the existing psychodynamic model was supplanted by a putative 'atheoretical' and medical model of psychiatry.

A2.3.2 Defining 'mental disorder'

Another major DSM-III innovation was the inclusion of an explicit definition for 'mental disorder'. According to Spitzer & Endicott (1978, p. 15), an attempt to define mental illness had not occurred in prior DSM and ICD editions, nor in "standard textbooks of medicine and psychiatry", hence, fashioning this definition represented an original undertaking in psychiatry. It also constituted a process that went to the problematic heart of reframing psychiatry as a medical profession and sought to answer several conjoint questions:

- What is a medical disorder?
- What is a mental disorder?
- In what ways might DSM-III mental disorders be construed as medical disorders?
- What are the professional boundaries of medical psychiatry?

Therefore, in 1975, the DSM-III task force decided to formulate a definition for mental disorder (Millon, 1983, p. 805). Beyond the apparent need to explicate the conceptual and ontological parameters of 'mental illness', a further and fundamental motivation for undertaking this task was to convince detractors that "psychiatry was a legitimate branch of medicine" (Spitzer, 1981, pp. 3, 33). The orchestrators of this initiative subsequently composed definitions for both 'medical disorder' and 'mental disorder', provided a rationale to support these definitions, and fashioned a model of proposed operational criteria for diagnostically distinguishing mental from non-mental medical disorders (ibid., pp. 18–30). Despite its seeming rigour, this proposal created a maelstrom of protest from psychologists who perceived it as an attempt by medical psychiatry to appropriate the domain of mental disorders as its professional purview, and was consequently rejected as "provocative" by formal vote at a 1978 APA meeting (Millon, 1983, pp. 805–806). Additionally, Moore (1978, p. 85) described the Spitzer-Endicott definition proposal as "stipulative" in that it prescriptively "focuses on how it ought to be used" rather than on implicit meaning. In 1980, the final definition was published in DSM-III, however, according to Millon (1983, p. 806), this was a modified version of the 1979 consensus definition, which had been altered "at the editorial level without task force approval". The final edited version included the term "biologic dysfunction" whereas the original did not.[148] When considering that DSM-III was published as a manual to guide the practice of a reinstituted medical model of psychiatry, and that a definition of mental illness delineates the essential nature of the psychiatric domain, then the obvious question raised is: For what possible purpose was this unauthorised change made?

In response to this question, it is apposite to suggest that the doctored DSM-III definition reflects the intentional insertion of a biomedical bias into the manual. Indeed, many commentators have expressed the view that the publication of DSM-III represented a switch to a biomedical model of psychiatry. For example, Arthur (1973, p. 846) observed that the advent of the DSM-III review project saw the emergence of a biomedical trend in American psychiatry that he variously described as: "a sudden

---

[148] The DSM-III glossary defines mental disorder as follows:

> A mental disorder is conceptualized as a clinically significant behavioral or psychologic syndrome or pattern that occurs in an individual and that typically is associated with either a painful symptom (distress) or impairment in one or more important areas of functioning (disability). In addition, there is an inference that there is a behavioral, psychologic, or *biologic dysfunction*, and that the disturbance is not only in the relationship between the individual and society. When the disturbance is limited to a conflict between an individual and society, this may represent social deviance, which may or may not be commendable, but is not by itself a mental disorder. (APA, 1980, p. 363, italics added)

The original and intended definition was as follows:

> No precise definition is available that unambiguously defines the boundaries of this concept. (This is also true of such concepts as physical disorder or mental or physical health.) However, in the DSM-III each of the mental disorders is conceptualized as a clinically significant behavioural or psychological syndrome or pattern of an individual that is associated, by and large, with either a painful symptom (distress) or impairment in one or more important areas of functioning (disability). (Millon, 1983, p. 806)

pullulation of basic biological research into mental illness"; "a neo-Kraepelinian revival of interest in typology"; and "a reaffirmation of the psychiatrist as medical specialist with problems clearly in the province of medicine rather than psychology, sociology, or anthropology". Similarly, Butler (1999, p. 21) maintained that the DSM-III project was governed by a covert biomedical agenda from the outset in that "the diagnostic project *intended* from its inception to lead to a progressive exclusion of non-biologically focused systems of explanation".[149] However, Spitzer vigorously and repeatedly refuted these claims. For instance, he asserted it was "nonsense" that "the focus of psychiatric physicians should be particularly on the biological aspects of mental illness" (Spitzer, 1982, p. 592). Indeed, twenty-one years after the publication of DSM-III he continued to argue that "it is not true that DSM-III … is covertly committed to a biological approach to explaining psychiatric disturbance" (Spitzer, 2001, p. 351).[150] Klerman, a key medical model proponent, contradicted Spitzer's rebuttals. For instance, he referred to the "biological concepts" of the "neokraepelinian view" (Klerman, 1971, p. 310), and observed that, "applied to schizophrenia, there is a greater attention to … biological causes and treatments of the disorder" in the proposed DSM-III (Klerman, 1978, p. 105). Despite this seeming impasse of opinion, it is evident that the DSM-III review process precipitated (either deliberately or inadvertently) a revival of biologically oriented psychiatry that has subsequently become integral to contemporary psychiatry and its fundamental understanding and definition of psychosis.

A2.3.3 Formulating operational diagnostic categories and criteria

The DSM-III task force believed the reliability crisis in American psychiatry was primarily due to DSM-II classifications being ambiguous and lacking formal definitions and operational criteria, resulting in psychiatrists making incongruent interpretations and diagnoses (Spitzer, Endicott & Robins, 1978, p. 773). As Spitzer (2001, p. 355) explains, "the brevity and general nature of these descriptions was of little help in indicating to the diagnostician which features of the disorder needed to be present in order to make the diagnoses". The embarrassing disparity between US and UK diagnoses of schizophrenia was primarily due to the vagueness of DSM-II classification descriptions, whereby American psychiatrists diagnosed the same people as schizophrenic that their British counterparts generally diagnosed as neurotic or depressed (Healy, 2002a, p. 298). While the DSM-I and DSM-II manuals provided a brief symptomatologic description of mental disorders, they did not include an operational system that prioritised and designated the number of symptoms required to make a diagnosis (Blashfield, 1984, p. 113). According to Spitzer, Endicott & Robins

---

[149] For further comments of a similar nature, see: Double, 2008, p. 332; Butler, 1999, p. 21; Wilson, 1993, p. 402; Gaines, 1992, p. 9; Klerman, 1978, p. 105; Romano, 1977, p. 798.

[150] For further comments by Spitzer of a similar nature, see: Spitzer & Williams, 1982, p. 23; Spitzer, 1981, p. 33; Spitzer & Endicott, 1978, pp. 17, 30; Spitzer et al., 1977, p. 6.

(1978, p. 773), this was a major source of unreliability due to diagnostic discordance resulting "when there are differences in the formal inclusion and exclusion criteria that clinicians use to summarize patient data into psychiatric diagnoses". Hence, the DSM-III authors focussed on "replacing vague descriptions of psychiatric disorders with precise definitions using specified criteria" (Spitzer, 1989) and established a tool that enabled clinicians "to determine the presence or absence of specific clinical phenomena, and then to apply the comprehensive rules provided for making the diagnosis" (Spitzer et al., 1977, p. 15). This innovation, coupled with the provision of descriptive diagnostic categories with information about clinical signs and symptoms for each disorder (Spitzer, 2001, p. 356), ostensibly worked to invest DSM-III diagnostic categories with empirical rigour and much improved reliability. Indeed, the DSM-III introduction attested that it had achieved "far greater reliability than had previously been obtained with DSM-II" (APA, 1980, p. 5), while Klerman (1984, p. 341) claimed that, in DSM-III, the reliability problem had been "solved". However, Klerman's claim was evidently overstated, for Spitzer explained in a 2005 interview that:

> To say that we've solved the reliability problem is just not true. It's been improved. But if you're in a situation with a general clinician it's certainly not very good. There's still a real problem, and it's not clear how to solve the problem. (Spitzer in Spiegel, 2005)

It therefore appears only a partial improvement of reliability was achieved in psychiatric diagnostics via this DSM-III development.

Indeed, while many DSM-III advocates have lauded the manual's enhanced diagnostic reliability, other commentators have contested this. Some assert that these claims to superior reliability are simply inaccurate. For example, after analysing studies upholding claims of high reliability in DSM-III diagnostic criteria, Caplan (1995, pp. 197–203) concluded that reliability was, in fact, "poor", while Kutchins & Kirk (1997, pp. 252–253), after a similar process, determined that "the evidence offered for this claim was lacking".[151] Others challenged the veracity of the process by which the diagnostic criteria were formulated. For instance, Millon (1983, p. 812) proffered the "insider's perspective" that DSM-III reliability was not "anchored to empirical research". This is a damning statement because, as a DSM-III task force member, his disclosure of this fact casts considerable doubt on the scientific soundness of DSM-III reliability measures. Millon's view is corroborated by American psychiatrist Mandel Cohen[152] who also spoke on the issue of DSM-III diagnostic criteria formulation:

---

[151] In their book *The Selling of DSM: The Rhetoric of Science in Psychiatry*, Kirk & Kutchins (1992, pp. 133–160) dedicate an entire chapter to a rigorous critical appraisal of studies claiming to corroborate high reliability.
[152] Mandel Cohen was an eminent American psychiatrist who championed a 'medical model' approach during the era when psychoanalytic psychiatry predominated. He was subsequently perceived by some as "deserving the credit for DSM-III" for his influential and founding role in mentoring a core group of like-minded psychiatrists who later became prime movers in formulating DSM-III (Healy, 2002b).

But you know the problem is that these people in DSM-III don't get their criteria now by research—they get a group of good people to sit around the table and discuss it all before they finally decide to accept whatever. (Healy, 2002b, p. 222)

It therefore appears that, rather than being the product of sound empirical research, the DSM-III diagnostic criteria were arrived at through a process of discussion and consensus.

In fact, descriptions of these diagnostic criteria formulation sessions indicate that they were more a process of unruly skirmish than of sage deliberation and debate. For instance, Millon (1983, p. 804) alludes to this in his reference to a process negotiated by "a highly diverse collection of outspoken and independently thinking professionals with clearly disparate views", while Spitzer (1985, p. 523) has admitted the "complicated and frequently heated interactions" when composing the DSM-III diagnostic content. British psychiatrist and DSM-III consultant, David Shaffer, also recalls that "whoever shouted the loudest tended to be heard ... it was more like a tobacco auction than a sort of conference" (Spiegel, 2003). Similarly, DSM-IV task force Chair, Allen Frances, retrospectively observes that "the loudest voices usually won out", and that Spitzer would synthesise these differing opinions into "some combination of the accepted wisdom of the group ... with a little added weight to the people he respected most" (Spiegel, 2005). It therefore seems that the validity of DSM-III diagnostic criteria and categories is tenuous, for they arguably reflect a process of heated wrangling rather than of objective empiricism. Furthermore, it seems that any improvement in reliability was not reflective of scientific rigour, but of a group of psychiatrists collectively memorising a set of agreed upon diagnostic criteria. As noted by Nathan (1979, p. 477), establishing reliability is simply a matter of consensus classification "given that clinicians can learn to agree on how to elicit and chronicle those criteria". The DSM-III operational criteria for diagnosing psychosis were also forged through this dubious process. It is consequently feasible to suggest that such criteria were more reflective of subjective opinions by psychiatrists about psychosis than of the actual nature of psychosis.

A2.3.4 Creating a multiaxial system

A final DSM-III innovation was the development of a multiaxial evaluation system. This consisted of five axes of evaluation, which formed a complete clinical picture when combined. Axis I pertained to "Clinical Syndromes", Axis II to "Personality Disorders", Axis III to "Physical Disorders and Conditions", Axis IV to "Severity of Psychosocial Stressors", and Axis V to "Highest Level of Adaptive Functioning Past Year". The first three axes constituted the "official diagnostic assessment" components, while the latter two axes provided additional information regarding possible related influences (APA, 1980, p. 23). Intriguingly, the influential role of psychosocial stressors in mental disorders that featured centrally in DSM-I, and were all but expunged from DSM-II, were resurrected in DSM-III as a seven-point rating system ranging in increasing severity from: 1 (None = "No apparent psychosocial stressor") through to 7 (Catastrophic = "Concentration camp experience; devastating natural disaster") (ibid., p. 27). This inclusion of psychosocial considerations within the diagnostic framework arguably counters accusations that DSM-III was biased towards a biomedical understanding of mental disorders. Indeed, Spitzer (2001, p. 357) claimed that the development of a multiaxial system "enabled DSM-III to be presented as within a broad biopsychosocial model—rather than the narrow diagnostic model that its critics feared".[153] However, with DSM-III the primary diagnosis was made in light of the first three axes only, which did not include psychosocial considerations. Such factors were secondary and not integral to making diagnosis. Therefore, it seems Spitzer's likening of DSM-III to a biopsychosocial model, due to its multiaxial system, was a rhetorical device employed to give the appearance of acknowledging psychosocial causes of mental disorders when, clearly, the chief aim was to enshrine psychiatry as a fundamentally medical discipline.

A2.4 Non-medical forces shaping DSM-III

In addition to the aforementioned embarrassments and factors that played an influential role in the DSM-III review project, sundry other socio-economic and political forces converged to shape the subsequent process, and the final published product. These are examined separately below as social, economic, and political forces, though, in fact, they worked together as a complex and synergistic whole.

A2.4.1 Social forces shaping DSM-III

The main social force that influenced the formulation of DSM-III was the alleged 'neo-Kraepelinian movement' driven by a group of medically oriented psychiatrists. According to Klerman (1978, pp. 104–105), this group championed key tenets of Kraepelinian thinking, particularly the categorisation of mental disorders, and also endorsed "a general movement of psychiatry towards greater integration with medicine". Decker (2007, p. 345) proffers the following description of the so-called neo-Kraepelinians:

> In the 1960s and early 1970s a small band of psychiatrists at Washington University in St Louis were dissatisfied with and critical of the state of American psychiatry. In their view, here was a psychiatry that dealt in non-psychiatric pursuits, had largely eschewed the medical model, did not value diagnosis and classification, rejected sharp distinctions between mental illness and mental health, and seemed unbothered by the abysmally low scores of inter-rater reliability—two or more

---

[153] The biopsychosocial model Spitzer alludes to here is that proposed by American psychiatrist, George Engel (1978; 1977), during the DSM-III review process, as a holistic alternative to medical psychiatry and its narrow diagnostic focus.

psychiatrists coming to the same conclusion about the diagnosis of a patient. The Washington University psychiatrists and their few sympathizers believed that only empirical psychiatric research with a strong focus on biology held any hope for the treatment and improvement of the mentally ill.

Blashfield (1984, pp. 43–45) maintained that the neo-Kraepelinian movement exemplified the notion from the sociology of science of an "invisible college", which has two fundamental features. First, it is similar to a college in that "the group represented a collection of intellectuals who had a sense of allegiance to each other and frequently interacted both professionally and socially", and second, it is 'invisible' in that the group's existence is generally not evident to those outside of it (Blashfield, 1982, p. 3). In sociological terms, although such groups can exercise considerable persuasive power, they are not actively clandestine, but emerge as a natural aspect of scientific progress (ibid.). This is arguably a fitting description of the DSM-III task force and others in psychiatric circles who worked closely with them.

The perceived existence of an invisible college of neo-Kraepelinian psychiatrists is more than conjecture, as their existence was substantiated by commentators at the time. For instance, Blashfield (1984, p. 36) created a sociogram to demonstrate that most neo-Kraepelinian members were employed at one of four networked institutions: Kings Hospital Institute (New York), New York State psychiatric Institute (New York), Washington University (St Louis), and University of Iowa (Iowa City). He also noted that, of the nineteen DSM-III task force members, ten were prominent figures within this neo-Kraepelinian network (ibid., p. 116). According to Klerman (1978, p. 105), the "founding" neo-Kraepelinian members were: Eli Robins, Sam Guze, and George Winokur from St Louis, who were task force consultants and/or advisory committee members, and co-authors of the Feigner paper that was pivotal to DSM-III's classification system and diagnostic criteria. He additionally named Donald Klein and Robert Spitzer from New York (both key task force members) as prominent neo-Kraepelinians (ibid.). It is pertinent to reiterate here that, at the time, Klerman ranked as one of America's leading psychiatrists and was renowned for his endorsement of reconstituting a medical model of psychiatry. Hence, his views pertaining to the identity of neo-Kraepelinian members hold considerable professional weight. Despite this body of evidence, Spitzer (1984b, p. 552) challenged the existence of such a consortium, which he derisively referred to as "the so-called neo-Kraepelinian group". Indeed, in an issue of *Schizophrenia Bulletin*, he lampooned the idea by stating that, "I take this opportunity, in the hallowed pages of this distinguished journal, to offer my resignation publically from the neo-Kraepelinian college" (Spitzer, 1982, p. 592). Regardless of Spitzer's aversion to the appellation 'neo-Kraepelinian', innumerable commentators have asserted the existence of such an elite group, and its prominent role in shaping DSM-III.

If the neo-Kraepelinians were the collective protagonist in the DSM-III move to medicalise psychiatry, and the task force spearheaded this venture, then Robert Spitzer was arguably the central driving force behind the entire mounting edifice.

In fact, Spiegel (2005; 2003) refers to Spitzer as being the man who "revolutionized the practice of psychiatry" and "revolutionized the Diagnostic and Statistical Manual", for he was a member of twelve of the fourteen Advisory Committees (APA, 1980)[154] and functioned as *the* executive dynamo in most aspects of developing DSM-III. For instance, DSM-III Advisory Committee member, David Shaffer (Spiegel, 2005), recalled that Spitzer made the final decisions concerning DSM-III classifications by consulting "some internal criteria" of his own. DSM-IV editor, Michael First, corroborates this view in stating that "a lot of what's in the *DSM* represents what Bob thinks is right ... He really saw this as *his* book, and if he thought it was right he would push very hard to get it in that way" (Spiegel, 2005). Indeed, Spitzer recalls with pride, "my fingers were on the typewriter that typed ... every word" of the diagnostic entities published in the manual (Spiegel, 2005). From this perspective, it is seemingly evident that the turning of the psychiatric tide back to a medical model in DSM-III was fundamentally influenced, not so much by hard science, but by a social force in the form of a neo-Kraepelinian clique that advocated a biogenic understanding of mental illness. This was further consolidated by the subjective sway of one man, Robert (Bob) Spitzer,[155] who intimately shaped the final DSM-III product.

Spitzer was also instrumental in advancing technological methodology in psychiatric diagnostics. For instance, due to his penchant for data-based diagnostics he consequently hand-picked "data-oriented people" as task force and Advisory Committee members (Spiegel, 2005), and also introduced computer programs to crunch data for diagnostic purposes (Endicott & Spitzer, 1978, p. 844). This operated as a powerful enabling force in furthering the DSM-III project, for, as retrospectively observed in a DSM-IV text:

> no technological advance has more significantly influenced the development of DSM-III and the way psychiatrists think about mental illness than the personal computer ... In subtle and often unacknowledged ways, modern psychiatry's devotion to the computer has determined its conception of the psyche. (LaBruzza & Mendez-Villarubia, 1994, p. 25)

Indeed, it appears that Spitzer's efforts to delineate mental illnesses into diagnostic units that could then be measured via technological methods was influenced by his personal uneasiness with the enigmatic and seemingly chaotic nature of the psyche. For instance, he admitted to having a poor understanding of people's emotions (Spiegel, 2003) and in harking back to his prior attempts to use a psychoanalytic

---

[154] The role of the Advisory Committees was to "come up with detailed descriptions of mental disorders" for each of the main categorical areas (Spiegel, 2005). Spitzer frankly admits his carte blanche role in selecting committee and task force members: "I was able to appoint anybody that I wanted, not only on the task force, but also on these you know, individual committees" (Spiegel, 2003).

[155] In fact, Spitzer was perceived by his contemporaries as being obsessed by the project, working up to eighty hours per week. He was consequently described by colleague Allen Frances as a "kind of an idiot savant of diagnosis—in a good sense, in the sense that he never tires of it" (Spiegel, 2005).

approach he confessed that: "I was uncomfortable with not knowing what to do with their messiness ... I don't think I was uncomfortable listening and empathizing; I just didn't know what the hell to do" (Spiegel, 2005). It seems he was more comfortable with a conception of the psyche that was conducive to the predictable diagnostic approach of structured observation, measurement, and categorisation exemplified in DSM-III. Consequently, the understandings of the psyche (and psychosis) in DSM-III are ostensibly more reflective of the authors' biomedical ideology, and Spitzer's personal technological preferences, than of robust scientific research, or deep phenomenological investigation into their nature.

Two further social forces that combined to foster the advance of DSM-III were the poor state of community mental health services in America in the late 1970s and the corresponding rise of pharmaceutical treatment approaches to mental disorders. During the 1960s, a policy of deinstitutionalisation was enacted in America whereby many people with psychiatric disorders were treated at Community Mental Health Centres (CMHC) rather state-run institutions (Mayes & Horwitz, 2005, p. 255). However, over the ensuing decade there was a concomitant trend in psychiatry towards private psychoanalytic practice, which resulted in the emergence of a "new cohort" of people with severe mental disorders in the understaffed community mental health system (ibid., p.256). Many CMHC psychiatrists felt ill-equipped to treat these people and progressively resorted to prescribing medications because of their apparent effectiveness in controlling or blunting psychiatric symptoms (ibid.). Consequently, a mutually beneficial relationship developed between the new DSM-III medical model and biological psychiatric approaches. On the one hand, "the symptom-based diseases" of the new manual helped spur growth in the psychiatric drug treatments market (Mayes & Horwitz, 2005, pp. 256, 266; Zung, 1975, p. 25), while correspondingly, the rising impetus of this biomedical enterprise bolstered the necessity for an empirical psychiatric manual (Wilson, 1993, p. 404). According to Healy (2002a, pp. 305–306), this heralded the birth of "a new psychiatry", which progressively consolidated into a biomedical model of psychiatric thinking and practice. In consideration of the abovementioned factors, it is evident that the formulation of DSM-III was powerfully influenced by various social forces.

A2.4.2 Economic forces shaping DSM-III

Economic imperatives also played a significant role in abetting the reestablishment of psychiatry as a medical discipline and the development of DSM-III as the official diagnostic guidebook. The foremost influence was pressure from health insurance companies for psychiatry to provide medically legitimate diagnoses. As Decker (2007, p. 345) explains, "third-party payers of psychotherapeutic treatment mounted a campaign to pay only for 'real diseases' ... psychotherapy was to them a bottomless pit". This concern was emphasised by the medical director of a major insurance company, who asserted in 1979 that "problems of living" treated by psychodynamic psychiatrists, such as "floundering marriages, trouble raising children, and the difficulties in finding meaning in life", were outside the principal remit of insurance coverage. He maintained that:

> Medical insurance should only be asked to cover medical mental disorders. Insurance is meant to pay for the sick, not the discontented who are seeking an improved lifestyle. We need your help in differentiating between those who have mental disorders and those who simply have problems. (Sharfstein, 1987, p. 533)

It appears there was a measure of desperation to this appeal, for according to Mayes & Horwitz (2005, p. 262), insurance companies "virtually begged Spitzer and his task force to standardize the manual's diagnostic criteria so that insurers could separate legitimate mental illness from nonpsychiatric problems". This development begs the question: Was DSM-III's ascendency chiefly due to the robust scientific validity of disorders included in the manual, or did serving national pecuniary interests help lend it legitimacy that it would not have achieved independently? When considering that the DSM-III task force frankly admits that all disorders therein are non-scientifically validated constructs, it appears that pecuniary interests were the more influential force. Indeed, as Kutchins & Kirk (1997, p. 256) observe, the interrelationship between economics and psychiatry was limited prior to 1980 but, since DSM-III, "a strange defacto institutional marriage" developed between health insurance companies and medical psychiatry. Others also attest to the emergent influence of economic forces upon psychiatry since the publication of DSM-III. For instance, McHugh (2006, p. 51) claims that "the new DSM approach of using experts and descriptive criteria in identifying psychiatric diseases has encouraged a productive industry", while Schacht (1985, p. 514) contends that DSM-III has become "an official document that participates in the organization and distribution of social and economic power". Hence, it seems economic forces not only shaped the DSM-III process and content, but also rendered the manual itself an economic force that precipitated the establishment of American psychiatry as a profitable industry.

Although the relationship between fiscal forces and psychiatry is a valid socio-economic reality from a certain perspective, there also exists the critical view that this alliance compromised the medical integrity of DSM-III. For example, while psychiatrist Ben Bursten (1981, p. 371) acknowledged the practical fact that "economics demand that we be medical", he also cautioned about "the danger ... that we will be forced to limit our activities to those that fit the popular concept of what is medical because that is what insurance companies will pay for". In a similar vein, just prior to DSM-III's publication, the ex-president of the American Psychological Association, George Albee (in Spitzer & Endicott, 1978, p. 36), expressed his concern that the manual was "turning every human problem into a disease, in anticipation of the shower of health plan gold that is over the horizon". Spitzer (1981, p. 3) vigorously rejected such suggestions as "nonsense" and "absurd", clarifying that:

> The only instance that I can recall in which 'economic' considerations influenced DSM-III was our reluctant decision to drop the term 'chronic minor affective disorders' because a group of clinicians insisted that insurance companies would not want to reimburse for the treatment of a condition that appeared to be both incurable and trivial.

This is a perplexing defence, for it openly admits what it aims to refute; for in at least one instance, a diagnostic entity was excluded from DSM-III due to economic considerations. Was this occurrence unique? It seems not. Task force member Henry Pinkser (in Wilson, 1993, p. 405) stated in a 1975 memorandum:

> I believe that many of what we now call disorders are really but symptoms ... Physicians diagnose these things, prescribe, and insurance companies reimburse. I don't believe the gastroenterologists have task forces to decide whether constipation and pylorospasm should be listed as diseases or not.

This statement implies the artificial construction of all DSM-III mental disorders as 'real' diseases in order to qualify, in part, for insurance reimbursement. Spitzer (in Wilson, 1993, p. 405) challenged this idea, warning that "reimbursement would be very difficult if the symptom clusters in the manual were not called 'syndromes' or 'disorders'". This arguably amounts to an admission that DSM-III entities are indeed symptom clusters, but presented as 'true' medical disorders for reasons of economic expediency. In sum, it appears economic forces played a pivotal role in enhancing the medical status of DSM-III, and economic considerations regulated the selection criteria for mental disorder inclusion in DSM-III more so than scientific veracity.

A2.4.3 Political forces shaping DSM-III

Political forces and factors also played a core role in shaping the DSM-III process and content. For instance, Schacht (1985, p. 516) argued that "political forces are an integral part of the rational-scientific knowledge-producing process", and explained that due to the prevailing and mistaken belief that scientific sanctity is preserved by separating it from politics, Spitzer was trapped into denying the political dimension of DSM-III, while simultaneously engaging in an ongoing process of politicking (ibid., pp. 518–520). Spitzer (1985, p. 524) rebutted this claim, stating, "I did not deny all political dimensions of DSM-III. I only denied certain specific allegations, such as that the politics of DSM-III compromised its scientific values for professional or economic gain". Regardless of these differing views as to the exact nature of political play in the DSM-III project, there appears to be general concurrence that, as Schacht (1985, p. 515) puts it, "DSM-III is a *political* document". Indeed, many commentators have used military terms to describe the success of the DSM-III project. For instance, the manual's inauguration is depicted by Houts (2000, p. 497) as "a successful palace coup within the APA", by Healy (2002a, p. 304) as being executed by an "army from nowhere, with the contest being over almost before anyone knew it had begun", and by others as a "revolution" (Decker, 2007, p. 350; Mayes & Horwitz, 2005; Rogler, 1997, p. 10). This raises the question: If a revolution did occur, then by whom was it instigated, and why?

My appraisal and distillation of the vast body of literature on the DSM-III phenomenon seems to provide a plausible answer to this question. Namely, that the DSM-III project was fundamentally a political struggle by a minority group of medically oriented neo-Kraepelinian psychiatrists against the prevailing force of psychodynamic psychiatry. The primary aims of this operation appear to be threefold:

1. To fight a battle of survival for the discipline of psychiatry generally.
2. To secure professional legitimacy for a medical model of psychiatry.
3. To establish a clear-cut jurisdictional arena for the practice of medical psychiatry.

These aims were mutually reinforcing in that: the perceived survival crisis was redressed by establishing professional legitimacy and jurisdiction; creating legitimacy advanced jurisdiction claims; and the status afforded by delineating a field of jurisdiction added further weight to medical psychiatry's legitimacy.

First, in terms of the perceived survival crisis, the 1976 APA President, Alan Stone, apprehensively noted that the socially oriented psychodynamic approach to psychiatry "had bought the profession to the edge of extinction" (Stone in Wilson, 1993, p. 402). Indeed, during the 1970s, the question loomed large among practitioners in the mental health field: What differentiates psychiatry from other mental health practices? For example, Hackett (1977, p. 434) observed at the time that "apart from their training in medicine, psychiatrists have nothing unique to offer that cannot be provided by psychologists, the clergy, or lay psychotherapists". Similarly, Mayes & Horwitz, (2005, p. 257) noted that "there was nothing explicitly *psychiatric* about dynamic psychiatry; nonmedical and medical professionals alike were equally able to learn and practice it". Hence, after two and a half decades of psychodynamic rule, psychiatry as a distinct discipline faced imminent redundancy by being absorbed into the nebulous matrix of psychological and mental health disciplines.

In response to this perceived survival crisis, members of the neo-Kraepelinian group of psychiatrists saw a need to concurrently establish empirical legitimacy and demarcate medical psychiatry's field of authority. In this political light, the DSM-III innovations of improving reliability, defining the concept of mental disorder, and developing a categorised, descriptive, operationalised, and multiaxial diagnostic system, served a twin purpose. One, it provided psychiatry with a stamp of empirical legitimacy, and two, it subsequently redefined psychiatry as belonging to the scientific field of medical disciplines. As Blashfield (1984, p. 77) observed, defining mental disorder in a medical context aimed to help "resolve the *demarcation problem* ... [and] draw a boundary between persons who should be seen by mental health professionals and persons who should not". This observation was corroborated by

Spitzer (1985, p. 525), who conceded that one of the "political advantages" of defining mental disorder was "justifying the professional activities of psychiatry as a branch of medicine". Arguably, such developments represent a case whereby the task force appropriated and used key tenets of medical science to develop an operational model of psychiatry that served the fundamental imperative of maintaining the discipline's survival. If so, then in this instance, it appears that survival, rather than science, was the primary factor driving the push for developing a medical model of psychiatry in DSM-III.

This move precipitated a strident backlash from psychoanalytic psychiatry that threatened to derail the review process. According to Spitzer (ibid., p. 523), as a consequence of proposed changes by the task force, there ensued:

> an extremely bitter political struggle between the DSM-III task force and a large number of psychiatrists within the American Psychiatric Association who believed that the task force was not representative of American psychiatry and was using DSM-III to expunge Freud's valuable contributions to the understanding of psychopathology.

This was particularly so when the task force attempted to remove the 'neurosis' category from DSM-III because it was deemed an ambiguous and theoretical notion (Bayer & Spitzer, 1985, p. 189). Healy (1997, p. 235) described the subsequent struggle as "a political skirmish ... [where] pitches made by both sides were based on what would secure votes rather than by appeals to the evidence". What had been, until then, a mostly undetected and well-orchestrated reform, suddenly became an open turf war. This conflict threatened to overthrow the DSM-III project, forcing Spitzer to negotiate a mutually acceptable compromise in 1979 (Bayer & Spitzer, 1985, p. 192), thus enabling the culmination of a turbulent transition from a psychodynamic to a medical model of psychiatry. A year later the neo-Kraepelinian coup was finally realised with the approval of DSM-III by majority vote at the 1980 APA annual meeting (Decker, 2007, p. 353). The formal publication of the new manual saw the reinstatement of a medical model of practice in American psychiatry, and arguably, the beginning of a concomitant trend towards biological determinism in understanding psychopathology and psychosis.

A2.5 DSM-III and psychosis

It stands to reason that the various dynamics and factors which shaped the production of DSM-III correspondingly shaped the construal of psychosis therein. Hence, in terms of aetiology, the DSM-II psychogenic understanding of psychosis as a reactive disorder precipitated by psychosocial stressors was superseded in DSM-III by an understanding of psychosis as a medical and ostensive biogenic disorder precipitated by yet-to-be-discovered anatomical aberrations. Additionally, it appears that the DSM-III construal of psychosis was not only shaped by empirical attempts to redress issues of diagnostic reliability and validity, but also by a raft of social, economic, and political factors. For instance, a precipitating social factor in the formulation of operationalised diagnostic criteria for psychotic disorders in DSM-III was the professional embarrassment caused to psychiatry by the Rosenhan experiment. Similarly, a failing community mental health system, coupled with fiscal pressure from insurance companies for psychiatric disorders to be differentiated from general psychological disorders, led to psychosis, and other forms of psychopathology, being diagnosed via a prescriptive medical diagnostic formula. All of this, in turn, was implemented through the medium of political manoeuvring and the pressing imperative, in the task force's view, for psychiatry to establish itself as a scientific and medical discipline in order to circumvent its own imminent demise. Finally, the quantitative development of diagnostic criteria for psychotic disorders was ultimately not born of objective science but by the subjective and political process of heated debate and voting. In composite, such factors have seemingly been instrumental in establishing a categorical and biogenic picture of psychosis in DSM-III. In light of all of this, it is apposite to suggest that the medical model for understanding psychosis in DSM-III and beyond has been radically shaped by socioeconomic and political expediency.

A2.6 Conclusion

This examination of the DSM-III review process has provided an informative window into the various factors and dynamics that have worked to shape not only a psychiatric diagnostic manual, but also to facilitate a sea-change transition from one model of psychiatry to another. In this instance, the transition was from a psychogenic-cum-psychodynamic to a biogenic-cum-biomedical model of understanding. The publication of DSM-III has been hailed for its purported science-based rigour and for supposedly investing psychiatry with the status of being a legitimate medical discipline. However, while it can be argued that DSM-III has the *appearance* of being a medical model due to its operationalised diagnostic criteria, descriptive diagnostic categories, multiaxial diagnostic system, definition of mental illness, and ostensibly improved diagnostic reliability, this does not make it a medical model per se. Indeed, in consideration of the material examined throughout this appendix, it can reasonably be argued that DSM-III was fundamentally shaped by a composite of social, economic, and political factors, with medical science factors playing a secondary role. The subsequent understanding of psychosis has been shaped by all of these factors.

APPENDIX 3

The many meanings of mysticism and related ramifications for better understanding psychosis

The term 'mysticism' has manifold meanings ranging from the universal to the specific. Consequently, the body of research relating to this subject is vast. Indeed, Feenstra & Tydeman (2011, p. 132) note that "a recently released encyclopaedia of mysticism written in Dutch took ten years, thirty-four collaborators and 1149 pages to bring together".[156] Hence, a thorough explication of the mystic domain is beyond the scope of this appendix and descriptions are limited to some key conceptualisations of mystical experience. Additionally, and importantly, the understanding of reality from a mystic perspective is seemingly at odds with conventional views of reality, and normal mystic experiences can mirror those which, from a psychiatric perspective, may appear to be psychotic. If the validity of mystic experience is accepted as possible then this calls for a reconsideration of what constitutes 'normal reality' versus 'psychotic unreality'.

In general, the word 'mystical' is a catchphrase referring to anything of an esoteric, magical, paranormal, or spiritual nature. This is evident in the manifold 'mystical' interests of the New Age spiritual movement, which is, itself, described as a "mystical" phenomenon (Hess, 1993, p. 159). However, in a theistic or spiritual sense, the term is mostly used to denote the path, the practices, and the experiences of psychospiritual development. Underhill (1912, pp. 113, 203) refers to this as "the Mystic Way", which consists of five general "states or stages of development", namely: "1) Awakening or Conversion; 2) Self-knowledge or Purgation; 3) Illumination; 4) Surrender, or the Dark Night; 5) Union". Hence, for the spiritual adherent, this development involves

---

[156] See Baers, J., Brinkman, G., Jelsma, A., & Steggink, O. (2003). *Encyclopedie van de mystiek, fundamenten, tradities, perspectieven*. Uitgeverij Kok.

a progressive vacillation between states of luminosity and dark suffering. Further to this, the philosopher-psychologist William James (1905, pp. 380–382) identifies four defining characteristics of mystical experience (see Table A1).

Table A1. James' four defining characteristics of mystical experience.

Characteristics of mystical experience

1. Ineffability – The handiest of the marks by which I classify a state of mind as mystical is negative. The subject of it immediately says that it defies expression, that no adequate report of its contents can be given in words. It follows from this that its quality must be directly experienced; it cannot be imparted or transferred to others. In this peculiarity mystical states are more like states of feeling than like states of intellect.
2. Noetic quality – Although so similar to states of feeling, mystical states seem to those who experience them to be also states of knowledge. They are states of insight into depths of truth unplumbed by the discursive intellect. They are illuminations, revelations, full of significance and importance, all inarticulate though they remain; and as a rule they carry with them a curious sense of authority for after-time.
3. Transiency – Mystical states cannot be sustained for long. Except in rare instances, half an hour, or at most an hour or two, seems to be the limit beyond which they fade into the light of common day. Often, when faded, their quality can but imperfectly be reproduced in memory; but when they recur it is recognized; and from one recurrence to another it is susceptible of continuous development in what is felt as inner richness and importance.
4. Passivity – Although the oncoming of mystical states may be facilitated by preliminary voluntary operations, as by fixing the attention, or going through certain bodily performances, or in other ways which manuals of mysticism prescribe; yet when the characteristic sort of consciousness once has set in, the mystic feels as if his own will were in abeyance, and indeed sometimes as if he were grasped and held by a superior power.

Source: James, 1905, pp. 380–382.

The first two characteristics he deemed to be the prominent and principal markers of a mystical state, while the latter two, though less common, were still indicative (ibid., p. 381). Indeed, Leonard (1999, p. 107) maintains that "mysticism is difficult to comprehend due in part to the pervasive difficulty of trying to say something meaningful about an awareness that mystics universally allege is ineffable". In fact, he suggests that ineffability is the "sine qua non for mystical experience" (ibid., p. 88). Hence, broadly speaking, the mystic experience is a non-ordinary state of consciousness that is ultimately impossible to elucidate in words.

The American philosopher-mystic Franklin Merrell-Wolff has also written profusely on the subject of mysticism. It is therefore apposite to examine some of his views, for as a contemporary Western mystic they are drawn from the process of his own experiences along the path to spiritual enlightenment. According to Merrell-Wolff (1995, pp. 222–223), conceptualisations of mysticism fall into three camps:

1. The religious view, which sees mystical "union" as the epitome of mysticism.
2. The epistemological view, which is concerned with definitions pertaining to "the instrumentality whereby the mystical consciousness is attained".
3. The psychological view, which "considers the state primarily as an 'experience' and hence something that may occur in the lives of empiric beings as they live in time".

He further notes that, from a psychological perspective, the subject of mysticism is "viewed from the outside, that is, as it can be observed by a consciousness that has no immediate acquaintance with the state" (ibid.). However, Merrell-Wolff (1994, p. 425) explains that true mystical experience is beyond the conventional understanding of 'experience':

> In the broadest sense, the Transcendent stands in radical contrast to the empirical. It is that which lies beyond experience. Hence, Transcendent Consciousness is non-experiential consciousness; and, since experience may be regarded as consciousness in the stream of becoming or under time, the form is of necessity a timeless Consciousness. The actuality of such Consciousness can never be proved directly from experience when the latter term is taken in this restricted sense. Thus, It is either a philosophic abstraction or a direct mystical Recognition.

The transcendent mystical event is experienced directly and not mediated via the sensory and conceptual modes of normal human cognition; or that which Merrell-Wolff calls "subject-object consciousness" (ibid., p. 13). In other words, while the subject-object act of cognition is comprised of an 'observer' and the 'observed', where the two seemingly exist as discrete phenomena, in the mystical 'experience' the observer and the observed become united. The conventional sense of distance or separation dissolves as subject-object consciousness is transcended (p. 199). However, because the core of mystical experience is inexpressible in language it can only be alluded to symbolically. Ultimately, mystic experience is transcendent and ineffable.

Aspects of Merrell-Wolff's mystic philosophy also have ostensible bearing on better understanding the psychotic experience. For example, his views on the relative nature of reality have significant implications for the psychiatric depiction of psychosis as a 'gross impairment in reality testing'. In regards to so-called 'hallucinations', Merrell-Wolff (pp. 331–332) argues that:

> modern psychology [and psychiatry] distinguishes between objects that it calls real and objects that it calls hallucinations … Some mystical states, probably the greater number, involve the experiencing of subtle objects of the type that the psychologist calls hallucination. Practically, this has the effect of classifying the mystic with

the psychotic, apparently with the intent of common depreciation. Such a course involves both intellectual laziness and a failure in discrimination.

He further holds that "there is no important difference" between 'consensual reality' and a 'hallucination' from the viewpoint of mystical enlightenment because the latter "merely means private experience as opposed to social experience" and subsequently "constitutes no true judgement of value" (pp. 331, 332). From this mystical perspective the notion of 'reality' becomes highly elastic, for 'hallucinations' are deemed to be as real as normal states of cognition. This view fundamentally challenges the binary model of psychiatric dualism. In fact, he argues that "in a given case, the so-called hallucination may far outreach any social object in the relative reality" (p. 332) and provocatively suggests "it is quite possible that some present inmate of a psychiatric institution may outdistance all the philistines in the world who pride themselves on their sanity" (p. 387). While these views do not assert the nonexistence of 'psychotic' states of consciousness, or suggest that all such experiences are actually mystical, they arguably indicate that investigating the phenomenon of psychosis, or apparent psychosis, from a mystical perspective may foster a greater understanding of this enigmatic experience, and concomitantly, foster a greater understanding of the nature of both physical and metaphysical reality.

APPENDIX 4

Franklin Merrell-Wolff: a mystic's critique of Dean's metapsychiatry

This appendix examines the appraisal of Dean's work on metapsychiatry by the American mystic Franklin Merrell-Wolff.[157] In 1974, Merrell-Wolff delivered a lecture in which he discussed the "difficulties that are connected with a scientific approach to an essentially religious subject matter" (Merrell-Wolff, 1974, p. 1) and, as a case in point, he critiqued Dean's (1974b) article titled 'Metapsychiatry: The confluence of psychiatry and mysticism'.[158] It is apposite to examine his critique of Dean's work for it offers a first-person mystic review of the merits and shortcomings of Dean's metapsychiatry project. This provides a rare and critical window of insight, from a mystic's perspective, into the idea of incorporating metaphysical realities into psychiatric practice.

Throughout his delivery Merrell-Wolf both endorses and challenges Dean's ideas. In terms of endorsement, his general response is to "commend wholeheartedly" Dean's proposal for its contribution towards furthering a dialogue between science and mysticism (Merrell-Wolff, 1974, p. 8). He also holds that Dean's word 'ultraconsciousness' is "a very excellent term for the higher consciousness" (ibid., p. 4), and offers positive appraisal on many other points. For instance, it is his opinion that considering Dean's lack of personal experience of psi or mystical states, he "attains an impressive and even astonishing degree of insight" (p. 3) in his compilation of psychic aphorisms. Two aphorisms in particular are highlighted for their insightful

---

[157] Merrell-Wolff achieved mystical enlightenment on 7 August 1936 and eschewed a promising academic career to pursue a path of mystical exploration and explication (Merrell-Wolff, 1976, p. 15). This included the production of a prodigious body of experiential and philosophical writings about mystic reality.

[158] It appears that Dean and other commentators were unaware of Merrell-Wolff's appraisal for it is mentioned nowhere in the literature pertaining to metapsychiatry.

significance. First, Merrell-Wolff affirms that Dean's aphorism "psychogeny recapitulates cosmogony"[159] is a "particularly impressive statement", in its succinct representation of the metaphysical principal that "development is synchronous in the different directions or forms of the development in nature, and in man, in apparent things, and in the states of consciousness" (p. 4). Hence, he concurs with Dean's notion of an evolutionary aspect to metaphysical human development whereby the gradual emergence of advanced states of consciousness supersedes normal modalities of human cognition. Second, he observes that Dean's aphorism "thought is a form of energy" is a "very important statement" because it characterises the mystic understanding that "thought is a power ... that can penetrate directly into the heart of things and that we are not restricted to the methods of scientific research which is oriented primarily to sensuous experience" (p.4). Dean's ten points pertaining to the nature of ultraconsciousness are also lauded by Merrell-Wolff as being "of particular interest" in that they are generally reflective of the mystical state of enlightenment (p. 5), however, he further stipulates that "many Awakenings include part of these but not all" (p. 6). Finally, in Merrell-Wolff's view, Dean "achieves his own particular orientation" (p. 7) in posing six questions to appraise the ramifications of ultraconsciousness theory for psychiatric thinking and practice.[160] Overall, his appraisal of Dean's project is mostly optimistic and he supports the idea of developing a confluence between psychiatry and mysticism.

In terms of challenge, Merrell-Wolff questions some of Dean's assumptions concerning the nature of a merger between psychiatry and mysticism. His main point of contention with metapsychiatry is that it posits mysticism as "subordinate to a discipline which is oriented to the pathological" (p. 3). This is a warranted criticism, for although Dean envisions metapsychiatry as a field that recognises the validity of and harnesses mystic knowledge, his depiction of mysticism as but one side of a pyramid, of which metapsychiatry forms the base, misrepresents the transcendental nature of ultraconsciousness. As Merrell-Wolff explains, mysticism is "that which belongs to the opening of another door of cognition which transcends the conceptual powers as it very definitely transcends the perceptual capacity of man" (p. 3). In other words, mystic reality cannot be sublimated to the status of a conceptual object within the rubric of a branch of psychiatry, for ultimately it transcends all conceptual constructs.

---

[159] See Dean (1974b, p. 9) for his list of aphorisms.
[160] These questions are:

1. Is the ultraconsciousness a gift of God, beyond human understanding? If so, it should be accepted as a matter of pure faith, and without further question.
2. Is it a pathological mental disorder? If so, how could it elicit genius in religion, literature, and the arts?
3. Is it hypnosis or suggestion?
4. Does self-mortification and sensory deprivation, as practiced by [the] ascetics, produce metabolic by-products with hallucinogenic properties similar to those of psychedelic drugs?
5. Is it all a matter of charlatanism?
6. *Is the ultraconscious experience a natural biological phenomenon latent in all of us?* (Merrell-Wolff, 1974, pp. 7–8; also, see Dean, 1974b).

Additionally, in framing the question "Is the ultraconscious experience a natural biological phenomenon latent in us all?", Dean apparently suggests the primacy of biology over spiritual experience. In response to this, Merrell-Wolff asserts:

> Indeed, I should say it is latent in all of us, but ... not of such a nature as to be called 'natural'. It is something that transcends nature and belongs to what we might call super-nature perhaps, or that which descends from on high into the consciousness. (p. 8)

From his own experience, Merrell-Wolff understands spiritual enlightenment, or mystical apotheosis, to be beyond confinement to a framework of psychiatric thinking. However, as indicated above, he believes Dean's metapsychiatric attempt to better understand mystic states of consciousness (as opposed to sublimating them) is a significant step towards bridging the gap between scientific and psychospiritual worldviews.

Another of Merrell-Wolff's key concerns is the tacit association of mystic experiences with pathology and disease via metapsychiatry. He notes that clinical psychiatry, by definition, is "a discipline concerned with the diseases of the mind", and consequently there exists "an overtone that is unavoidably denigrating when one associates a type of consciousness which transcends the normal consciousness as being related to disease" (p. 2). In fairness, when conceptualising metapsychiatry, Dean made no pathological inferences about ultraconscious phenomena; however, the potential for mysticism to be appropriated under the umbrella of psychiatry's psychopathology-centred remit is arguably a valid concern. In fact, Merrell-Wolff stresses that the transcendent states of consciousness characteristic of mysticism "should not be viewed from the angle of disease; rather, it is becoming essentially well" (p. 2); and he affirms that "I wish to underscore this as powerfully as I can. It is not disease. It is becoming at last truly well" (p. 9). It appears this assertion inversely suggests that normal human consciousness is somehow 'not fully well'. Indeed, Merrell-Wolff (p. 3) contends that from the viewpoint of mystic enlightenment, "our so-called normal state ... is the norm of an asylum". This speaks to the important issue of the relativity of defining insanity, particularly in the attempt to better understand psychosis.

In sum, while Merrell-Wolff's appraisal of Dean's work does not address psychiatric illnesses per se, he offers some potentially valuable insights into the efficacy of incorporating psychospiritual knowledge into better understanding psychotic experiences. For instance, he affirms the existence of modes of cognition that 'are not restricted to the methods of scientific research' which, nevertheless, provide valid insights into the nature of life and its multifarious phenomena. Also, his allusion to the danger of materialist reductionism, and the related conflation of spiritual and psychopathological experiences, has also been expressed by commentators in the field of psychopathology. Indeed, Newberg & Lee (2005, pp. 481–482) exhort that "care must be taken to avoid referring to spiritual experience only in pathological terms or as associated with pathological conditions and also to avoid reducing spiritual experiences only to neurophysiological mechanisms". Finally, Merrell-Wolff's discussion on two of Dean's aphorisms (i.e., 'psychogeny recapitulates cosmogony' and 'thought is a form of energy') depicts consciousness as holistically integral with, rather than epiphenomenal to, the physical body. This has considerable ramifications for the prevailing psychiatric view that psychotic states of consciousness are the product of a yet-to-be-discovered anatomical aberration. What if this view is incorrect? What if states of consciousness are interrelated with, but not epiphenomenal to, anatomical processes? How might this influence the quest to understand the causes and nature of psychosis? Such questions reflect the challenge that psychospiritual considerations can pose to conventional psychiatric assumptions and beliefs.

APPENDIX 5

List of texts examined in my content analysis

Table A2 below lists, in alphabetical order, the seventy texts examined in my Chapter Nine content analysis, all of which contributed to my findings. Hence, this list depicts the nature and scope of the material from which my topmost nine criteria discerning psychotic from psychospiritual experiences have been drawn. Many of these texts are cited throughout Chapters Nine and Ten, and also elsewhere throughout this book, and are included in my general reference list. However, not all are cited in this book and consequently do not appear in the end-of-text references, therefore it is apposite to list all seventy citations here.

Table A2. List of texts examined in my context analysis.

Citation
Arieti, S. (1961). The loss of reality. *Psychoanalysis and the Psychoanalytic Review, 48*(3), 3–24.
Arieti, S. (1976). *Creativity: The magic synthesis.* Basic Books.
Assagioli, R. (1965). *Psychosynthesis: A manual of principles and techniques.* Penguin Books.
Austin, J. (1998). *Zen and the brain: Toward an understanding of meditation and consciousness.* MIT Press.
Boisen, A. (1936). *The exploration of the inner world: A study of mental disorder and religious experience.* Willett, Clark & Company.

(Continued)

Table A2. (Continued)

Citation

Bomford, R. (2014). Mystical theology, mysticism and madness. In J. Gale, M. Robson & G. Rapsomatioti (Eds.), *Insanity and divinity: Studies in psychosis and spirituality* (pp. 173–190). Routledge.

Bragdon, E. (2006). *A sourcebook for helping people in spiritual emergency*. Lightening Up.

Brett, C. (2002a). Psychotic and mystical states of being: Connections and distinctions. *Philosophy, Psychiatry and Psychology, 9*(4), 321–342.

Brett, C. (2002b). Spiritual experience and psychopathology: Dichotomy or interaction. *Philosophy, Psychiatry, and Psychology, 9*(4), 373–380.

Brown, J. (2005). *Inquiry into the understanding and applications of DSM-IV category Religious or Spiritual Problem, V-Code 62.89 by American Psychological Association (APA) psychologists* [Unpublished Doctoral thesis]. Institute of Transpersonal Psychology.

Buckley, P. (1981). Mystical experience and schizophrenia. *Schizophrenia Bulletin, 7*(3), 516–521.

Butler, C. (1926). *Western mysticism: The teaching of Saints Augustine, Gregory and Bernard on contemplation and the contemplative life*. E. P. Button.

Cantlie, A. (2014). The tantric ascetics of West Bengal. In J. Gale, M. Robson & G. Rapsomatioti (Eds.), *Insanity and divinity: Studies in psychosis and spirituality* (pp. 90–111). Routledge.

Carroll, M. (2007). *Am I going mad? The unsettling phenomena of spiritual evolution*. Inner Peace.

Chadwick, P. (2001). Sanity to supersanity to insanity: A personal journey. In I. Clarke (Ed.), *Psychosis and spirituality: Exploring the new frontier* (pp. 75–89). Whurr.

Clarke, I. (2000). Madness and mysticism: Clarifying the mystery. *Network: The Scientific and Medical Network Review, 72*, 11–14.

Clarke, I. (2001). Psychosis and spirituality: The discontinuity model. In I. Clarke (Ed.), *Psychosis and Spirituality: Exploring the New Frontier* (pp. 129–142). Whurr.

Crowley, N. (2006). Psychosis or spiritual emergence? Consideration of the transpersonal perspective within psychiatry. *Spirituality and Psychiatry Special Interest Group.* https://www.rcpsych.ac.uk/docs/default-source/members/sigs/spirituality-spsig/spirituality-special-interest-group-publications-nicki-crowley-psychosis-or-spiritual-emergence.pdf?sfvrsn=5685d4c1_2

de Menezes Junior, A. & Moreira-Almeida, A. (2009). Differential diagnosis between spiritual experiences and mental disorders of religious content. *Revista de Psiquiatria Clínica, 36*(2), 75–82.

DeHoff, S. (2012). *Distinguishing mystical religious experience from psychotic experience in the Presbyterian Church (USA)* [Unpublished Doctoral thesis]. Boston University.

Deikman, A. (1971). Bimodal consciousness. *Archives of General Psychiatry, 25*(6), 481–489.

(Continued)

Table A2. (Continued)

Citation

Drazenovich, G. (2007). *An exploration of the value of spirituality in the field of mental health* [Unpublished Masters thesis]. University of South Africa.

Eeles, J., Lowe, T., & Wellman, N. (2003). Spirituality or psychosis? An exploration of the criteria that nurses use to evaluate spiritual-type experiences reported by patients. *International Journal of Nursing Studies, 40*(2), 197–206.

Goretzki, M., Thalbourne, M., & Storm, L. (2009). The questionnaire measurement of spiritual emergency. *Journal of Transpersonal Psychology, 41*(1), 81–97.

Greeley, A. (1974). *Ecstasy: A way of knowing.* Prentice-Hall.

Greenberg, D., Witztum, E., & Buchbinder, J. (1992). Mysticism and psychosis: The fate of Ben Zoma. *British Journal of Medical Psychology, 65,* 223–235.

Greenwell, B. (2002). *Diagnostic criteria comparing kundalini awakening to other DSM diagnoses* [Unpublished manuscript]. Institute of Transpersonal Psychology.

Greyson, B. (1993). The physio-kundalini syndrome and mental illness. *Journal of Transpersonal Psychology, 25*(1), 43–58.

Grof, C., & Grof, S. (1995). *The stormy search for the self: Understanding and living with spiritual emergency.* Thorsons.

Hunt, H. (2007). 'Dark nights of the soul': Phenomenology and neurocognition of spiritual suffering in mysticism and psychosis. *Review of General Psychology, 11*(3), 209–234.

Jackson, M., & Fulford, K. (1997). Spiritual experience and psychopathology. *Philosophy, Psychiatry and Psychology, 4*(1), 41–65.

Jackson, M., & Fulford, K. (2002). Psychosis good and bad: Values-based practice and the distinction between pathological and nonpathological forms of psychotic experience. *Philosophy, Psychiatry and Psychology, 9*(4), 387–394.

Jackson, M. (2001). Psychotic and spiritual experience: A case study comparison. In I. Clarke (Ed.), *Psychosis and spirituality: Exploring the new frontier* (pp.165–190). Whurr.

James, W. (1905). *The varieties of religious experience: A study in human nature.* Longmans, Green, and Co.

Johnson, C., & Friedman, H. (2008). Enlightened or delusional? Differentiating religious, spiritual, and transpersonal experiences from psychopathology. *Journal of Humanistic Psychology, 48*(4), 505–527.

Jung, C. (1966). *Collected works: Volume 7: Two essays on analytical psychology.* Routledge & Kegan Paul.

Jung, C. (1969). *Collected works: Volume 8: The structure and dynamics of the psyche.* Princeton University Press.

Jung, C. (2009). *The red book: Liber novus: A reader's edition.* S. Shamdasani (Ed.). W. W. Norton & Co.

(Continued)

Table A2. (Continued)

Citation
Kant, I. (1964 [1798]). *The classification of mental disorders.* Doylestown Foundation.
Kemp, D. (2000). A Platonic delusion: The identification of psychosis and mysticism. *Mental Health, Religion & Culture, 3*(2), 157–172.
Kingdon, D., Siddle, R., Naeem, F., & Rathod, S. (2010). Spirituality, psychosis and the development of normalising rationales. In I. Clarke (Ed.), *Psychosis and spirituality: Consolidating the new paradigm* (pp. 239–247). John Wiley & Sons Ltd.
Koenig, H. (2007). Religion, spirituality and psychotic disorders. *Revista de Psiquiatria Clínica, 34*(supplement 1), 95–104.
Koenig, H. (2011). Schizophrenia and other psychotic disorders. In J. Peteet, F. Lu & W. Narrow (Eds.), *Religious and spiritual issues in psychiatric diagnosis: A research agenda for DSM-V* (pp. 31–51). American Psychiatric Publishing.
Lacan, J. (1993). *The psychoses: The seminar of Jacques Lacan: Book III 1955–1956,* Routledge.
Lukoff, D. (1985). Diagnosis of mystical experiences with psychotic features. *The Journal of Transpersonal Psychology, 17*(2), 155–181.
McGhee, M. (2002). Mysticism and psychosis: Descriptions and distinctions. *Philosophy, Psychiatry and Psychology, 9*(4), 343–347.
Meher Baba. (1988). The difference between ordinary madness and Mast states. In W. Donkin (Ed.), *The wayfarers: An account of the work of Meher Baba with the God-intoxicated, and also with advanced souls, sadhus, and the poor* (pp. 1–11). Sheriar Press.
Nelson, J. (1994). *Healing the split: Integrating spirit into our understanding of the mentally ill.* State University of New York Press.
Noll, R. (1983). Shamanism and schizophrenia: A state-specific approach to the 'schizophrenia metaphor' of shamanic states. *American Ethnologist, 10*(3), 443–459.
Pahnke, W., & Richards, W. (1966). Implications of LSD and experimental mysticism. *Journal of Religion and Health, 5*(3), 175–208.
Perceval, J. (1840). *A narrative of the treatment experienced by a gentleman, during a state of mental derangement.* Effingham Wilson.
Peters, E. (2001). Are delusions on a continuum? The case of religious and delusional beliefs. In I. Clarke (Ed.), *Psychosis and spirituality: Exploring the new frontier* (pp. 191–207). Whurr Publications.
Podvoll, E. (1979). Psychosis and the mystic path. *Psychoanalytic Review, 66*(4), 571–590.
Robbins, M. (2011). *The primordial mind in health and illness: A cross-cultural perspective.* Routledge.
Sannella, L. (1987). *The kundalini experience: Psychosis or transcendence?* Integral Publishing.
Sekida, K. (1985). *Zen training: Methods and philosophy.* Shambala.

(Continued)

Table A2. (Continued)

Citation

Shamdasani, S. (2009). Introduction. In S. Shamdasani (Ed.), *The red book: Liber novus: A reader's edition* (pp. 1–98). W. W. Norton& Co.

Siddle, R., Haddock, G., Tarrier, N., & Faragher, E. (2002). Religious delusions in patients admitted to hospital with schizophrenia. *Social Psychiatry and Psychiatric Epidemiology, 37*(3), 130–138.

Siegler, M., Osmond, H., & Mann, H. (1969). Laing's models of madness. *The British Journal of Psychiatry, 115*(525), 947–958.

Siglag, M. (1986). *Schizophrenic and mystical experience: Similarities and differences* [Unpublished Doctoral thesis]. University of Detroit.

Silverman, J. (1967). Shamans and acute schizophrenia. *American Anthropologist, 69*(1), 21–31.

Sims, A. (1997). Commentary on 'spiritual experience and psychopathology'. *Philosophy, Psychiatry and Psychology, 4*(1), 79–81.

Stephen, M., & Suryani, L. (2000). Shamanism, psychosis and autonomous imagination. *Culture, Medicine and Psychiatry, 24*(1), 5–38.

Stifler, K., Greer, J., Sneck, W., & Dovenmuehle, R. (1993). An empirical investigation of the discriminability of reported mystical experiences among religious contemplatives, psychotic inpatients, and normal adults. *Journal for the Scientific Study of Religion, 32*(4), 366–372.

Tobert, N. (2010). The polarities of consciousness. In I. Clarke (Ed.), *Psychosis and spirituality: Consolidating the new paradigm* (pp. 37–48). John Wiley & Sons Ltd.

Wapnick, K. (1969). Mysticism and schizophrenia. *Journal of Transpersonal Psychology, 1*(2), 49–67.

Watkins, J. (2010). *Unshrinking psychosis: Understanding and healing the wounded soul.* Michelle Anderson Publishing.

Wilber, K. (1975). Psychologia perennis: The spectrum of consciousness. *Journal of Transpersonal Psychology, 7*(2), 105–132.

Wulff, D. (2000). Mystical experience. In E. Cardeña, S. Lynn & S. Krippner (Eds.), *Varieties of anomalous experience: Examining the scientific evidence* (pp. 397–439). American Psychological Association.

Zaehner, R. (1961). *Mysticism sacred and profane: An inquiry into some varieties of praeternatural experiences.* Oxford University Press.

Typologies proposed by various authors for differentiating psychotic from psychospiritual experiences

D iscerning psychotic from psychospiritual experiences is a complex undertaking. Indeed, I argue in Focal Setting Four that, ultimately, it is a seemingly impossible task, and the diversity of views throughout the tabled models below seem to support this argument. However, they also provide a comprehensive and unique compilation of resources from this field of study. To my knowledge, such a list has not been previously composed. Despite the complex and diverse nature of these collective views, they also constitute a valuable body of phenomenological research into both psychotic and psychospiritual states of consciousness.

Table A3. Austin's comparisons between the mystical path and schizophrenic reactions.

	Mystical path	Schizophrenic psychosis
General nature and duration	An ongoing, more orderly development	May be compressed, disorderly and disorganized
Hallucinatory phenomena	In general, more visual; not threatening	In general, more auditory; can be threatening
Ideas of self-reference	Enlightenment cuts off the personal connotations of stimuli	Stimuli generate ideas of self-reference, especially in paranoid schizophrenia
A gap is experienced which splits outer social reality from inner personal reality	1*	3

(Continued)

293

Table A3. (Continued)

	Mystical path	Schizophrenic psychosis
Inhabiting only the inner world and being fearful of it	0–1	3
Degree of tolerance for inner experiences	Trained for and well-tolerated	May be overwhelmed by them
Simplification of lifestyle and renunciation of worldliness	More under conscious control	More under unconscious control
Dissolution of social achievements	1	3
Re-entry into society, improved by experience	The usual goal	Less common
Subsequent ongoing fruitful, well-integrated contacts with society	2	1 or 0
Sense of unity with the environment	2 (partially cultivated)	Less commonly perceived
Driving by craving and aversions	Reduced	May be enhanced
Continued conscious control	Usual	Less effective

* 0 = none; 5 = maximal.
Source: Austin, 1998, p. 31.

Table A4. Chadwick's parallels between mystical and psychotic states.

Mystical intuitions	Psychotic intuitions
I am in touch with everyone	Everyone can hear my thoughts
The world is not as it is commonly seen	The world has changed, there's a war on
There is great harmony and oneness between all things	People and the world are all together in communication against me
Nothing is trivial	Everything means something, even street signs and car number plates
No one is a stranger	Everyone knows me and is plotting against me
I am both supreme and insignificant	I am the Christ and the Devil
I am passive, floating, at one with the universe, open to all	I am dissolving, decaying, penetrated by rays, penises
Meaning is everywhere/all is meaning	Everything that I do or that happens has double, triple or quadruple meanings

(Continued)

Table A4. (Continued)

Mystical intuitions	Psychotic intuitions
I do not think, I am thought	I do not think, thoughts are planted in my head by computers/hypnotherapy at a distance

Source: Chadwick, 2001, p. 86.

Table A5. DeHoff's psychotic experience versus mystical experience.

Psychotic experiences	Mystical experiences
Fearing others conspiring against oneself	Experiencing a visceral sense of God's presence
Person out of touch with reality	Seeing a bright, white light
Using language not connected with [sic]	Hearing God's voice internally
Using incohesive language	Seeing Jesus
Claiming to be Jesus or the Virgin Mary	Experiencing God's physical, psychological healing
Hearing voices telling one to harm self or others	Feeling God's hands
Lacking insight	Hearing God's voice externally
Exhibiting flat affect	Experiencing God's inner presence
Focusing on self, not others	God leading so that "everything works out"
Avoiding of eye contact	God communicating through coincidences in nature
Exhibiting poor self-care, inability to function	One person instrumental in healing another
Lacking positive relationships	Experiencing God in secular life

Source: DeHoff, 2012, p. 195.

Table A6. Eeles et al.'s main indicators of mental illness versus well being.

	Nature of the experience	Outcome of the experience	Context of the experience
Indicators of illness	Similarity to common symptoms of mental illness Negative content	Risk to self or others Negative emotional outcome or grandiosity	Concern from people close to the individual
Indicators of well being	This did not feature predominantly	Good functioning at work and in relationships	This did not feature predominantly

Source: Eeles et al., 2003, p. 204.

Table A7. Greenwell's diagnostic criteria comparing kundalini symptoms with other DSM conditions.

Psychosis/Schizophrenia	Kundalini
General history/characteristics	
Onset is usually during adolescence or early adulthood. Pre-morbid history usually indicates poor adaptability in work and relationships. Usually personality was suspicious, introverted, withdrawn or eccentric before the break. In some cases they had a schizotypal or borderline personality disorder prior to the break. During acute stages the person may lack the ability and/or interest in eating and grooming. DSM 3 states that full recovery is considered so rare that many clinicians question the diagnosis of anyone who recovers. For a true diagnosis of schizophrenia the person should have continuous signs of illness for six months, including psychotic symptoms.	Usually very positive premorbid history, sometimes exceptional. Success in school, work, personal relationships. Healthy sense of self. Possibly someone who has searched for the meaning of life or the nature of God, or followed some kind of proactive spiritual practices, body therapies, martial arts or psychotherapy. Prior to onset may recently have had a traumatic physical or emotional event in their life or a strong personal encounter with a guru or spiritual teacher.
Loss of boundaries or consensus reality	
Person is flooded most of the time with the inability to differentiate information from the unconscious mind from consensus reality. It is hard to distinguish what is imaginal (and often paranoid) from what is actually happening. Delusions are usually multiple, fragmented and bizarre (i.e. thoughts are being broadcast from the head into others or from the TV set). One is unable to organize thoughts or to use insight to determine the meaning of events. May engage in bizarre repetitive rituals. Little awareness of needs or opinions of others. Likely to be compulsive, irrational, unreliable.	May occasionally have had an experience of expanded awareness, as if they are out of their body, their consciousness is spreading into space, or they are merged with another place or person (even inside a painting). Such events may be reported as frightening or awesome but the person recognizes them as distinctly altered from ordinary states. May feel once or twice a need to perform a ritual, which is usually seen as having significant meaning spiritually (i.e. taking a bath in salt, or balancing masculine and feminine energies in the house). These are not repetitive or compulsive, and a person can break the activity (e.g. to answer the front door) if need be. Usually there is conscious concern about what others will think and an effort to keep behavior compartmentalized in a way that it will not cause any problems in their life. There is often an enhanced sensitivity to the feelings of others.

(Continued)

Table A7. (Continued)

Psychosis/Schizophrenia	Kundalini
Hallucinatory visions and voices	
Hearing voices from outside the head is the most common hallucination, and usually they are insulting or threatening. May be flooded and driven by visions or inner voices, interpreting them with inflation (I am God) or ominous meaning (I am going to be destroyed or I must destroy someone else). Feels helpless in the face of these recurrent messages. DSM 3 lists auditory and tactile hallucinations i.e. electrical, tingling or burning sensations, and the sensation of snakes crawling inside the abdomen.	May receive an inner voice or perceive a vision occasionally. Most often these are positive and affirming experiences, with helpful advice, such as 'peace' or 'call to commitment'. Sometimes they come in a foreign language … or they are Biblical quotes. Visions may be in the form of symbolic or geometric shapes, images of spiritual beings, images of deceased loved ones or strangers, depict images of another lifetime or point in history, or seem to be predictors of future events. They are random, infrequent, and a person will describe them in a way that you get a felt sense of their genuine experience and their rational thoughts and concerns about the event.
Communication with others	
Affect is often blunted, flattened or inappropriate, with little facial expression. In some cases people believe you can read their mind, or are having the same experiences and are holding out on them. In others there is extreme distrust and an unwillingness to tell you what they are experiencing. But if you talk to a person in psychosis long enough some of the distortions in their thinking will be revealed. You often cannot understand what they actually said. Writing is often convoluted and ideas are mixed up in incongruent pictures. Sometimes speech is garbled, the person is unable to accomplish clear connection interpersonally, and has delusions about the intentions of others. There is a 'loosening of association' to the point that speech may become incomprehensible. Your counter-transference—often you feel confused and uncomfortable, unable to feel a genuine connection.	Good affect and sociability is most common. People express a relief and happiness in finding someone they can tell their story to who is not labelling them. Speech is normal although the person may become slightly dissociated or weepy when talking of the events. They usually relate some positive associations and feelings and are seeking a way to make these events more meaningful in their life, while managing or reducing the uncomfortable symptoms. Counter-transference—you are interested and often touched deeply by their presence and what they are telling you.

(Continued)

Table A7. (Continued)

Psychosis/Schizophrenia	Kundalini
Regression and connection to self	
Ability to function at mature adult level is seriously impaired most of the time and person acts compulsively out of defensive patterns. Logic is convoluted, bringing in data that seems to have no basis in objective reality.	Occasionally the person feels regressed or overwhelmed by memories, past-life images, strong emotions or hypersensitivity to others, but is usually able to pull together and function appropriately if they need to. Often they need to relieve stresses in their life and avoid toxic relationships for a while. Some go through stages of avoiding television and newspapers, and want to be more in a nature environment. But there is a sense of progression, rather than regression in these decisions, a sense they are connecting more deeply to who they are.
Religious ideation	
May have spiritual visions while deeply regressed and become confused, believing this means he/she is a god, the mother Mary, or Jesus. May see the devil in others. These experiences become alienating and may lead to inappropriate expectations and actions. If there is a unitive experience it is felt as regressive—wanting to coil up and retreat, be embraced into the connection, or feel special and that only they have such experiences, so they must be a saint.	May have spiritual visons while deeply regressed, and become confused. May have spiritual visons of any denomination, or light experiences, and are profoundly moved by these, possibly humbled, filled with joy or ecstasy. They may sense what is happening is a life-changing event, and find shifting interests and priorities in their life. They may be fearful that others will label this 'crazy' and will likely be cautious about who they tell about these experiences. May describe unitive experiences or transcendent awareness, a perception of merging or being scattered into something all-encompassing and greater than oneself. Following this event they usually describe peace, understanding, bliss.

(Continued)

Table A7. (Continued)

Psychosis/Schizophrenia	Kundalini
Changed affect	
Some of the consequences can be confusion, depression, dark foreboding, fear, convoluted information, paranoia, sense of inner chaos, sexual and aggressive fantasies.	Touched with awe, seeking understanding, reports ecstasy or joy, insight, sense of a deep wisdom guiding their life, feelings of unconditional love. They may seem naïve in their level of trust, or they fear death or insanity.
Attempt at transformation	
The psychological structure is collapsing and needs to be rebuilt with a new ego structure if there is to be hope of cure. Usually there is simply management with medication and the quality of life is dependent on the circumstances the person is in related to family and economic support.	The sense of self is realising limitations and growing into a greater sense of connection with the cosmic whole. Once there is understanding and acceptance of this as a spiritual process these is a calming and working-through phase of personal growth.

Source: Greenwell, 2002.

Table A8. Jackson's distinctions between spiritual and psychotic experience according to content, form and process.

Content	Spiritual experience	Psychotic experience
Content		
Religious or paranormal content	Sub-culturally based, socially accepted	Idiosyncratic, bizarre, alienating
Belief in personal mission, divine calling	Humility, recognition of personal fallibility	Grandiosity, sense of infallibility
Experience of discarnate entities, 'sense of presence'	Benign, recognised entity	Malignant, idiosyncratic entity
Sense of being guided by external power	Volitional control is retained	Involitional
Form		
Hallucinations—visions and voices	Pseudo hallucinations	True hallucinations
	Visual modality	Auditory modality
	Mood congruent, coherent, friendly	'First rank', chaotic, critical hallucinations
Delusions/revelations	Corrigible beliefs	Incorrigible beliefs
	Comprehensible beliefs	Bizarre beliefs
	Presence of 'insight'	Absence of 'insight'

(Continued)

Table A8. (Continued)

Content	Spiritual experience	Psychotic experience
Process		
Duration	Transient in time	Extended in time
Creative problem solving process (impasse—insight —resolution)	Spiritual fruits (humility, altruism, creativity)	Mental illness (self-centredness, inability to function)

Source: Jackson, 2001, p. 170.

Table A9. Jackson & Fulford's criteria for distinguishing between spiritual and pathological forms of psychotic experience.

Spiritual experience	Psychosis
Doctrinal orthodoxy—content acceptable to sub-cultural group	Bizarre content—particularly claims of divine status or special powers
Sensory elements are "intellectual" (experienced as mental contents)	Sensory elements are "corporeal" (experienced as veridical perceptions)
Predominantly visual hallucinations	Predominantly auditory hallucinations
Beliefs formed with possibility of doubt. Insight present	Incorrigible beliefs. Insight absent
Brief duration	Extended duration
Volitional control over experiences	Experiences are involitional
Other oriented	Self-oriented
"Self actualizing"; life enhancing; spiritual fruits	Disintegrative; deterioration in life functioning

Source: Jackson & Fulford, 1997, p. 62.

Table A10. Kemp's comparison between the healthy, the mystic, and the psychotic person.

Healthy	Mystic	Psychotic
Independent	Dependent on God	Dependent on a 'controlling force'; thought insertion
Conform to social roles and position	Only conform if it is 'right'	Conform to their own interpretation of the world. Adoption of Messiah/Saint stance
Communication with speech	Communication with God through prayer	Communication with others through telepathy; broadcasting of thoughts

(Continued)

Table A10. (Continued)

Healthy	Mystic	Psychotic
'Self-assertive': i.e. neither introverted nor extraverted	Oscillates between being meek and humble, and claiming to be a child of God	Delusions of grandeur, e.g. claims to be Christ, coupled with intense feeling of shame or guilt
Imaginative and creative	Believes in supernatural phenomena	Receives visions or signs
Not compulsive; spontaneous	Follows divine rules	Obsessive about apparently mundane matters
Mood equilibrium	Sinner/saved polarity	Intense polarity of moods: overjoyed/damned
Able to adapt to new situations	Adapts new situations to unchanging laws	Mission to change the world
Reason as source of knowledge	Revelation	Voices
Stability between life- (eros) and death- (thanatos) libido	Claims to be born again, be dead to the old life and have eternal life	Wants to die/believes to be already dead
In control of thoughts at all times	Seeks to gradually lose control of thoughts through following God's will	Sudden, passive experience of loss of control of thoughts
Sociable	Loves strangers and enemies	Everyone knows me and is plotting against me

Source: Kemp, 2000, p. 162.

Table A11. Nelson's signs for distinguishing regression in the service of transcendence (RIST) from schizophrenia.

RIST	Schizophrenia
Begins abruptly	Insidious onset
Precipitated by stressful life event	Usually unrelated to specific life events
Affect and feeling-tone is preserved and often wildly exaggerated	Bleak greyness
Shock of self-recrimination and guilt	No shock of self-recrimination and guilt
Can occur any time of life	Usually occurs during the second and third decades of life
Hallucinated voices never command	Hallucinated voices do command

(Continued)

Table A11. (Continued)

RIST	Schizophrenia
May be dramatically extroverted in its presentation or take an introspective turn	Almost always leads to withdrawal
Can maintain some insight into one's disordered state	No insight
Can try to restrain behaviour	Impulsive
Paranoid ideas absent or in context of a global terror of the unknown	Paranoid ideas present and in context of a specifically defined conspiracy
Tells a meaningful story composed of archetypal or mythic themes	Tells an incomprehensible story

Source: Nelson, 1994, pp. 248–249.

Table A12. Siegler et al.'s differences between psychedelic and psychotic experiences.

Psychedelic experience	Psychotic experience
Time dimension	
Liberation from time.	Frozen in time: nothing will ever change.
Expansion of time dimensions.	Shrinkage and collapse of time dimensions.
Internal or external time may speed up, increasing possibility of quick and decisive action.	Internal and external time may slow down, inhibiting action and creating despair.
Ability to modify past, present, future.	Inability to influence any of the temporal categories.
The future is the realm of ambition and motivation.	The future is the realm of anxiety and danger.
Space dimension	
Expanded depth.	Reduced depth.
Enhanced distance.	Reduced distance.
Distance perception stable.	Distance perception highly variable.
Distances so vast that one feels liberated.	Distances so vast that one feels isolated and alienated.
Affect	
Feeling that everything is meaningful and exhilarating.	Feeling that everything contains hidden, threatening meanings.
Feelings of love, empathy, consideration, affection.	Feelings of isolation, fear, hatred, suspicion.
Euphoria.	Depression.
Feeling of delight with oneself.	Feeling of disgust with oneself.

(Continued)

Table A12. (Continued)

Psychedelic experience	Psychotic experience
Thought processes	
Thought changes are sought for, expected, valued.	Thought changes come unawares, are not welcome, are seen as accidental.
Seeing more possibilities that can be acted upon, which makes life exciting.	Seeing so many possibilities that action is impossible.
Seeing beyond the usual categories.	Seeing only fragments or parts of the usual categories.
Seeing new connections which have always been possible.	Seeing connections which are not possible.
Ability to see things objectively.	No objectivity, inability to disengage from total involvement.
Ability to see things subjectively.	No subjectivity, estrangement from self.
Ability to explain thought changes.	Desperate attempts (delusions) to explain thought changes.
Perceptions	
Clear and distinct vision.	Blurred and distorted vision.
Augmentation of perception.	Diminution of perception.
Unusual perceptions seem to emanate from greater-than-human spirit or force.	Unusual perceptions seem to emanate from mechanical or sub-human forces.
Perceptual changes may be experienced as exhilarating, exciting, novel.	Perceptual changes may be experienced as frightening, threatening, dangerous.
Identity	
Feeling of unity with people and material objects.	Feeling of invasion by people and material objects.
Experience of the self.	Experience of the no-self ego fragmentation.
Feeling of being at one with the world.	Feeling of being opposed to and in conflict with oneself and the world.
Feelings of humility and awe as one sees oneself as part of the universe.	Feelings of smallness and insignificance as one feels at the mercy of the universe.
Feelings of integrity and identity.	Loss of integrity and identity.
Pleasant, creative fantasies that one can control.	Nightmarish fantasies that one cannot control.
Feeling that one can join the company of other enlightened people.	Feeling that one is less and less human, more and more isolated.

Source: Siegler et al., 1969, p. 956.

Table A13. Siglag's similarities and differences between schizophrenic individuals who claim to have had a mystical experience and other schizophrenic individuals.

Similarities	Differences
Do not feel any greater control over their experiences	Are more likely to have experienced a sense of unity, oneness, connectedness in the world
Do not feel a greater sense of coping ability	Report more of a range of affective experiences, and are more likely to have experienced joyful, peaceful states of consciousness
Do not experience any more improvement in their relationships	Are more likely to report time-space distortions
Experience terror, fear, depression, and a sense of insecurity	Experience more of a sense of sacredness or holiness

Source: Siglag, 1986, p. 138.

Table A14. Watkins' criteria for discerning authentic from erroneous spiritual experiences and practices.

Discerning criteria	Authentic spiritual experiences and beliefs	Erroneous spiritual experiences and beliefs
Peace versus agitation	Contribute to enhancement of mental peace, serenity, and an abiding state of emotional equanimity.	Tend to foster impulsiveness, impatience, seriousness, inflexibility and lack of reflection … Likely to exacerbate fear, guilt, anger, and despair in the long-term.
Growth versus stagnation	Are life-enhancing. Nourish the spirit, inspire and guide in a positive way, help people love and accept themselves and others, foster inner strength and personal responsibility, facilitate acceptance of reality and an ability to deal with complexity and uncertainty, enhance enjoyment and appreciation of life.	Preoccupation with erroneous ideas fosters misguided or inflexible behaviour which impairs adaptation and inhibits personal growth. In extreme cases may condemn a person to limited, unproductive, socially impoverished way of life.

(Continued)

Table A14. (Continued)

Discerning criteria	Authentic spiritual experiences and beliefs	Erroneous spiritual experiences and beliefs
Humility versus inflation	Promote humility and an attitude of reverence for life in all its myriad forms. Foster selflessness and willing acceptance of limitations and shortcomings. Accommodate a sense of humour that helps counteract pride or tendencies to take oneself too seriously.	May foster an attitude characterised by pride, arrogance, and an inflated or grossly exaggerated sense of self-importance that culminates in development of grandiose delusional beliefs.
Balance versus preoccupation	Are kept in perspective and understood to be but one facet of life. Are consistent with beliefs held before the psychotic crisis occurred and capable of being integrated into a harmonious, life-affirming personal belief system.	Lack of appropriate balance and perspective may result in a tendency to overemphasize irrational notions or become preoccupied with trivial issues. Phenomena with the power to dominate and entrance the mind often possess an addictive quality and may readily become the predominant focus of a person's life.
Free will versus compulsion	Do not impair free will. Person may surrender to certain legitimate beliefs of experiences but is able to exercise choice and demonstrate mature self-control. Good 'reality testing' is maintained, enabling person to question and critically evaluate his or her beliefs and experiences.	May be so compelling and mesmerising that choice, free will, and self-control are compromised. Certain phenomena (e.g. voices) may involve specific orders or demand unquestioning obedience. In extreme cases person may become enslaved by phenomena that obsess and possess them to such an extent they are unwilling or unable to question or challenge them.

(Continued)

Table A14. (Continued)

Discerning criteria	Authentic spiritual experiences and beliefs	Erroneous spiritual experiences and beliefs
Legitimacy versus eccentricity	While varying in specific form and content from one person to another nonetheless meet legitimacy criteria established by recognised authorities, e.g. religious tradition, respected teachers, sacred texts. Novel ideas, insights or beliefs are consistent with those of others with a comparable religious and/or spiritual philosophy and world view.	Are often highly idiosyncratic, eccentric, or bizarre and diverge substantially from generally accepted standards. Some ideas may be patently irrational, self-contradictory or incomprehensibly 'autistic', i.e. person concerned understands them but nobody else can.
Inclusiveness versus isolation	Build bridges between people by fostering awareness of the fundamental unity of life and sense of trust in the universe. Enhance the capacity for love and intimacy in relationships which may grow into genuine compassion for the whole of humanity and all living beings.	Fanatical ideas create barriers that shut a person off from others in increasing isolation, exclusiveness, and self-absorption. May devolve into narcissistically constricted 'all about me' attitude that results in ever-diminishing sensitivity to the feelings and needs of others.

Source: Watkins, 2010, pp. 216–218.

An overview of Emanuel Swedenborg's theory of mind

The content of this appendix enables a deeper appreciation of Swedenborg's metaphysical theory of mind, which informed van Dusen's unique research into the ostensible relationship between psychotic voice hearing and spirit possession. Here, I explicate Swedenborg's understanding of the intrinsic interconnectedness between human thoughts, affects, and spirit beings.

During the earlier half of his life, Swedenborg's empirical investigation into the nature of reality involved an exhaustive immersion into the physical sciences of the time. However, in failing to find the answers he was seeking through exploring the physical sciences, he turned his focus inwards to conduct an equally thorough empirical investigation of the metaphysical world. Like Jung, two hundred years later, he saw both science and metaphysics as empirical pursuits, because each involved the investigation of observable phenomena: the material via physical sense faculties and the metaphysical via latent inner senses. From the perspective of materialist science, Swedenborg's explication of the nature of mind and self may appear outrageous, if not psychotic. Therefore, it is apposite to note that as far-fetched or 'psychotic' as his theory of mind may appear, he maintained a highly functional life until he died at the age of eighty-four, well-respected by his gentry peers. Soon after his death, the Swedenborgian New Church was founded as a religion, and has since expanded to many countries around the world (Williams-Hogan, 2005a; 2005b). These factors suggest that his views are of a mystical rather than delusional nature.

As a mystic, Swedenborg's theory of mind did not emerge from a process of abstract conceptualisation, but from direct personal experience of transpersonal states, or realms, of consciousness. According to van Dusen (1974, p. 115) his writings constituted a "theological psychology". From his forays into realms of reality existing beyond the conscious apprehension of most people, he came to understand that thought derives from feeling, or, as he put it "the thought is nothing other than the form of the affection" (Swedenborg, 1892 [1764], p. 124). For van Dusen (1974, p. 101), means that thoughts are the product and expression of underlying affective states: "The affective side of thought can be felt as a tone or as the background of feeling from which thought arises. Thought gives feeling form and is part of its actualising". By and large, this idea is congruent with many models of modern psychological thinking, however, his further views on this issue go beyond the bounds of Western epistemology, both secular and religious.

While it is beyond the scope of this overview to describe the manifold dynamics and intricacies of Swedenborg's theory of mind, in general terms he saw humans and spirits as intrinsically, though unconsciously, interconnected in affect and thought. For instance, he asserts that "spirits are affections, and therefore in a human form similar to their affections" (Swedenborg, 1905 [1758], p. 474) and, elsewhere, that "a man's spirit is nothing else than affection ... after death he becomes an affection, an angel of heaven if he is an affection for a good use, a spirit of hell if an affection for an evil use" (Swedenborg, 1942 [1763], p. 18). Here he appears to be saying that spirits *are* affects and their existence is analogous to the affective states of human experience. Yet he goes further to seemingly suggest an intrinsic interrelationship between humans and spirits and affect-thoughts:

> With every man there are good spirits and evil spirits ... When these spirits come to man, they enter into all his memory, and thus into his entire thought, evil spirits into the evil things of his memory and thought, and good spirits into the good things of his memory and thought. (Swedenborg, 1905 [1758], pp. 229–230)

Indeed, he holds that humans and spirits can unconsciously share a common affect-thought experience, with each being unaware of the other, and believing the experience to be uniquely their own. As he explains, "these spirits have no knowledge whatever that they are with man; but when they are with him they believe that all things of his memory and thought are their own" (ibid., p. 230). In other words, humans and spirits are intrinsically and unknowingly connected through the experience of affect-thought.

How, then, does psychotic experience fit into Swedenborg's theory of mind? Although his writings predate the advent of psychiatry and the formulation of diagnostic categories such as 'psychosis' and 'schizophrenia', he did allude to issues of madness in places. For instance, he speaks of people who "labor under an infirmity of mind" when they grandiosely believe in and become fixated by "illusions" that are fabricated by spirits (Swedenborg, 2010a [1747–1765]), and also of psychotic-like spirit possession whereby a spirit will "enter into his body, and occupy all his senses, and speak through his mouth, and act through his members" (Swedenborg, 1905 [1758], p. 192). Interestingly, however, he predominantly construes insanity as the existential state in which a person, despite outward appearances, is principally driven by secular desires and selfish appetites, so that "each one is insane in accord with his own lusts" (ibid., p. 460). He maintains that such a person is subject to "insanities and phantasies of various kinds" and although he (or she) may be "sane in outward appearance" and presents as "a rational man", the ultimate truth is that when "stripped of his externals his insanities are revealed" (pp. 534, 457). This mystical view of insanity subverts the usual meaning of the term. Rather than juxtaposing secular normality against psychopathology, it sets a measure by which many so-called normal people would qualify as insane. Indeed, this idea is common to many mystical traditions. Arguably, then, it proffers a challenge to the conventional psychiatric understanding of psychopathology; here, sanity is not relative to apparent normality, but to the degree that psychospiritual maturity has been achieved. Thus, from this perspective, psychosis and secular normality may be seen as different types of insanity.

van Dusen's phenomenological description of lower and higher order voices (spirits)

The phenomenological descriptions below, of lower and higher order spirit voices, are excerpted verbatim from van Dusen's journal article titled 'Hallucinations as the world of spirits' (1970, pp. 62–63). They complement the typology of van Dusen's higher order and lower order voices in Chapter Twelve, Section 12.4.4.1 (see Table 11). In regards to his work with voice hearers, van Dusen explains that "in my dialogues with patients I learned of two orders of experience, borrowing from the voices themselves, called the higher and the lower order" (ibid., p. 62). This material exemplifies how psychospiritual research can open new investigative paths to identifying possible determinants in the experience of voice hearing and to better understanding the mysteries of both psychosis and being human.

Lower order voices

(Quoted verbatim from van Dusen (1970, pp. 62–63).)

Lower order voices are as though one is dealing with drunken bums at a bar who like to tease and torment just for the fun of it. They will suggest lewd acts and then scold the patient for considering them. They find a weak point of conscience and work on it interminably. For instance one man heard voices teasing him for three years over a ten-cent debt he had already paid. They call the patient every conceivable name, suggest every lewd act, steal memories or ideas right out of consciousness, threaten death, and work on the patient's credibility in every way. For instance they will brag that they will produce some disaster on the morrow and then claim honor for one in the daily paper. They suggest foolish acts (such as: Raise your right hand in the air and stay that way) and tease if he does it and threaten him if he doesn't. The lower order

311

can work for a long time to possess some part of the patient's body. Several worked on the ear and the patient seemed to grow deafer. One voice worked two years to capture a patient's eye which visibly went out of alignment. Many patients have heard loud and clear voices plotting their death for weeks on end, an apparently nerve-wracking experience. One patient saw a noose around his neck which tied to "I don't know what" while voices plotted his death by hanging. They threaten pain and can cause felt pain as a way of enforcing their power. The most devastating experience of all is to be shouted at constantly by dozens of voices. When this occurred—the patient had to be sedated. The vocabulary and range of ideas of the lower order is limited, but they have a persistent will to destroy. They invade every nook and cranny of privacy, work on every weakness and credibility, claim awesome powers, lie, make promises and then undermine the patient's will. They never have a personal identity though they accept most names or identities given them. They either conceal or have no awareness of personal memories. Though they claim to be separate identities they will reveal no detail that might help to trace them as separate individuals. Their voice quality can change or shift, leaving the patient quite confused as to who might be speaking. When identified as some friend known to the patient they can assume this voice quality perfectly. For convenience many patients call them by nick-names, such as "Fred," "The Doctor," or "The Old Timer." I've heard it said by the higher order that the purpose of the lower order is to illuminate all of the person's weaknesses. They do that admirably and with infinite patience. To make matters worse they hold out promises to patients and even give helpful sounding advice only to catch the patient in some weakness. Even with the patient's help I found the lower order difficult to relate to because of their disdain for me as well as the patient.

The limited vocabulary and range of ideas of the lower order is striking. A few ideas can be repeated endlessly. One voice just said "hey" for months while the patient tried to figure out what "hey" or "hay" was meant. Even when I was supposedly speaking to an engineer that a woman heard, the engineer was unable to do any more arithmetic than simple sums and multiplication the woman had memorized. The lower order seems incapable of sequential reasoning. Though they often claim to be in some distant city they cannot report more than the patient sees, hears, or remembers. They seem imprisoned in the lowest level of the patient's mind, giving no real evidence of a personal world or any higher order thinking or experiencing.

All of the lower order are irreligious or anti-religious. Some actively interfered with the patients' religious practices. Most considered them to be ordinary living people, though once they appeared as conventional devils and referred to themselves as demons. In a few instances they referred to themselves as from hell. Occasionally they would speak through the patient so that the patient's voice and speech would be directly those of the voices. Sometimes they acted through the patient. One of my female patients was found going out the hospital gate arguing loudly with her male voice that she didn't want to leave, but he was insisting. Like many, this particular hallucination claimed to be Jesus Christ, but his bragging and argumentativeness rather gave him away as of the lower order. Sometimes the lower order is embedded in physical concerns, such as a lady who was tormented by "experimenters" painfully treating her joints to prevent arthritis. She held out hope they were helping her, though it was apparent to any onlooker they had all but destroyed her life as a free and intelligent person.

Higher order voices

(Quoted verbatim from van Dusen (1970, p. 63).)

In direct contrast stands the rarer higher order hallucinations. In quantity they make up perhaps a fifth or less of the patients' experiences. The contrast may be illustrated by the experience of one man. He had heard the lower order arguing a long while how they would murder him. He also had a light come to him at night like the sun. He knew it was a different order because the light respected his freedom and would withdraw if it frightened him. In contrast, the lower order worked against his will and would attack if it could see fear in him. This rarer higher order seldom speaks, whereas the lower order can talk endlessly. The higher order is much more likely to be symbolic, religious, supportive, genuinely instructive, and communicate directly with the inner feelings of the patient. I've learned to help the patient approach the higher order because of its great power to broaden the individual's values. When the man was encouraged to approach his friendly sun he entered a world of powerful numinous experiences, in some ways more frightening than the murderers who plotted his death. In one scene he found himself at the bottom of a long corridor with doors at the end behind which raged the powers of hell. He was about to let out these powers when a very powerful and impressive Christlike figure appeared and by direct mind-to-mind communication counseled him to leave the doors closed and follow him into other experiences which were therapeutic to him. In another instance the higher order appeared to a man as a lovely woman who entertained him while showing him thousands of symbols. Though the patient was a high-school educated gas-pipe fitter, his female vision showed a knowledge of religion and myth far beyond the patient's comprehension. At the end of a very rich dialogue with her (the patient reporting her symbols and responses) the patient asked for just a clue as to what she and I were talking about.

In general the higher order is richer than the patient's normal experience, respectful of his freedom, helpful, instructive, supportive, highly symbolic and religious. It looks most like Carl Jung's archetypes, whereas the lower order looks like Freud's id. In contrast to the lower order, it thinks in something like universal ideas in ways that are richer and more complex than the patient's own mode of thought. It can be very powerful emotionally and carry with it an almost inexpressible ring of truth. The higher order tends to enlarge a patient's values, something like a very wise and considerate instructor. Some patients experience both the higher and lower orders at various times and feel caught between a private heaven and hell. Many only know the attacks of the lower order. The higher order claims power over the lower order and indeed shows it at times, but not enough to give peace of mind to most patients. The higher order itself has indicated that the usefulness of the lower order is to illustrate and make conscious the patients' weaknesses and faults.

APPENDIX 9

Methodological approaches and processes

Heuristic approach

This book aims to examine and critically appraise a broad spectrum of views on psychosis, ranging from the materialist to the metaphysical. Doing so necessitates utilising an open investigative approach that is not bound by any particular model or methodology of understanding. A heuristic methodological approach meets this requirement.

Etymologically, the term 'heuristic' derives from the Greek '*heuriskein*', meaning "to discover or to find" (Moustakas, 1990, p. 9). During the 1960s, heuristics was developed as a methodology for furthering "processes of understanding" (Lauer, 2004, p. 8) and has since been adopted as a theoretical and research model by a raft of disciplines (Gilovich & Griffin, 2002, p. 2). Although formally recognised as a research methodology, from a certain perspective, heuristics is essentially, and paradoxically, non-methodological. As Douglass & Moustakas (1985, p. 44) note, a heuristic approach to research ideally operates "free from external methodological structures that limit awareness or channel it". Therefore, as an unbounded research medium it provides me with the flexibility to examine a variety of perspectives on psychotic and psychotic-like experiences.

This approach especially enables the critical investigation of understandings of psychosis within and beyond the epistemological horizons of psychiatric diagnostics and scientific materialism. As Segen (1992, p. 294) contends, a heuristic approach is:

> a form of problem-solving based, not on scientific proof but rather on plausible, possible, or creative conclusions to questions that cannot be answered in the context of, or the 'logic' of which lies outside of, a currently accepted scientific paradigm.

Hence, it allows a critical examination of materials and worldviews pertaining to psychosis that medical science perceive to be unscientific, irrational, or unreal. In this sense, I use a heuristic approach to bridge the perceived gap between materialist and metaphysical worldviews, because its open-ended nature enables phenomenological investigation in both domains. While psychiatry has been described as a phenomenological discipline in its attention to the details of psychopathological symptomatology (Bürgy, 2008; Nelson et al., 2008; Andreasen; 2007; Owen & Harland, 2007),[161] this is limited to considering only that which can be physically observed. A heuristic approach creates the scope to extend beyond this limitation to investigate and understand the possible play of psychospiritual phenomena in psychosis.

A further advantage in using this approach is that its mutable nature enables me to formulate innovative ideas that attempt to reconcile some of the ambiguities and paradoxes that abound in the quest to better understand psychosis. Heuristic research is renowned for its usefulness in tackling the complex issues of being human (Greig et al., 2007, p. 45). For instance, the psychiatric understanding of psychosis is replete with binary tensions such as normal versus mad, pathological versus healthy, physical versus psychological, scientific versus irrational (i.e. metaphysical), psychotic versus sane, and so on. Jablin & Putnam (2001, p. 388) refer to these conundrums as "intersecting dualisms" that are heuristically valuable for "making sense of opposing views" and establishing new lines of research. Similarly, Saukko (2003, pp. 180, 178) advocates heuristic investigation "that is capable of doing justice to difference and to point to unities across differences" and which enables the researcher:

> to break up what appears inevitable or common sense by illuminating that the same phenomenon may be attached to very different social agendas in different locations and contexts, to the extent it may begin to look as if one is no longer talking about the same phenomenon.

This reflects my heuristic use of focal settings to systematically examine, and extend beyond, various viewpoints concerning the nature and genesis of psychosis. According to psychiatrist and Native American healer Lewis Mehl-Madrona (2005, p. 189) "mind, body, spirit, and community are one, and … our modern boundaries between self and others, self and nature, self and spirit are artificial constructions of a restricted materialist vision". This book aims to demonstrate that this holistic view applies also to psychotic experiences and a heuristic approach provides an apt medium for doing so.

Finally, my investigative process does not aim to arrive at any reified or ultimate understanding of psychosis. As Abbott (2004, p. 160) asserts, *"heuristics should not be reified. They are not about the true and the untrue but about finding new ideas. They*

---

[161] The psychiatric observation of physical symptomatology is exemplified in Karl Jaspers' phenomenological approach (see Chapter Four, Section 4.3).

should be taken as aids to reflection, not as fixed things". Similarly, Mehl-Madrona (2007, p. 200) contends that our knowledge about things does not represent absolute truth, but serves the function of fashioning "experience into interpretive frameworks". He subsequently asserts that:

> there are no privileged stories except those that work, when and where they do work. Within medicine, this means challenging the sanctity of the randomized, controlled clinical trial as the only valid way to obtain knowledge. It provides a fresh critique of what has been called 'evidence–based medicine', from the understanding that acceptable evidence is itself determined by a story about the world that can be challenged. (ibid.)

Hence, although I examine various models for conceptualising psychosis, my aim is not to generate an ultimate model for understanding psychosis, but to orchestrate an open-ended inquiry that includes, yet supersedes, the epistemological limits of the biomedical model. Doing so intrinsically challenges the conventional medical and materialist–based model of psychiatry, yet also opens other prospective lines of inquiry for future research into better understanding psychosis and developing apposite therapeutic practices.

Explication on focal settings

This book is structured in four progressive and interrelated parts, each of which represents a particular 'focal setting', a notion adopted from the philosophy of the Tibetan Buddhist teacher Tarthang Tulku. According to Tulku (1977, p. 12) the development of human understanding can be profoundly impeded by "different 'focal' or epistemic settings". He maintains that:

> throughout history, we have been maintaining a fixed and limiting 'focal setting' without even being aware of doing so. Yet, although our familiar world seems to depend upon this 'setting', if we become able to change the 'setting', fantastic new knowledge and appreciation of life can be gained. (Ibid., pp. 4–5)

Hence, a 'focal setting' constitutes a certain worldview about reality beyond which investigation does not usually ensue. An exemplary case in point is the materialist-based focal setting that scopes psychiatric research, and which proscribes the exploration of possible psychospiritual determinants in psychosis. However, while a focal setting is, by nature, conceptually restrictive, it can also be extended to enable new paradigms of investigation. Tulku (1984, p. 25) expresses this with simple eloquence:

> By accepting provisional answers as conclusive, we close off the possibility of deeper knowing. We trap ourselves in a vast unknown realm that we do not even

know is unknown. Paradoxically, it will remain unknown as long as we already 'know' it. To begin to know something new, we must first realise that there is something we do not know.

Throughout this book, then, I aim to systematically reveal 'something new' about psychosis in order to better understand it. The use of focal settings works as a heuristic tool that enables a deeper, broader, and progressive investigation of this phenomenon. As my trajectory of inquiry unfolds, each successive focal setting introduces a broader epistemological paradigm, thus establishing new investigative pathways for better understanding psychosis, and related notions concerning its assumed psychopathological and incomprehensible nature. Each focal setting sequentially investigates the construal of psychosis in the context of various paradigms of psychospiritual understanding.

Focal setting one

Focal Setting One undertakes a historical overview of depictions of psychosis by mainstream psychiatry since the term's inception. Within this purview, where scientific materialist theory sets psychiatric research parameters, psychosis is construed as psychopathological, and the consideration of psychospiritual determinants in understanding psychosis is absent. The challenge to psychiatry here is in highlighting and critically appraising its ambiguous depictions of, and its predominant bias towards, a biogenic understanding of psychosis.

Focal setting two

Focal Setting Two examines significant instances within mainstream psychiatry whereby psychospiritual matters have been viewed as important to better understanding psychopathology. As a focal setting, this moves beyond psychiatry's conventional materialist strictures to bring metaphysical concerns into its epistemological fold. Doing so challenges and repudiates the prevailing view that such matters have no place in psychiatric research and epistemology. It demonstrates that psychiatry *can* investigate psychospiritual considerations in psychosis research. Establishing this prepares for the in-depth critical investigation of the psychosis-psychospiritual nexus throughout Focal Settings Three and Four.

Focal setting three

Here psychospiritual determinants are presented as central to the task of better understanding and diagnosing psychosis. In examining and conducting a content analysis of literature on the issue of discerning psychotic from psychotic-like psychospiritual experiences, Focal Setting Three represents a significant paradigm shift. Demonstrating the pertinence of psychospiritual considerations in diagnostic practice challenges psychiatry to reassess its understanding of psychosis and psychopathology, and to extend its epistemological borders to incorporate metaphysical matters.

Focal setting four

Focal Setting Four undertakes a deeper critical appraisal of cross-cultural and psychospiritual matters in the context of psychiatric psychopathology. Here I argue that discerning psychotic from psychotic-like psychospiritual experiences is seemingly impossible. This constitutes a further paradigm shift, whereby the validity of key psychosis diagnostic criteria is further contested, as is the veracity of psychiatry's modus operandi of psychopathology-seeking. Cross-cultural conundrums and considerations are also examined, including the phenomenon of spirit possession and its practical application in Tibetan Buddhist psychiatry. Psychiatry is subsequently challenged to supersede its prescriptive psychopathological approach with a heuristic-phenomenological approach in order to foster deeper insights into the psychotic-psychospiritual nexus of human experience.

Content analysis

In Focal Setting Three of this book, I undertake a comprehensive content analysis of literature that engages the problem of symptomatically discerning psychotic from psychospiritual experiences. Krippendorff (2004, p. 18) broadly defines content analysis as a methodology that "provides new insights [and] increases a researcher's understanding of particular phenomena", while Pfarrer (2012) notes that "by systematically evaluating texts ... qualitative data can be converted into quantitative data". These descriptions essentially reflect my objective for using this tool. Analysing the various ways in which numerous commentators understand the differences and similarities between psychotic and psychospiritual phenomena enables me to elicit quantitative data on the nine foremost differentiation criteria identified by authors. Further details pertaining to this investigative undertaking are provided in Chapter Nine.

REFERENCES

Abbott, A. (2004). *Methods of discovery: Heuristics for the social sciences*. W. W. Norton & Company.

Ackerknecht, E. (1943). Psychopathology, primitive medicine and primitive culture. *Bulletin of the History of Medicine, 14*, 30–67.

Albers, P. (2003). *The home of the bison: An ethnographic and ethnohistorical study of traditional cultural affiliations to Wind Cave National Park*. University of Nebraska. https://digitalcommons.unl.edu/cgi/viewcontent.cgi?article=1150&context=natlpark

Alexander, F. (1931). Buddhistic training as an artificial catatonia. *Psychoanalytic Review, XVIII*(2), 129–145.

Allardyce, J., Gaebel, W., Zielasek, J., & van Os, J. (2010). Deconstructing Psychosis Conference February 2006: The validity of schizophrenia and alternative approaches to the classification of psychosis. In C. Tamminga, P. Sirovatka, D. Regier & J. van Os (Eds.), *Deconstructing Psychosis: Refining the Research Agenda for DSM-V* (pp. 1–10). American Psychiatric Publishing.

American Press. (1984, January 10). Medical schools are urged to teach psychic phenomena. *Observer-Reporter: Washington*, p. 16.

American Psychiatric Association. (2021). *DSM-5 development: Frequently asked questions*. American Psychiatric Association. https://psychiatry.org/psychiatrists/practice/dsm/frequently-asked-questions

—— (2013). *Diagnostic and statistical manual of mental disorders: Fifth edition*. American Psychiatric Publishing.

—— (2000). *Diagnostic and statistical manual of mental disorders: Fourth edition, Text revision*. American Psychiatric Association.

—— (2006). *Resource document on religious/spiritual commitments and psychiatric practice*. The Corresponding Committee on Religion, Spirituality and Psychiatry. https://www.psychiatry.org/File%20Library/Psychiatrists/Directories/Library-and-Archive/resource_documents/rd2006_Religion.pdf

—— (1999). *Position statement on diversity*. American Psychiatric Association. https://www.psychiatry.org/file%20library/about-apa/organization-documents-policies/policies/position-1999-diversity.pdf

—— (1994). *Diagnostic and statistical manual of mental disorders: Fourth edition*. American Psychiatric Association.

—— (1987). *Diagnostic and statistical manual of mental disorders: Third edition, revised*. American Psychiatric Association.

—— (1980). *Diagnostic and statistical manual of mental disorders: Third edition*. American Psychiatric Association.

—— (1968). *Diagnostic and statistical manual of mental disorders: Second edition*. American Psychiatric Association.

—— (1952). *Diagnostic and statistical manual of mental disorders: First edition*. American Psychiatric Association.

American Psychiatric Association, Committee on Public Information, & Frazier, S. (1975). *A psychiatric glossary: The meaning of terms frequently used in psychiatry*. Basic Books.

American Psychological Association. (2011, October 23). *Open letter to the DSM-5*. Society for Humanistic Psychology, Division 32 of the American Psychological Association. http://www.ipetitions.com/petition/dsm5/?utm_medium=social&utm_source=facebook&utm_campaign=button

Anderson, E. (1959). Preface. In K. Schneider (Ed.), *Clinical psychopathology* (pp. v–xiii). Grune & Stratton.

Andreasen, N. (2007). DSM and the death of phenomenology in America: An example of unintended consequences. *Schizophrenia Bulletin, 33*(1), 108–112.

—— (2005). The spirit doctor. *New Scientist, 188*(2526), 50–53.

—— (1997a). What is psychiatry? *The American Journal of Psychiatry, 154*(5), 591–593.

—— (1997b). The evolving concept of schizophrenia: From Kraepelin to the present and future. *Schizophrenia Research, 28*(2–3), 105–109.

Andreasen, N., & Flaum, M. (1991). Schizophrenia: The characteristic symptoms. *Schizophrenia Bulletin, 17*(1), 27–49.

Appelbaum, P. (2017). DSM-5.1: Perspectives on continuous improvement in diagnostic frameworks. In K. Kendler & J. Parnas (Eds.), *Philosophical issues in psychiatry IV: Classification of psychiatric illness* (pp. 392–402). Oxford University Press.

Arieti, S. (1961). The loss of reality. *Psychoanalysis and the Psychoanalytic Review, 48*(3), 3–24.

Arthur, R. (1973). Social psychiatry: An overview. *The American Journal of Psychiatry, 130*(8), 841–849.

Assagioli, R. (1989). Self-realisation and psychological disturbances. In S. Grof & C. Grof (Eds.), *Spiritual emergency: When personal transformation becomes a crisis* (pp. 28–48). Jeremy P. Tarcher/Putnam.

—— (1965). *Psychosynthesis: A manual of principles and techniques*. Penguin Books.

Austin, J. (1998). *Zen and the brain: Toward an understanding of meditation and consciousness*. MIT Press.

Avdibegović, E. (2012). Contemporary concepts of dissociation. *Psychiatria Danubina, 24*(3), 367–372.

Ayto, J. (1994). *Dictionary of word origins*. Columbia Marketing.

Azaunce, M. (1995). Is it schizophrenia or spirit possession? *Journal of Social Distress and the Homeless, 4*(3), 255–263.

Baers, J., Brinkman, G., Jelsma, A., & Steggink, O. (2003). *Encyclopedie van de mystiek, fundamenten, tradities, perspectieven*. Uitgeverij Kok.

Barnhart, R. (Ed.) (1988). *The Barnhart dictionary of etymology*. The H.W. Wilson Company.

Barton, W. (1987). *The history and influence of the American Psychiatric Association*. American Psychiatric Press.

Baruš, I. (2007). *Science as a spiritual practice*. Imprint Academic.

Bayer, R., & Spitzer, R. (1985), Neurosis, psychodynamics, and DSM-III: A history of the controversy. *Archives of General Psychiatry, 42*(2), 187–196.

Beauregard, M. (2012). *Brain wars: The scientific battle over the existence of the mind and the proof that will change the way we live our lives*. HarperOne.

Beauregard, M., & O'Leary, D. (2007). *The spiritual brain: A neuroscientist's case for the existence of the soul*. HarperCollins Publishers.

Beauregard, M., & Paquette, V. (2006). Neural correlates of a mystical experience in Carmelite nuns. *Neuroscience Letters, 405*(3), 186–190.

Beavan, V. (2007). *Angels at our tables: New Zealanders' experiences of hearing voices* [Unpublished Doctoral thesis]. University of Auckland.

Beavan, V., de Jager, A., & dos Santos, B. (2017). Do peer-support groups for voice-hearers work? A small scale study of Hearing Voices Network support groups in Australia. *Psychosis, 9*(1), 57–66.

Beddow, M. (2004). *Telepathy, parapsychology and psychiatry*. Spirituality and Psychiatry Special Interest Group. https://web.archive.org/web/20060924205741/https://www.rcpsych.ac.uk/pdf/MarkBeddow1.11.04.pdf

Beer, M. (1996a). Psychosis: A history of the concept. *Comprehensive Psychiatry, 37*(4), 273–291.

—— (1996b). The endogenous psychoses: A conceptual history. *History of Psychiatry, 7*(25), 1–29.

—— (1996c). The dichotomies: Psychosis/neurosis and functional/organic: A historical perspective. *History of Psychiatry, 7*(26 Pt 2), 231–255.

—— (1995a). Psychosis: From mental disorder to disease concept. *History of Psychiatry, 6*(22), 177–200.

—— (1995b). The importance of the social and intellectual contexts in a discussion of the history of the concept of psychosis. *Psychological Medicine, 25*(2), 317–321.

Begley, S. (1994). Tibetan Buddhist medicine: A transcultural nursing experience. *Journal of Holistic Nursing, 12*(3), 323–342.

Benedict, R. (1934). Anthropology and the abnormal. *The Journal of General Psychology, 11*, 59–82.

Bentall, R. (2004). *Madness explained: Psychosis and human nature*. Penguin Books.

—— (1993). Deconstructing the concept of 'schizophrenia'. *Journal of Mental Health, 2*(3), 223–238.

Berman, L. (1981). Letters to the Editor: Putting psychic studies to the test. *The American Journal of Psychiatry, 138*(3), 395.

Berrios, G. (2008). Descriptive psychiatry and psychiatric nosology during the nineteenth century. In E. Wallace & J. Gach (Eds.), *History of psychiatry and medical psychology* (pp. 353–380). Springer.

Berrios, G., & Beer, D. (1994). The notion of unitary psychosis: A conceptual history. *History of Psychiatry, 5*(17), 13–36.

Betty, S. (2005). The growing evidence for demonic possession: What should psychiatry's response be? *Journal of Religion and Health, 44*(1), 13–30.

Beveridge, A. (2011). *Portrait of the psychiatrist as a young man: The early writing and work of R.D. Laing, 1927–1960.* Oxford University Press.

Binet-Sanglé, C. (1910–1915). *La folie de Jésus.* A. Maloine.

Black, A. (2008). Psychosis and the community of the question: Training therapists in therapeutic community. In J. Gale, A. Realpe & E. Pedriali (Eds.), *Therapeutic communities for psychosis: Philosophy, history and clinical practice* (pp. 73–89). Routledge.

Black, D., & Grant, J. (2014). *DSM-5 guidebook: The essential companion to the Diagnostic and Statistical Manual of Mental Disorders, Fifth edition.* American Psychiatric Publishing.

Blashfield, R. (1984). *The classification of psychopathology: Neo-Kraepelinian and quantitative approaches.* Plenum Press.

—— (1982). Feighner et al., invisible colleges, and the Matthew effect. *Schizophrenia Bulletin, 8*(1), 1–6.

Blavatsky, H. (1889). *The key to theosophy: Being a clear exposition, in the form of question and answer, of the ethics, science, and philosophy for the study of which the Theosophical Society has been founded.* Theosophical Publishing Society.

—— (1888a). *The secret doctrine: The synthesis of science, religion and philosophy: Volume 1: Cosmogenesis.* Theosophical Publishing Society.

—— (1888b). *The secret doctrine: The synthesis of science, religion and philosophy: Volume 2: Anthropogenesis.* Theosophical Publishing Society.

Bleuler, E. (1950). *Dementia praecox or the group of schizophrenias.* International Universities Press.

—— (1911). *Dementia praecox oder die gruppe der schizophrenien.* Deuticke.

Boisen, A. (1936). *The exploration of the inner world: A study of mental disorder and religious experience.* Willett, Clark & Company.

Borges, P., & Tomlinson, K. (2017). *CRAZYWISE.* [Documentary]. https://crazywisefilm.com/#home

Bourguignon, E. (1973). Introduction: A framework for the comparative study of altered states of consciousness. In E. Bourguignon (Ed.), *Religion, altered states of consciousness, and social change* (pp. 3–38). Ohio State University Press.

Bowen, D. (1981). Letters to the Editor: Applause for psychic studies. *The American Journal of Psychiatry, 138*(4), 540.

Bowman, K., & Rose, M. (1951). A criticism of the terms 'psychosis', 'psychoneurosis' and 'neurosis'. *The American Journal of Psychiatry, 108*(3), 161–166.

Boyle, M. (2002). *Schizophrenia: A scientific delusion?* Routledge.

Braceland, F. (1957). Psychiatry and the science of man. *The American Journal of Psychiatry, 114*, 1–9.

Bragdon, E. (1990). *The call of spiritual emergency: From personal crisis to personal transformation.* Harper & Row.

Brandon, B. (2010). *Symptoms of spiritual crisis and the therapeusis of healing.* Spirituality and Psychiatry Special Interest Group. https://www.rcpsych.ac.uk/docs/default-source/members/sigs/spirituality-spsig/spirituality-special-interest-group-publications-beatrice-brandon-symptoms-of-spiritual-crisis.pdf?sfvrsn=2f12d0bb_2

Brett, C. (2010). Transformative crisis. In I. Clarke (Ed.), *Psychosis and Spirituality: Consolidating the New Paradigm* (pp. 155–174). John Wiley & Sons Ltd.

—— (2002). Psychotic and mystical states of being: Connections and distinctions. *Philosophy, Psychiatry and Psychology, 9*(4), 321–342.

Brett, C., Peters, E., Johns, L., Tabraham, P., Valmaggia, L., & McGuire, P. (2007). Appraisals of Anomalous Experiences Interview (AANEX): A multidimensional measure of psychological responses to anomalies associated with psychosis. *The British Journal of Psychiatry, 191*(51), s23–s30.

Brill, H. (1962). Reappraisal of attitudes with regard to schizophrenia: A clinical view. *Annals of the New York Academy of Sciences, 96*(1), 487–490.

British Psychological Society. (2011). *Response to the American Psychiatric Association: DSM-5 development*. The British Psychological Society. https://web.archive.org/web/20110626015643/http://apps.bps.org.uk/_publicationfiles/consultation-responses/DSM-5%202011%20-%20BPS%20response.pdf

Brown, J. (2005). *Inquiry into the understanding and applications of DSM-IV category Religious or Spiritual Problem, V-Code 62.89 by American Psychological Association (APA) psychologists* [Unpublished Doctoral thesis]. Institute of Transpersonal Psychology.

Bruijnzeel, D., & Tandon, R. (2011). The concept of schizophrenia: From the 1850s to the DSM-5. *Psychiatric Annals, 41*(5), 289–295.

Bucke, R. (1901). *Cosmic consciousness: A study in the evolution of the human mind*. E.P. Dutton and Company.

—— (1897). Mental evolution in man: A paper read before the American Medico-Psychological Association in Philadelphia, 18 May, 1894, by Dr. R. M. Bucke. *The British Medical Journal, 2*(1915), 643–645.

—— (1894). *Cosmic consciousness: A paper read before the American Medico-Psychological Association in Philadelphia, 18 May, 1894, by Dr. R. M. Bucke*. The Conservator.

Buckley, P. (1981). Mystical experience and schizophrenia. *Schizophrenia Bulletin, 7*(3), 516–521.

Bundy, W. (1922). *The psychic health of Jesus*. The Macmillan Company.

Burang, T. (1974). *Tibetan art of healing*. Watkins Publishing.

Bürgy, M. (2008). The concept of psychosis: Historical and phenomenological aspects. *Schizophrenia Bulletin, 34*(6), 1200–1210.

Bursten, B. (1981). Rallying 'round the medical model. *Psychiatric Services, 32*(6), 371.

Butler, P. (1999). Diagnostic line-drawing, professional boundaries, and the rhetoric of scientific justification: A critical appraisal of the American Psychiatric Association's DSM project. *Australian Psychologist, 34*(1), 20–29.

Cameron, V. (2012). The college internationally. *Royal College of Psychiatrists: Annual Review*, p. 15.

Campbell, J. (1972). *Myths to live by*. Viking.

Campbell, R. (2009). *Campbell's psychiatric dictionary: The definitive dictionary of psychiatry*. Oxford University Press.

Canadian Press. (1976, March 17). Packed house for first parapsychology symposium. *The Montreal Gazette*, p. 11.

Canstatt, C. (1843). *Handbuch der medicinischen klinik: Die specielle pathologie und therapie*. Ekne.

—— (1841). *Handbuch der medizinischen klinik*. Enke.

Cantlie, A. (2014). The Tantric ascetics of West Bengal. In J. Gale, M. Robson & G. Rapsomatioti (Eds.), *Insanity and divinity: Studies in psychosis and spirituality* (pp. 90–111). Routledge.

Caplan, P. (1995). *They say you're crazy: How the world's most powerful psychiatrists decide who's normal.* Addison-Wesley Publishing Company.

Capriles, E. (1990, March 26–30). Science, shamanism and metashamanism [Paper presentation]. *Second Venezuelan Seminar on Ethnomedicine and Religion, Mérida, Venezuela.*

Carroll, M. (2007). *Am I going mad? The unsettling phenomena of spiritual evolution.* Inner Peace Publishing.

Carpenter, W., Bustillo, J., Thaker, G., van Os, J., Krueger, R., & Green, M. (2009). The psychoses: Cluster 3 of the proposed meta-structure for DSM-V and ICD-11. *Psychological Medicine, 39*(12), 2025–2042.

Carson, R. (1991). Dilemmas in the pathway of the DSM-IV. *Journal of Abnormal Psychology, 100*(3), 302–307.

Casstevens, W., Cohen, D., Newman, F., & Dumaine, M. (2006). Evaluation of a mentored self-help intervention for the management of psychotic symptoms. *International Journal of Psychosocial Rehabilitation, 11*(1), 37–49.

Casher, M. (1981). Letters to the Editor: Putting psychic studies to the test. *The American Journal of Psychiatry, 138*(3), 395–396.

Cashwell, C., Bentley, P., & Yarborough, J. (2007). The only way out is through: The peril of spiritual bypass. *Counseling and Values, 51*(2), 139–148.

Caygill, M., & Culbertson, P. (2010). Constructing identity and theology in the world of Samoan and Tongan spirits. In E. Wainwright, P. Culbertson & S. Smith (Eds.), *Spirit possession, theology, and identity: A pacific exploration* (pp. 25–60). ATF Theology.

Chadwick, P. (2010). On not drinking soup with a fork. In I. Clarke (Ed.), *Psychosis and spirituality: Consolidating the new paradigm* (pp. 65–73). John Wiley & Sons Ltd.

—— (2001). Sanity to supersanity to insanity: A personal journey. In I. Clarke (Ed.), *Psychosis and spirituality: Exploring the new frontier* (pp. 75–89). Whurr.

Chapman, S. (2011). *Erasing the interface between psychiatry and medicine (DSM-5).* DSM-5 and ICD-11 Watch. https://web.archive.org/web/20110216152657/https://dsm5watch. wordpress.com/2011/02/13/erasing-the-interface-between-psychiatry-and-medicine/

Child, L. (2010). Spirit possession, seduction and collective consciousness. In B. Schmidt & L. Huskinson (Eds.), *Spirit Possession and Trance* (pp. 53–70). Continuum International Publishing Group.

Citizens Commission on Human Rights. (2010, 21 May). *DSM panel members still getting pharma funds.* Citizens Commission on Human Rights International. http://www. cchrint.org/2010/05/21/dsm-panel-members-still-getting-pharma-funds/

—— (2009). *Shrinks for sale: Psychiatry's conflicted alliance.* Citizens Commission on Human Rights. https://www.cchrint.org/issues/the-corrupt-alliance-of-the-psychiatric-pharmaceutical-industry/

Clark, W. (1966). Discussion of paper by Prince and Savage. *Psychedelic Review, 8,* 76–81.

Clarke, I. (Ed.) (2010). *Psychosis and spirituality: Consolidating the new paradigm.* John Wiley & Sons Ltd.

—— (2006, June 21). Psychosis and spirituality: The journey of an idea. *Spirituality and Psychiatry Special Interest Group Newsletter,* 1–5.

—— (Ed.) (2001). *Psychosis and spirituality: Exploring the new frontier.* Whurr Publications.

—— (2000). Madness and mysticism: Clarifying the mystery. *Network: The Scientific and Medical Network Review, 72,* 11–14.

Clifford, T. (1984). *Tibetan Buddhist medicine and psychiatry: The diamond healing.* Samuel Weiser Inc.

Coghlan, C. (2007). *The snake and the chalice.* Spirituality and Psychiatry Special Interest Group. https://www.rcpsych.ac.uk/docs/default-source/members/sigs/spirituality-spsig/spirituality-special-interest-group-publications-cherrie-coghlan-the-snake-and-the-chalice.pdf?sfvrsn=779363c3_2

—— (2003). *'May your God go with you!': Spiritual themes and issues in a general psychiatric setting.* Spirituality and Psychiatry Special Interest Group. https://www.rcpsych.ac.uk/docs/default-source/members/sigs/spirituality-spsig/spirituality-special-interest-group-publications-dr-cherrie-coghlan-may-your-god-go-with-you.pdf?sfvrsn=52eb7841_2

Cohen, R. (2005). Response: The circle without a center: Rethinking religious authority in India. *Journal of the American Academy of Religion, 73*(1), 133–150.

Cole, J. & Gerard, R. (Eds.) (1959). Psychopharmacology: Problems in evaluation. In *Proceedings of a Conference on the Evaluation of Pharmacotherapy in Mental Illness.* 18–22 September 1956. National Academy of Sciences, National Research Council: Washington, DC.

Coleman, R., & Smith, M. (2006). *Working with voices: Victim to victor.* P&P Ltd. Press.

Congressional Record. (1971, November 17). Metapsychiatry and the ultra-conscious. *Congressional Record 17, 117*(176).

Cook, C. (2012). *Spirituality and Psychiatry Special Interest Group: Annual Report 2012.* Spirituality and Psychiatry Special Interest Group. https://web.archive.org/web/20130313154922/http://www.rcpsych.ac.uk/pdf/SPSIG%20Annual%20Report%202012.pdf

—— (2011). *Recommendations for psychiatrists on spirituality and religion.* Royal College of Psychiatrists. https://www.merseycare.nhs.uk/media/1862/rcpsych-position-statement.pdf

—— (2004). Psychiatry and mysticism. *Mental Health, Religion & Culture, 7*(2), 149–163.

Cornwall, M. (2002). *Alternative treatment of psychosis: A qualitative study of Jungian medication-free treatment at Diabasis* [Unpublished Doctoral thesis]. California Institute of Integral Studies.

Corstens, D., Longden, E., & May, R. (2012). Talking with voices: Exploring what is expressed by the voices people hear. *Psychosis, 4*(2), 95–104.

Cosgrove, L., Krimsky, S., Vijayaraghavan, M., & Schneider, L. (2006). Financial ties between DSM-IV panel members and the pharmaceutical industry. *Psychotherapy and Psychosomatics, 75*(3), 154–160.

Coyte, M., Gilbert, P., & Nicholls, V. (Eds.) (2007). *Spirituality, values and mental health: Jewels for the journey.* Jessica Kingsley Publishers.

Crichton, P. (1996). First-rank symptoms or rank-and-file symptoms? *The British Journal of Psychiatry, 169*(5), 537–540.

Crowley, N. (2007). *Psychotic episode or spiritual emergency? The transformative potential of psychosis in recovery.* Spirituality and Psychiatry Special Interest Group. https://www.rcpsych.ac.uk/docs/default-source/members/sigs/spirituality-spsig/spirituality-special-interest-group-publications-nicki-crowley-psychotic-episode-or-spiritual-emergency.pdf?sfvrsn=d64fcd69_2

—— (2006). *Psychosis or spiritual emergence?—Consideration of the transpersonal perspective within psychiatry.* Spirituality and Psychiatry Special Interest Group. https://www.rcpsych.ac.uk/docs/default-source/members/sigs/spirituality-spsig/spirituality-special-interest-group-publications-nicki-crowley-psychosis-or-spiritual-emergence.pdf?sfvrsn=5685d4c1_2

Cunningham, P. (2015). Transpersonality disorders. *Research Gate.* https://www.research-gate.net/publication/317613496_Transpersonality_Disorders

—— (2011a). *Bridging psychological science and transpersonal spirit: A primer of transpersonal psychology.* https://www2.rivier.edu/faculty/pcunningham/Research/A%20Primer%20of%20Transpersonal%20Psychology.pdf

—— (2011b). Are religious experiences really localized within the brain? The promise, challenges, and prospects of neurotheology. *Journal of Mind and Behavior, 32*(3), 223–250.

Cutting, J., Mouratidou, M., Fuchs, T., & Owen, G. (2016). Max Scheler's influence on Kurt Schneider. *History of Psychiatry, 27*(3), 336–344.

Czaplicka, M. (1914). *Aboriginal Siberia: A study in social anthropology.* Oxford University Press.

d'Aquili, E., & Newberg, A. (1999). *The mystical mind: Probing the biology of religious experience.* Fortress Press.

Dean, S. (1981). Letters to the Editor: Dr. Dean replies. *The American Journal of Psychiatry, 138*(3), 396–397.

—— (1978). Metapsychiatry and psychosocial futurology. *MD,* December, 11–13.

—— (1977). Metapsychiatry: The confluence of psychiatry and mysticism. In B. Wolman (Ed.), *International encyclopedia of psychiatry, psychology, psychoanalysis and neurology* (pp. 214–215). Aesculapius Publishers.

—— (1976). A quest for purpose in psychic research. *Mental Health and Society, 3*(1–2), 114–121.

—— (1975a). Metapsychiatry: Part II. *Science of Mind, 48*(4), 43–48.

—— (1975b). Metapsychiatry: The confluence of psychiatry and mysticism. In S. Dean (Ed.), *Psychiatry and Mysticism* (pp. 3–17). Nelson-Hall.

—— (1975c). Section I. In S. Dean (Ed.), *Psychiatry and Mysticism* (pp. 1–2). Nelson-Hall.

—— (1975d). Introduction. In S. Dean (Ed.), *Psychiatry and Mysticism* (pp. xix–xxii). Nelson-Hall.

—— (1974a). The ultraconscious mind. In J. White (Ed.), *Frontiers of Consciousness* (pp. 15–26). Avon Books,.

—— (1974b). Metapsychiatry: The confluence of psychiatry and mysticism. *Fields Within Fields, 11,* 3–11.

—— (1973). Metapsychiatry: The interface between psychiatry and mysticism. *American Journal of Psychiatry, 130*(9), 1036–1038.

—— (1971). Metapsychiatry and the ultraconscious. *The American Journal of Psychiatry, 128*(5), 662–663.

—— (1970a). The ultraconscious mind. *Behavioral Neuropsychiatry, 1–2*(1), 32–36.

—— (1970b). Is there an ultraconscious beyond the unconscious? *Canadian Psychiatric Association Journal, 15*(1), 57–62.

—— (1965). Beyond the unconscious: The ultraconscious. *The American Journal of Psychiatry, 122*(4), 471.

Dean, S., & Thong, D. (1975). Transcultural aspects of metapsychiatry: Focus on shamanism in Bali. In S. Dean (Ed.), *Psychiatry and Mysticism* (pp. 271–282). Nelson-Hall.

—— (1972). Shamanism versus psychiatry in Bali, 'Isle of the Gods': Some modern implications. *The American Journal of Psychiatry, 129*(1), 59–62.

Dean, S., Plyer, C., & Dean, M. (1980). Should psychic studies be included in psychiatric education?: An opinion survey. *The American Journal of Psychiatry, 137*(10), 1247–1249.

Deane, S. (2014). From sadness to madness: Tibetan perspectives on the causation and treatment of psychiatric illness. *Religions, 5*(2), 444–458.

De Boismont, A. (1859). *On hallucinations: A history and explanation of apparitions, visions, dreams, ecstasy, magnetism, and somnambulism.* Henry Renshaw.

Decker, H. (2010). *A moment of crisis in the history of American psychiatry.* h-madness. http://historypsychiatry.wordpress.com/2010/04/27/a-moment-of-crisis-in-the-history-of-american-psychiatry/

—— (2007). How Kraepelinian was Kraepelin? How Kraepelinian are the neo-Kraepelinians?—from Emil Kraepelin to DSM-III. *History of Psychiatry, 18*(3), 337–360.

DeHoff, S. (2012). *Distinguishing mystical religious experience from psychotic experience in the Presbyterian Church (U.S.A.)* [Unpublished Doctoral thesis]. Boston University.

Deikman, A. (2012). *Dr. Arthur J. Deikman.* Arthur J. Deikman Website. http://www.deikman.com/index.html

—— (1978). Comments on the GAP report on mysticism. *Association for Humanistic Psychology Newsletter*, January, 16–19.

—— (1971). Bimodal consciousness. *Archives of General Psychiatry 25*(6), 481–489.

Dein, S., Cook, C., Powell, A., & Eagger, S. (2010). Religion, spirituality and mental health. *Psychiatric Bulletin, 34*(2), 63–64.

De Loosten, G. (1905). *Jesus Christus von standpunkte des psychiaters.* Handels-Druckerei.

de Menezes Junior, A., & Moreira-Almeida, A. (2009). Differential diagnosis between spiritual experiences and mental disorders of religious content. *Revista de Psiquiatria Clínica, 36*(2), 75–82.

Densmore, F. (1918). *Teton Sioux music.* Government Printing Office.

Devereux, G. (1956). Normal and abnormal: The key problem of psychiatric anthropology. In J. Casagrande & T. Gladwin (Eds.), *Some uses of anthropology: Theoretical and applied* (pp. 23–48). Anthropological Society of Washington.

Dillon, J. (2010). The personal is political. In S. Benamer (Ed.), *Telling stories?: Attachment-based approaches to the treatment of psychosis* (pp. 23–50). Karnac Books.

Dillon, J., & Hornstein, G. (2013). Hearing voices peer support groups: A powerful alternative for people in distress. *Psychosis, 5*(3), 286–295.

Dodds, E. (1951). *The Greeks and the irrational.* University of California Press.

Dos Santos, B., & Beavan, V. (2015). Qualitatively exploring Hearing Voices Network support groups. *The Journal of Mental Health Training, Education and Practice, 10*(1), 26–38.

Double, D. (2008). Adolf Meyer's psychobiology and the challenge for biomedicine. *Philosophy, Psychiatry, & Psychology, 14*(4), 331–339.

Douglas-Smith, B. (1971). An empirical study of religious mysticism. *The British Journal of Psychiatry, 118*(546), 549–554.

Douglass, B., & Moustakas, C. (1985). Heuristic inquiry: The internal search to know. *Journal of Humanistic Psychology, 25*(3): pp. 9–55.

D'souza, R., & George, K. (2006). Spirituality, religion and psychiatry: Its application to clinical practice. *Australasian Psychiatry, 14*(4), 408–412.

Dyga, K., & Stupak, R. (2015). Meditation and psychosis: trigger or cure? *Archives of Psychiatry and Psychotherapy, 3*, 48–58.

Eagger, S. (2006). *Spirituality and Psychiatry Special Interest Group: Annual Report 2006.* Spirituality and Psychiatry Special Interest Group. https://web.archive.org/web/20071011193316/http://www.rcpsych.ac.uk/pdf/Annual%20Report%202006x.pdf

Eagger, S., & Ferdinando, S. (2013). *Exploring spirituality with people who use mental health services.* Royal College of Psychiatrists. https://web.archive.org/web/20130909030755/http://www.psychiatrycpd.co.uk/learningmodules/exploringspiritualitywithpe.aspx

Edelston, H. (1949). Differential diagnosis of some emotional disorders of adolescence (with special reference to early Schizophrenia). *Journal of Mental Science, 95*(401), 960–967.

Eeles, J., Lowe, T., & Wellman, N. (2003). Spirituality or psychosis?: An exploration of the criteria that nurses use to evaluate spiritual-type experiences reported by patients. *International Journal of Nursing Studies, 40*(2), 197–206.

Ehrenwald, J. (1973). Letters to the Editor: Psyching out psi. *The American Journal of Psychiatry, 138*(3), 328–329.

Eisenmann, G. (1835). *Die vegetativen krankheiten und die entgiftende heilmethode.* Palm & Enke.

Eliade, M. (1964). *Shamanism: Archaic techniques of ecstasy.* Penguin Books.

—— (1958). *Rites and symbols of initiation: The mysteries of birth and rebirth.* Harper & Brothers.

Endicott, J., & Spitzer, R. (1978). A diagnostic interview: The schedule for affective disorders and schizophrenia. *Archives of General Psychiatry, 35*, 837–844.

Engel, G. (1978). The biopsychosocial model and the education of health professionals. *Annals of the New York Academy of Sciences, 310*(1), 169–181.

—— (1977). The need for a new medical model: A challenge for biomedicine. *Science, 196*(4286), 129–136.

Epstein, M., & Topgay, S. (1982). Mind and mental disorders in Tibetan medicine. *Revision, 5*(1), 67–79.

Escher, S., & Romme, M. (2012). The hearing voices movement. In J. Blom & I. Sommer (Eds.), *Hallucinations: Research and practice* (pp. 385–393). Springer.

Esima, E. (2017). *My story.* Sangoma Healing. https://web.archive.org/web/20170922162346/http://www.sangomahealing.com/about/

Esquirol, J. (1845). *Mental maladies: A treatise on insanity.* Lea & Blanchard.

Esterberg, M., & Compton, M. (2006). Causes of schizophrenia reported by family members of urban African American hospitalized patients with schizophrenia. *Comprehensive Psychiatry, 47*(3), 221–226.

Estroff, S. (1989). Self, identity, and subjective experiences of schizophrenia: In search of the subject. *Schizophrenia Bulletin, 15*(2), 189–196.

Ethnic Health Initiative. (2013, September 20). *Spirit possession and mental health* [Paper presentation]. Ethnic Health Initiative Conference. London: https://web.archive.org/web/20130810202315/http://bmehealth.org/userfiles/SPIRIT%20POSSESSION_BROCHURE.pdf

Evans-Wentz, W. (1968). *The Tibetan book of the great liberation, or, the method of realizing Nirvana through knowing the mind.* Oxford University Press.

Fabrega Jr, H. (2000). Culture, spirituality and psychiatry. *Current Opinion in Psychiatry* (WPA Forums), *13*(6). https://web.archive.org/web/20120525123024/http://www.wpanet.org/uploads/Publications/WPA_Books/Additional_Publications/WPA_Forums_on_Current_Opinion/culture-spirituality-psychiatry.pdf

Farmer, A. (1997). Current approaches to classification. In R. Murray, P. Hill & P. McGuffin (Eds.), *The essentials of postgraduate psychiatry* (pp. 53–64). Cambridge University Press.

Faust, D., & Miner, R. (1986). The empiricist and his new clothes: DSM-III in perspective. *The American Journal of Psychiatry, 143*(8), 962–967.

Feenstra, L., & Tydeman, N. (2011). Mystical experience as an empirical fact. Perception, meaning, insight. *Ludus Vitalis, 19*(35), 131–144.

Feighner, J., Robins, E., Guze, S., Woodruff Jr, R., Winokur, G., & Munoz, R. (1972). Diagnostic criteria for use in psychiatric research. *Archives of General Psychiatry, 26*(1), 57–63.

Fenwick, P. (2011). *The neuroscience of spirituality.* Royal College of Psychiatrists: Spirituality and Psychiatry Special Interest Group. https://www.rcpsych.ac.uk/docs/default-source/members/sigs/spirituality-spsig/spirituality-special-interest-group-publications-peter-fenwick-the-neuroscience-of-spirituality.pdf?sfvrsn=f5f9fed8_2

—— (2009). Neuroscience of the spirit. In C. Cook, A. Powell & A. Sims (Eds.), *Spirituality and psychiatry* (pp. 169–189). Royal College of Psychiatrists.

—— (2004). *Scientific evidence for the efficacy of prayer.* Spirituality and Psychiatry Special Interest Group. https://citeseerx.ist.psu.edu/viewdoc/download?doi=10.1.1.559.3438&rep=rep1&type=pdf

Feuchtersleben, E. (1847 [1845]). *The principles of medical psychology, being the outlines of a course of lectures.* The Sydenham Society.

—— (1845). *Lehrbuch der ärztlichen seelenkunde, als skizze zu vorträgen.* Gerold.

Flemming, C. (1859). *Die pathologie und therapie der psychosen nebst anhang: Über das gerichtsärztliche verfahren bei enforschung krankhafter seelenzustände.* Hirschwald.

Frances, A. (2013a). *Saving normal: An insider's revolt against out-of-control psychiatric diagnosis, DSM-5, Big Pharma, and the medicalization of ordinary life.* William Morrow.

—— (2013b). *DSM 5 boycotts and petitions: Too many, too sectarian.* Psychology Today. https://www.psychologytoday.com/blog/saving-normal/201302/dsm-5-boycotts-and-petitions

—— (2010). Opening Pandora's box: The 19 worst suggestions for DSM5. *Psychiatric Times, 27*(2), 1–10.

—— (2009, June 26). A warning sign on the road to DSM-V: Beware of its unintended consequences. *Psychiatric Times.* https://web.archive.org/web/20100815051224/http://www.psychiatrictimes.com/print/article/10168/1425378?printable=true

Frances, A., & Cooper, A. (1981). Descriptive and dynamic psychiatry: A perspective on DSM-III. *The American Journal of Psychiatry, 138*(9), 1198–1202.

Frances, A., First, M., Widiger, T., Miele, G., Tilly, S., Davis, W., & Pincus, H. (1991). An A to Z guide to DSM-IV conundrums. *Journal of Abnormal Psychology, 100*(3), 407–412.

Francis, A., Widiger, T., First, M., Pincus, H., Tilly, S., Miele, G., & Davis, W. (1991). DSM-IV: Toward a more empirical diagnostic system. *Canadian Psychology, 32*(2), 171–173.

Frank, J. (1977). Mysticism: Spiritual quest or psychic disorder? Report 97. *The American Journal of Psychiatry, 134*(9), 1057–1058.

Freeman, D. (2006). Delusions in the nonclinical population. *Current Psychiatry Reports. 8*(3), 191–204.

Funnell, A. (2014, August 19). Psychiatrists split on whether to ditch DSM. *ABC Radio National.* http://www.abc.net.au/radionational/programs/futuretense/the-psychiatrists-are-revolting/5680842

Fusar-Poli, P. (2013). One century of Allgemeine Psychopathologie (1913 to 2013) by Karl Jaspers. *Schizophrenia Bulletin, 39*(2), 268–269.

Gach, J. (2008). Biological psychiatry in the nineteenth and twentieth centuries. In E. Wallace & J. Gach (Eds.), *History of psychiatry and medical psychology* (pp. 381–418). Springer.

Gaines, A. (1992). From DSM-I to III-R: Voices of self, mastery and the other: A cultural constructivist reading of US psychiatric classification. *Social Science & Medicine, 35*(1), 3–24.

Gallagher, E., Wadsworth, A., & Stratton, T. (2002). Religion, spirituality, and mental health. *The Journal of Nervous and Mental Disease, 190*(10), 697–704.

Ghaemi, S. (2008). On the nature of mental disease: The psychiatric humanism of Karl Jaspers. *Existenz, 3*(2), 1–9.

Gilbert, P., Nicholls, V., McCulloch, A., & Sheehan, A. (2003). *Inspiring hope: Recognising the importance of spirituality in a whole person approach to mental health.* National Institute for Mental Health in England.

Gilman, S. (2008). Constructing schizophrenia as a category of mental illness. In E. Wallace & J. Gach (Eds.), *History of psychiatry and medical psychology* (pp. 461–484). Springer.

Gilovich, T., & Griffin, D. (2002). Introduction—Heuristics and biases: Then and now. In T. Gilovich, D. Griffin & D. Kahneman (Eds.), *Heuristics and biases: The psychology of intuitive judgment* (pp. 1–17). Cambridge University Press.

Giorgi, A. (1997). Humanistic psychology and the humanism of Karl Jaspers. *The Humanistic Psychologist, 25*(1), 15–29.

Gleig, A. (2010). Psychospiritual. In D. Leeming, K. Madden & S. Marlan (Eds.), *Encyclopedia of psychology and religion: L–Z* (pp. 738–739). Springer.

Glynn, S., Marder, S., Cohen, A., Hamilton, A., Saks, E., Hollan, D., & Brekke, J. (2010, August 12–15). *How do some people with schizophrenia thrive* [Paper presentation]. American Psychological Association. APA 118th Annual Convention. San Diego. https://web.archive.org/web/20170428215158/https://www.apa.org/practice/leadership/serious-mental-illness/glynn.pdf

Goddard, D. (1938). *A Buddhist bible.* E. P. Dutton & Co.

Goethe, J. (2001). *Faust: A tragedy.* WW Norton & Co.

Goldsmith, L. (2012). A discursive approach to narrative accounts of hearing voices and recovery. *Psychosis, 4*(3), 235–245.

Goretzki, M. (2007). *The differentiation of psychosis and spiritual emergency* [Unpublished Doctoral thesis]. University of Adelaide.

Goretzki, M. Thalbourne, M., & Storm, L. (2009). The questionnaire measurement of spiritual emergency. *Journal of Transpersonal Psychology, 41*(1), 81–97.

Granet, R. (1981). Letters to the Editor: Metapsychiatry and psychiatric education. *The American Journal of Psychiatry, 138*(5), 703.

Greeley, A. (1974). *Ecstasy: A way of knowing.* Prentice-Hall.

Greenberg, G. (2010). *Inside the battle to define mental illness.* Wired Magazine. https://www.wired.com/2010/12/ff-dsmv/

Greenwell, B. (2002). *Diagnostic criteria comparing kundalini awakening to other DSM diagnoses* [Unpublished manuscript]. Institute of Transpersonal Psychology.

Greig, A., Taylor, J., & MacKay, T. (2007). *Doing research with children.* SAGE Publications Ltd.

Greyson, B. (1993). The Physio-Kundalini Syndrome and mental illness. *Journal of Transpersonal Psychology, 25*(1), 43–58.

Grof, C., & Grof, S. (1995). *The stormy search for the self: Understanding and living with spiritual emergency.* Thorsons.

Grof, S. (2008a). *Spiritual emergencies: Understanding and treatment of psychospiritual crises.* Reality Sandwich. http://realitysandwich.com/1800/spiritual_emergencies/

—— (2008b). A brief history of transpersonal psychology. *International Journal of Transpersonal Studies, 27,* 46–54.

—— (2000). *Psychology of the future: Lessons from modern consciousness research.* State University of New York Press.

—— (1994). Alternative cosmologies and altered states. *Noetic Sciences Review, 32,* 21–29.

—— (1983). East and West: Ancient wisdom and modern science. *Journal of Transpersonal Psychology, 15*(1), 13–36.

—— (1975). *Realms of the human unconscious: Observations from LSD research.* The Viking Press.

—— (1972). Varieties of transpersonal experiences: Observations from LSD psychotherapy. *Journal of Transpersonal Psychology, 4*(1), 45–80.

Grof, S., & Grof, C. (c2007). *Understanding and treatment of psychospiritual crises ('spiritual emergencies').* Wisdom University. https://web.archive.org/web/20180712185703/https://www.wisdomuniversity.org/grof/module/week5/pdf/Spiritual%20Emergencies.pdf

—— (Eds.). (1989). *Spiritual emergency: When personal transformation becomes a crisis.* Jeremy P. Tarcher/Putnam.

—— (1977). The concept of spiritual emergency: Understanding and treatment of transpersonal crises [Unpublished mimeographed manuscript].

Group for the Advancement of Psychiatry. (1976). *Mysticism: Spiritual quest or psychic disorder?* [Formulated by the Committee on Psychiatry and Religion]. Group for the Advancement of Psychiatry.

Groves, P. (2014). Buddhist approaches to addiction recovery. *Religions, 5*(4), 985–1000.

Gruenberg, A., Goldstein, R., & Pincus, H. (2005). Classification of depression: Research and diagnostic criteria: DSM-IV and ICD-10. In J. Licinio & M. Wong (Eds.), *Biology of depression. From novel insights to therapeutic strategies: Volume 1* (pp. 1–12). Wiley-VCH.

Gruenberg, E. (1969). How can the new diagnostic manual help? *International Journal of Psychiatry, 7*(6), 368–374.

Gur, R., Keshavan, M., & Lawrie, S. (2010). Deconstructing psychosis with human brain imaging. In C. Tamminga, P. Sirovatka, D. Regier & J. van Os (Eds.), *Deconstructing psychosis: Refining the research agenda for DSM-V* (pp. 109–129). American Psychiatric Publishing.

Gurney, E., Myers, F., & Podmore, F. (1886a). *Phantasms of the living: Volume 1.* Rooms of the Society for Psychic Research.

—— (1886b). *Phantasms of the living: Volume 2*. Rooms of the Society for Psychic Research.

Gutberlet, C. (1913). Materialism. In C. Herbermann, E. Pace, C. Pallen, T. Shahan & J. Wynne (Eds.), *The Catholic encyclopedia: An international work of reference on the constitution, doctrine, discipline and history of the Catholic Church: Volume X* (pp. 41–46). The Encyclopedia Press, Inc.

Gutmann, P. (2008). Julius Ludwig August Koch (1841–1908): Christian, philosopher and psychiatrist. *History of Psychiatry, 19*(2), 202–214.

Guze, S. (1982). Comments on Blashfield's article. *Schizophrenia Bulletin, 8*(1), 6–7.

Hackett, A. (1977). The psychiatrist: In the mainstream or on the banks of medicine? *The American Journal of Psychiatry, 134*(4), 432–434.

Haddock, G., Benthall, R., & Slade, P. (1996). Psychological treatments for auditory hallucinations, focussing or distraction? In G. Haddock & P. Slade (Eds.), *Cognitive behavioural interventions with psychotic disorders* (pp. 45–71). Routledge.

Hamilton, M. (Ed.) (1985). *Fish's clinical psychopathology*. John Wright & Sons.

Harakas, M. (1985, October 2). Psychiatrist: Put mysticism in med school. *Sun Sentinal*, p. 1.

Harrowes, W. (1929). Personality and psychosis: A study in schizophrenia. *Journal of Neurology and Psychopathology, 10*(37), 14–20.

Havis, D. (2001). An inquiry into the mental health of Jesus: Was he crazy? *San Francisco Atheists*. https://web.archive.org/web/20130620085105/http://www.sfatheists.com/Essays/Documents/An%20Inquiry%20into%20the%20Mental%20Health%20of%20Jesus.pdf

Healy, D. (2002a). *The creation of psychopharmacology*. Harvard University Press.

—— (2002b). Mandel Cohen and the origins of the Diagnostic and Statistical Manual of Mental Disorders: DSM-III. *History of Psychiatry, 13*(50), 209–230.

—— (1997). *The antidepressant era*. Harvard University Press.

Hearing Voices Network. (2013). *Hearing Voices Network: England's position statement on DSM 5 & psychiatric diagnoses*. Hearing Voices Network. http://www.hearing-voices.org/wp-content/uploads/2013/05/HVN-Position-Statement-on-DSM5-and-Diagnoses.pdf

—— (2012). *Hearing voices: Coping strategies*. Hearing Voices Network. http://www.hearing-voices.org/wp-content/uploads/2012/05/Hearing_Voices_Coping_Strategies_web.pdf

Hearing Voices Network Australia. (2013). *Strategies for coping with distressing voices*. Hearing Voices Network WA. https://web.archive.org/web/20170425162900/http://hearingvoiceswa.org.au/wp-content/uploads/2013/04/Coping_Stratigies_Poster.pdf

Heinimaa, M. (2008). *The grammar of psychosis* [Unpublished Doctoral thesis]. University of Turku.

Henriksen, M. (2013). On incomprehensibility in schizophrenia. *Phenomenology and the Cognitive Sciences, 12*, 105–129.

Herrick, K. (2008). *Naming spiritual experiences* [Unpublished Doctoral thesis]. Union Institute and University.

Hess, D. (1993). *Science in the new age: The paranormal, its defenders and debunkers, and American culture*. University of Wisconsin Press.

Hirsch, W. (1912). *Religion and civilization: The conclusions of a psychiatrist*. The Truth Seeker Company.

Ho, D. (2016). Madness may enrich your life: A self-study of unipolar mood elevation. *Psychosis, 8*(2), 180–185.

Hoenig, J. (1983). The concept of schizophrenia: Kraepelin-Bleuler-Schneider. *The British Journal of Psychiatry, 142*(6), 547–556.

Hoff, P. (2003). Emile Kraepelin's concept of clinical psychiatry. In T. Hamanaka & G. Berrios (Eds.), *Two millennia of psychiatry in west and east: Selected papers from the International Symposium History of Psychiatry on the Threshold to the 21st Century, 20–21 March 1999, Nagoya, Japan* (pp. 65–79). Gakuju Shoin.

Horgan, J. (2004). *Rational mysticism: Spirituality meets science in the search for enlightenment.* Houghton Mifflin Company.

Horopciuc, M., & Petrea, C. (1994). *Spiritual approach to psychology and psychiatry.* Jean-Marc Mantel Website. http://jmmantel.net/int/eng/texts/archives/psychiatry2.html

Horwitz, A. (2010). *DSM-V: Getting closer to pathologizing everyone?* h-madness. http://historypsychiatry.wordpress.com/2010/03/15/dsm-v-getting-closer-to-pathologizing-everyone/

Houts, A. (2000). Fifty years of psychiatric nomenclature: Reflections on the 1943 War Department Technical Bulletin, Medical 203. *Journal of Clinical Psychology, 56*(7), 935–967.

Howard, A., Forsyth, A., Spencer, H., Young, E., & Turkington, D. (2013). Do voice hearers naturally use focusing and metacognitive coping techniques? *Psychosis, 5*(2), 119–126.

Huber, G. (2002). The psychopathology of K. Jaspers and K. Schneider as a fundamental method for psychiatry. *World Journal of Biological Psychiatry, 3*(1), 50–57.

Huguelet, P., Mohr, S., Borras, L., Gillieron, C, & Brandt, P. (2006). Spirituality and religious practices among outpatients with schizophrenia and their clinicians. *Psychiatric Services, 57*(3), 366–372.

Hunt, H. (2007). 'Dark nights of the soul': Phenomenology and neurocognition of spiritual suffering in mysticism and psychosis. *Review of General Psychology, 11*(3), 209–234.

Huskinson, L. (2010). Analytical psychology and spirit possession: Towards a non-pathological diagnosis of spirit possession. In B. Schmidt & L. Huskinson (Eds.), *Spirit possession and trance* (pp. 71–96). Continuum International Publishing Group.

Huskinson, L., & Schmidt, B. (2010). Introduction. In B. Schmidt & L. Huskinson (Eds.), *Spirit possession and trance* (pp. 1–15). Continuum International Publishing Group.

Hyman, S. (2010). The diagnosis of mental disorders: The problem of reification. *Annual Review of Clinical Psychology, 6*, 155–179.

International Association for Spiritual Psychiatry (2005). *International Association for Spiritual Psychiatry.* International Association for Spiritual Psychiatry. https://web.archive.org/web/20051231054204/http://www.essence-euro.org/iasp/

Intervoice. (2021a). *National networks.* Intervoice: The International Hearing Voices Network. http://www.intervoiceonline.org/about-intervoice/national-networks-2

—— (2021b). *Values and vision.* Intervoice: The International Hearing Voices Network. https://www.intervoiceonline.org/about-intervoice/values-vision

Interuniversity Consortium for Political and Social Research (ICPSR). (2016). *Epidemiologic catchment area study, 1980–1985.* ICPSR. http://www.icpsr.umich.edu/icpsrweb/ICPSR/studies/6153

Jablensky, A. (2013). Karl Jaspers: Psychiatrist, philosopher, humanist. *Schizophrenia Bulletin, 39*(2), 239–241.

—— (1987). Multicultural studies and the nature schizophrenia: A review. *Journal of the Royal Society of Medicine 80*(3), 162–167.

Jablin, F., & Putnam, L. (2001). *The new handbook of organizational communication.* SAGE Publications, Inc.

Jackson, B. (1969). Reflections on DSM-II. *International Journal of Psychiatry, 7*(6), 385–392.

Jackson, M. (2010). The paradigm-shifting hypothesis. In I. Clarke (Ed.), *Psychosis and spirituality: Consolidating the new paradigm* (pp. 139–153). John Wiley & Sons Ltd.

—— (2001). Psychotic and spiritual experience: A case study comparison. In I. Clarke (Ed.), *Psychosis and spirituality: Exploring the new frontier* (pp. 165–190). Whurr Publications.

—— (1991). *A study of the relationship between psychotic and religious experience* [Unpublished Doctoral thesis]. University of Oxford.

Jackson, M., & Fulford, K. (1997). Spiritual experience and psychopathology. *Philosophy, Psychiatry and Psychology, 4*(1), 41–65.

Jackson, S. (2008). A history of melancholia and depression. In E. Wallace & J. Gach (Eds.), *History of psychiatry and medical psychology* (pp. 443–460). Springer.

James, W. (1905). *The varieties of religious experience: A study in human nature.* Longmans, Green, and Co.

Jansson, L., & Parnas, J. (2007). Competing definitions of schizophrenia: What can be learned from polydiagnostic studies? *Schizophrenia Bulletin, 33*(5), 1178–1200.

Janzarik, W. (2003). The concept of psychosis and psychotic qualities. *Der Nervenarzt, 74*(1), 3–11.

Jaspers, K. (1997 v1). *General psychopathology: Volume 1.* John Hopkins University Press.

—— (1997 v2). *General psychopathology: Volume 2.* John Hopkins University Press.

—— (1968 [1912]). The phenomenological approach in psychopathology. *The British Journal of Psychiatry, 114*(516), 1313–1323.

—— (1963). *General psychopathology.* Manchester University Press.

—— (1913). *Allgemeine psychopathologie.* Springer.

—— (1912). 'Die phänomenologische forschungsrichtung in der psychopathologie. *Zeitschrift für die Gesamte Neurologie und Psychiatrie, 9,* 391–408.

Jastrow, R. (1978). *God and the astronomers.* W.W. Norton.

Jeans, J. (1984). Sir James Jeans: A universe of pure thought. In K. Wilber (Ed.), *Quantum questions: Mystical writings of the world's greatest physicists* (pp. 140–144). Shambhala Publications.

Jenkins, J. (1998). Diagnostic criteria for schizophrenia and related psychotic disorders: Integration and suppression of cultural evidence in DSM-IV. *Transcultural Psychiatry, 35*(3), 357–376.

Johnson, C., & Friedman, H. (2008). Enlightened or delusional?: Differentiating religious, spiritual, and transpersonal experiences from psychopathology. *Journal of Humanistic Psychology, 48*(4), 505–527.

Jones, N., Marino, C. K., & Hansen, M. (2016). The Hearing Voices Movement in the United States: Findings from a national survey of group facilitators. *Psychosis, 8*(2), 106–117.

Jones, N., Shattell, M., Kelly, T., Brown, R., Robinson, L., Renfro, R., Harris, B., & Luhrmann, T. (2016). 'Did I push myself over the edge?': Complications of agency in psychosis onset and development. *Psychosis, 8*(4), 324–335.

Jones, S., & Fernyhough, C. (2008). Talking back to the spirits: The voices and visions of Emanuel Swedenborg. *History of the Human Sciences, 21*(1), 1–31.

Jones, S., Guy, A., & Ormrod, J. (2003). A Q-methodological study of hearing voices: A preliminary exploration of voice hearers understanding of their experiences. *Psychology and Psychotherapy: Theory, Research and Practice, 76*(2), 189–209.

Jung, C. (2009). *The red book: Liber novus.* W. W. Norton & Co.

—— (1970). *Collected works: Volume 14: Mysterium conjunctionis: An inquiry into the separation and synthesis of psychic opposites in alchemy.* Routledge & Kegan Paul.

—— (1969). *Collected works: Volume 8: The structure and dynamics of the psyche.* Princeton University Press.

—— (1968). *Collected works: Volume 9, Part 1: The archetypes and the collective unconscious.* Routledge & Kegan Paul.

—— (1966). *Collected works: Volume 7: Two essays on analytical psychology.* Routledge & Kegan Paul.

—— (1965). *Memories, dreams, reflections.* Vintage Books.

—— (1960). *Collected works: Volume 3: The psychogenesis of mental illness.* Routledge & Kegan Paul.

—— (1939). On the psychogenesis of schizophrenia. *The British Journal of Psychiatry, 85*(358), 999–1011.

—— (1914). On the importance of the unconscious in psychopathology. *The British Medical Journal, 2*(2814), 964–968.

Kant, I. (1964 [1798]). *The classification of mental disorders.* Doylestown Foundation.

Kantjuriny, N., Tjilari, A., & Burton, M. (2013, May 18). Super powers of central Australia's traditional healers. *The Australian: Magazine,* p. 20.

Katschnig, H. (2010). Are psychiatrists an endangered species? Observations on internal and external challenges to the profession. *World Psychiatry, 9*(1), 21–28.

Keks, N., & D'Souza, R. (2003). Spirituality and psychosis. *Australasian Psychiatry, 11*(2), 170–171.

Kelleher, I., Connor, D., Clarke, M., Devlin, N., Harley, M., & Cannon, M. (2012). Prevalence of psychotic symptoms in childhood and adolescence: A systematic review and meta-analysis of population-based studies. *Psychological Medicine, 42*(9), 1857–1863.

Kemp, D. (2000). A Platonic delusion: The identification of psychosis and mysticism. *Mental Health, Religion & Culture, 3*(2), 157–172.

Kendler, K., Spitzer, R., & Williams, J. (1989). Psychotic disorders in DSM-III-R. *The American Journal of Psychiatry, 146*(8), 953–962.

Kimura, Y. (2008). *Consciousness, space, and the foundation of new science.* Vision in Action. [Not available online as of 22 July 2022].

Kingdon, D., Siddle, R., Naeem, F., & Rathod, S. (2010). Spirituality, psychosis and the development of 'normalising rationales'. In I. Clarke (Ed.), *Psychosis and spirituality: Consolidating the new paradigm* (pp. 239–247). John Wiley & Sons Ltd.

Kiran Kumar, S., Raj, A., Murthy, P., Parimala, N., Rekha, K., & Gaur, S. (2005). Concept *ahamkara*: Theoretical and empirical analysis. In K. Rao & S. Marwaha (Eds.,) *Towards a spiritual psychology: Essays in Indian psychology* (pp. 97–122). Samvad India Foundation.

Kirk, S., & Kutchins, H. (1992). Reliability and the remarkable achievement. In S. Kirk & H. Kutchins., *The Selling of DSM: The Rhetoric of Science in Psychiatry* (pp. 133–160). Aldine de Gruyter.

Klerman, G. (1984). A debate on DSM-III—Gerald L. Klerman: The advantages of DSM-III. *The American Journal of Psychiatry, 141*(4), 539–542.

—— (1978). The evolution of a scientific nosology. In J. Shershow (Ed.), *Schizophrenia: Science and Practice* (pp. 99–121). Harvard University Press.

—— (1971). Clinical research in depression. *Archives of General Psychiatry, 24*, 305–319.

Knight, T. (2010). Beyond Belief: An interview with Dr. Tamasin Knight on alternative responses to unusual beliefs. *ENUSP Bulletin—Newsletter of the European Network of (ex-) Users and Survivors of Psychiatry, 1*, 21–23.

—— (2009). *Beyond belief: Alternative ways of working with delusions, obsessions and unusual experiences*. Peter Lehmann Publishing.

Koch, J. (1891). *Die psychopathischen minderwertigkeiten*, Maier.

Kohls, N., & Walach, H. (2008). *Lack of spiritual practice—an important risk factor for suffering from distress*. Spirituality and Psychiatry Special Interest Group. https://web.archive.org/web/20150930082031/http://www.rcpsych.ac.uk/pdf/Niko%20Kohls%20and%20Harald%20Walach%20Lack%20of%20Spiritual%20Practice.x.pdf

Kraemer, H. (2008). DSM categories and dimensions in clinical research contexts. In J. Helzer, H. Kraemer, R. Krueger, H. Wittchen, P. Sirovatka & D. Regier (Eds.), *Dimensional approaches in diagnostic classification: Refining the research agenda for DSM-V* (pp. 5–17). American Psychiatric Association.

Kraepelin, E. (1921). Psychological work experiments. *Zeitschrift fur die Gesamte Neurologie und Psychiatrie, 70*, 230–240.

—— (1920). Die erscheinungsformen des irreseins. *Zeitschrift der gesamten Psychiatrie und Neurologie, 62*, 1–29.

—— (1902). *Clinical psychiatry: For students and physicians*. The Macmillan Company.

—— (1899). *Psychiatrie. Ein lehrbuch für studirende und aerzte*. Abel.

Krippendorff, K. (2004). *Content analysis: An introduction to its methodology*. Sage Publications.

Krippner, S. (2007). Humanity's first healers: Psychological and psychiatric stances on shamans and shamanism. *Archives of Clinical Psychiatry (São Paulo), 34*(1), 17–24.

Krishna, G. (1977). *Kundalini: The evolutionary energy in man*. Shambala.

Kroeber, A. (1940). Psychotic factors in shamanism. *Character and Personality, 8*(3), 204–215.

Kupfer, D., First, M., & Regier, D. (Eds.) (2002). *A research agenda for DSM-V*. American Psychiatric Association.

Kutchins, H., & Kirk, S. (1997). *Making us crazy: DSM: The psychiatric bible and the creation of mental disorders*. Constable.

LaBruzza, A., & Mendez-Villarrubia, J. (1994). *Using DSM-IV: A clinician's guide to psychiatric diagnosis*. Jason Aronson.

Lacan, J. (1993). *The psychoses: The seminar of Jaques Lacan: Book III 1955–1956*. Routledge.

Laibelman, A. (2004). *Going against the flow: An exercise in ethical syncretism*. Peter Lang Publishing.

Laing, R. (1990). *The divided self: An existential study of sanity and madness*. Penguin Books.

—— (1972). Metanoia: Some experiences at Kingsley Hall, London. In Ruitenbeek, H. (Ed.), *Going crazy: The radical therapy of R. D. Laing and others* (pp. 11–21). Bantam.

—— (1967). *The politics of experience and the bird of paradise*. Penguin Books.

—— (1965). Transcendental experience in relation to religion and psychosis. *Psychedelic Review, 6*, 7–15.

Lama Govinda. (1969). *Foundations of Tibetan mysticism*. Rider and Company.

Lama Yeshe. (2003). *Becoming your own therapist: and introduction to the Buddhist way of thought … and … make your mind an ocean: Aspects of Buddhist psychology*. N. Ribush (Ed.). Lama Yeshi Wisdom Archive.

Lambrecht, I. (2017). *Shamanic spiritual emergencies: The dialectic of distress and spirituality.* [Video]. https://www.youtube.com/watch?v=crqeauJI2bg

—— (2015). A shamanic tale of death and Unbehagen. *The Candidate, 6,* 1–10.

—— (2009). *Shamans as expert voice hearers.* Hearing Voices Network Aotearoa NZ: Te Reo Orooro. http://www.hearingvoices.org.nz/attachments/article/14/Shamans%20as%20Expert%20Voice%20Hearers%20By%20Ingo%20Lambrecht.pdf

Laplanche, J., & Pontalis, J. (1980). *The language of psycho-analysis.* Hogarth Press.

Laszlo, E. (2003). *The connectivity hypothesis: Foundations of an integral science of quantum, cosmos, life, and consciousness.* State University of New York Press.

Lauer, J. (2004). *Invention in rhetoric and composition.* Parlor Press and The WAC Clearinghouse.

Lawrence, R. (2002). *'God's place' in psychiatry: Spirituality in psychiatric education and training.* Spirituality and Psychiatry Special Interest Group. https://www.rcpsych.ac.uk/docs/default-source/members/sigs/spirituality-spsig/lawrence.pdf?sfvrsn=7217cf2f_2

Leff, J., Williams, G., Huckvale, M., Arbuthnot, M., & Leff, A. (2014). Avatar therapy for persecutory auditory hallucinations: What is it and how does it work? *Psychosis, 6*(2), 166–176.

Leonard, R. (1999). *The transcendental philosophy of Franklin Merrell-Wolff.* State University of New York Press.

Lidz, T. (1966). Adolf Meyer and the development of American psychiatry. *The American Journal of Psychiatry, 123*(3), 320–332.

Loewenthal, K. (2012). *Spirit possession: Jews don't do that, do they?* Spirituality and Psychiatry Special Interest Group. https://www.rcpsych.ac.uk/docs/default-source/members/sigs/spirituality-spsig/jews-don't-do-that-do-they-kate-loewenthal.pdf?sfvrsn=b12a6d7_4

Long, G., & Macleane, A. (Eds.) (1868). *The Phaedrus of Plato.* Whittaker and Co.

Longden, E., Read, J., & Dillon, J. (2018). Assessing the impact and effectiveness of Hearing Voices Network self-help groups. *Community Mental Health Journal, 54*(2), 184–188.

López Piñero, J. (1983). *Historical origins of the concept of neurosis.* Cambridge University Press.

Louchakova, O. (2005). On advantages of the clear mind: Spiritual practices in the training of a phenomenological researcher. *The Humanistic Psychologist, 33*(2), 87–112.

Louchakova, O., & Warner, A. (2003). Via kundalini: Psychosomatic excursions in transpersonal psychology. *The Humanistic Psychologist, 31*(2), 115–158.

Lu, F., Lukoff, D., & Turner, R. (1997a). Commentary on 'Spiritual experience and psychopathology'. *Philosophy, Psychiatry and Psychology, 4*(1), 75–77.

—— (1997b). Religious or spiritual problems. In T. Widiger, A. Frances, H. Pincus, R. Ross, M. First & W. Davis (Eds.), *DSM-IV sourcebook: Volume 3* (pp. 1001–1016). American Psychiatric Association.

Lukoff, D. (2009). Kundalini awakening. In G. Khalsa, K. Wilber, S. Radha, G. Krishna & J. White (Eds.), *Kundalini rising: Exploring the energy of awakening* (pp. 127–140). Sounds True.

—— (2007). Visionary spiritual experiences. *Southern Medical Journal, 100*(6), 635–641.

—— (2001). *DSM-IV religious and spiritual problems.* Spiritual Competency Resource Centre. http://www.spiritualcompetency.com/dsm4/dsmrsproblem.pdf

—— (1988). Transpersonal perspectives on manic psychosis: Creative, visionary, and mystical states. *Journal of Transpersonal Psychology, 20*(2), 111–139.

—— (1985). Diagnosis of mystical experiences with psychotic features. *The Journal of Transpersonal Psychology, 17*(2), 155–181.

Lukoff, D., Cloninger, C., Galanter, M., Gellerman, D., Glickman, L., Koenig, H., Lu, F., Narrow, W., Peteet, J., Thielman, S., & Yang, C. (2010). Religious and spiritual considerations in psychiatric diagnosis: Considerations for the DSM-V. In P. Verhagen, H. Van Praag, J. López-Ibor Jr, J. Cox & D. Moussaoui (Eds.), *Religion and psychiatry: Beyond boundaries* (pp. 423–444). Wiley-Blackwell.

Lukoff, D., & Lu, F. (1999). Cultural competence includes religious and spiritual issues in clinical practice. *Psychiatric Annals, 29*(8), 469–472.

Lukoff, D., Lu, F., & Turner, R. (1998). From spiritual emergency to spiritual problem: The transpersonal roots of the new DSM-IV category. *Journal of Humanistic Psychology, 38*(2), 21–50.

—— (1996). Diagnosis: A transpersonal clinical approach to religious and spiritual problems. In B. Scotton, A. Chinen & R. Battista (Eds.). *Textbook of transpersonal psychiatry and psychology* (pp. 231–249). Basic Books.

—— (1995). Cultural considerations in the assessment and treatment of religious and spiritual problems. *Psychiatric Clinics of North America, 18*(3), 467–485.

—— (1992). Toward a more culturally sensitive DSM-IV: Psychoreligious and psychospiritual problems. *The Journal of Nervous and Mental Disease, 180*(11), 673–682.

Lukoff, D., Lu, F., & Yang, C. (2011). DSM-IV religious and spiritual problems. In J. Peteet, F. Lu & W. Narrow (Eds.), *Religious and spiritual issues in psychiatric diagnosis: A research agenda for DSM-V* (pp. 171–198). American Psychiatric Publishing.

Lukoff, D., Provenzano, R., Lu, F., & Turner, R. (1999). Religious and spiritual case reports on MEDLINE: A systematic analysis of records from 1980 to 1996. *Alternative Therapies in Health and Medicine, 5*(1), 64–70.

Lukoff, D., Turner, R., & Lu, F. (1993). Transpersonal psychology research review: Psychospiritual dimensions of healing. *Journal of Transpersonal Psychology, 25*(1), 11–28.

—— (1992). Transpersonal psychology research review: Psychoreligious dimensions of healing. *Journal of Transpersonal Psychology, 24*(1), 41–60.

Magier, I. (1972). Letters to the Editor: Metapsychiatry in the United States. *The American Journal of Psychiatry, 129*(4), 486.

Mails, T. (1990). *Fools Crow*. Bison Books.

Mantel, J. (2004). *A spiritual psychiatry: Challenge or heresy?* Royal College of Psychiatrists: Spirituality and Psychiatry Special Interest Group. https://www.rcpsych.ac.uk/docs/default-source/members/sigs/spirituality-spsig/jm-mantel1-11-04.pdf?sfvrsn=ebf5be36_2

Maritain, J. (1964). *Moral philosophy: An historical and critical survey of the great systems, Volume 1*. Scribner.

Marohn, S. (2003). *The natural medicine guide to bipolar disorder*. Hampton Roads Publishing Company.

Marriot, M. (2008). *Personal religious or spiritual beliefs, and the experience of hearing voices, having strong beliefs, or other experiences affecting mental well-being and general functioning*. Spirituality and Psychiatry Special Interest Group. https://web.archive.org/web/20130425212545/http://rcpsych.ac.uk/pdf/Marriot%20Spirituality%20and%20psychosis.pdf

Martindale, B. (2015). Commentary from a psychodynamic perspective. *Psychosis*, *7*(1), 59–62.

Marzanski, M., & Bratton, M. (2002). Psychopathological symptoms and religious experience: A critique of Jackson and Fulford. *Philosophy, Psychiatry and Psychology*, *9*(4), 359–371.

Maslow, A. (1963). Fusions of facts and values. *The American Journal of Psychoanalysis*, *23*(2), 117–131.

—— (1962). Notes on being-psychology. *Journal of Humanistic Psychology*, *2*(2), 47–71.

Masserman, J. (1979). Presidential address: The future of psychiatry as a scientific and humanitarian discipline in a changing world. *The American Journal of Psychiatry*, *136*(8), 1013–1019.

May, R. (2007a). Working outside the diagnostic frame. *The Psychologist*, *20*(5), 300–301.

—— (2007b). Reclaiming mad experience: Establishing unusual belief groups and evolving minds public meetings. In P. Stastny & P. Lehmann (Eds.), *Alternatives beyond psychiatry* (pp. 117–127). Peter Lehmann Publishing.

Mayes, R., & Horwitz, A. (2005). DSM-III and the revolution in the classification of mental illness. *Journal of the History of the Behavioral Sciences*, *41*(3), 249–267.

McDonald, A. (1981). Letters to the Editor: Putting psychic studies to the test. *The American Journal of Psychiatry*, *138*(3), 396.

McGhee, M. (2002). Mysticism and psychosis: Descriptions and distinctions. *Philosophy, Psychiatry and Psychology*, *9*(4), 343–347.

McGuire, W. (Ed.) (1974). *The Freud/Jung letters: The correspondence between Sigmund Freud and C. J. Jung*. Hogarth Press and Routledge & Kegan Paul.

McHugh, P. (2006). *The mind has mountains: Reflections on society and psychiatry*. The John Hopkins University Press.

McIntyre, J. (1994). Psychiatry and religion: A visit to Utah. *Psychiatric News*, *29*(4 March), 3, 25.

McLaren, N. (2007). *Humanizing madness: Psychiatry and the cognitive neurosciences*. Future Psychiatry Press.

Mechler, A. (1965). Über den begriff der psychose. *Jahrbuch der Psychologie und Psychotherapie*, *XII*, 67–74.

Meddings, S., Walley, L., Collins, T., Tullett, F., & McEwan, B. (2006, September). The voices don't like it. *Mental Health Today*, pp. 26–30.

Meddings, S., Walley, L., Collins, T., Tullet, F., McEwan, B., & Owen, K. (2004). *Are hearing voices groups effective? A preliminary evaluation*. Intervoice: The International Hearing Voices Network. http://www.intervoiceonline.org/wp-content/uploads/2011/03/Voiceseval.pdf

Medicine Grizzlybear Lake. (1991). *Native healer: Initiation into an ancient art*. Quest Books.

Meher Baba. (1988). The difference between ordinary madness and Mast states. In W. Donkin (Ed.), *The wayfarers: An account of the work of Meher Baba with the God-intoxicated, and also with advanced souls, sadhus, and the poor* (pp. 1–11). Sheriar Press.

Mehl-Madrona, L. (2007). *Narrative medicine: The use of history and story in the healing process*. Bear & Company.

—— (2005). *Coyote wisdom: The power of story in healing*. Bear & Company.

Mellor, C. (1970). First rank symptoms of schizophrenia. *The British Journal of Psychiatry*, *117*(536), 15–23.

Menninger, K. (1969). Sheer verbal Mickey Mouse. *International Journal of Psychiatry, 7*(6), 415.

Menninger, K., Mayman, M., & Pruyser, P. (1977). *The vital balance: The life process in mental health and illness.* Penguin Books.

Mental Health Foundation. (2002). *Taken seriously: Report of the Somerset Spirituality Project.* Mental Health Foundation.

Merrell-Wolff, F. (1995). *Transformations in consciousness: The metaphysics and epistemology.* State University of New York Press.

—— (1994). *Experience and philosophy: A personal record of transformation and a discussion of transcendental consciousness.* State University of New York Press.

—— (1976). *Pathways through to space: A personal report of transformation in consciousness.* Warner Books.

—— (1974). 'Abstract of the philosophy: Part 4 of 14'. *The Franklin Merrell-Wolff Fellowship.* Retrieved from http://www.merrell-wolff.org/sites/default/files/M170.pdf

—— (1938). *The Chicago Lectures: September 4–18, 1938.* The Franklin Merrell-Wolff Fellowship. https://www.merrell-wolff.org/sites/default/files/55.pdf

Meyer, A. (1957). *Psychobiology: A science of man.* Charles C. Thomas.

—— (1941). Spontaneity. *Sociometry, 4*(2), 150–167.

—— (1940). Mental health. *Science, 92*(2387), 271–276.

—— (1908). The problems of mental reaction-type, mental causes and diseases. *Psychological Bulletin, 5*(8), 245–261.

Mezzich, J., Kirmayer, L., Kleinman, A., Fabrega Jr, H., Parron, D., Good, B., Lin, K., & Manson, S. (1999). The place of culture in DSM-IV. *The Journal of Nervous and Mental Disease, 187*(8), 457–464.

Middleton, W., Dorahy, M., & Moskowitz, A. (2008). Historical conceptions of dissociation and psychosis: Nineteenth and early twentieth century perspectives on severe psychopathology. In A. Moskowitz, I. Schafer & M. Dorahy (Eds.), *Psychosis, trauma, and dissociation: Emerging perspectives on severe psychopathology* (pp. 9–20). Wiley-Blackwell.

Miller, I. (2001, July 19–22). *Extrasensory science: Human response to modulated electromagnetic energy* [Paper presentation]. Consciousness Technologies II Conference, Sisters, Oregon.

Milligan, D., McCarthy-Jones, S., Winthrop, A., & Dudley, R. (2013). Time changes everything? A qualitative investigation of the experience of auditory verbal hallucinations over time. *Psychosis, 5*(2), 107–118.

Millon, T. (1983). The DSM-III: An insider's perspective. *American Psychologist, 38*(7), 804–814.

Mishara, A., & Fusar-Poli, P. (2013). The phenomenology and neurobiology of delusion formation during psychosis onset: Jaspers, Truman symptoms, and aberrant salience. *Schizophrenia Bulletin, 39*(2), 278–286.

Mitchell, S. (2010). *Spiritual aspects of psychosis and recovery.* Spirituality and Psychiatry Special Interest Group. https://www.rcpsych.ac.uk/docs/default-source/members/sigs/spirituality-spsig/susan-mitchell-spiritual-aspects-of-psychosis-and-recovery-edited.pdf?sfvrsn=23c8dab0_2

Moerchen, F. (1908). *Die psychologie der heiligkeit: Eine religionswissenschaftliche studie.* C. Marhold.

Moore, M. (1978). Discussion of the Spitzer-Endicott and Klein proposed definitions of mental disorder (illness). In R. Spitzer & D. Klein (Eds.), *Critical issues in psychiatric diagnosis* (pp. 85–104). Raven Press.

Moran, M. (2007). Their religion may differ, but goals are the same. *Psychiatric News, 42*(6), 10–27.

Morris, W. (Ed.) (1969). *The American heritage dictionary of the English language.* Hougton Mifflin.

Moustakas, C. (1990). *Heuristic research: Design, methodology, and applications.* SAGE Publications, Inc.

Mullen, P. (2007). A modest proposal for another phenomenological approach to psychopathology. *Schizophrenia Bulletin, 33*(1), 113–121.

Muller, R. (2008, May 1). Neurotheology: Are we hardwired for God? *Psychiatric Times, 25*(6). https://www.psychiatrictimes.com/view/neurotheology-are-we-hardwired-god

Mundt, C. (1993). Images in psychiatry: Karl Jaspers. *The American journal of Psychiatry, 150*(8), 1244–1245.

Murray, E., Cunningham, M., & Price, B. (2012), The role of psychotic disorders in religious history considered. *The Journal of Neuropsychiatry and Clinical Neurosciences, 24*(4), 410–426.

Nathan, P. (1979). DSM-III and schizophrenia: Diagnostic delight or nosological nightmare? *Journal of Clinical Psychology, 35*(2), 477–479.

Nazir, S. (2010). *What proportion of psychiatrists take a spiritual history?* Spirituality and Psychiatry Special Interest Group. https://www.rcpsych.ac.uk/docs/default-source/members/sigs/spirituality-spsig/saliha-nazir-what-proportion-of-psychiatrists-take-a-spiritual-history-edited-x.pdf?sfvrsn=c39defe_2

Nelson, B., Yung, A., Bechdolf, A., & McGorry, P. (2008). The phenomenological critique and self-disturbance: Implications for ultra-high risk ('prodrome') research. *Schizophrenia Bulletin, 34*(2), 381–392.

Nelson, J. (1994). *Healing the split: Integrating spirit into our understanding of the mentally ill.* State University of New York Press.

Newberg, A. (2010). *The principles of neurotheology.* Ashgate Publishing Limited.

Newberg, A., d'Aquili, E., & Rause, V. (2002). *Why God won't go away: Brain science and the biology of belief.* Ballantine Books.

Newberg, A., & Lee, B. (2005). The neuroscientific study of religious and spiritual phenomena: Or why God doesn't use biostatistics. *Zygon, 40*(2), 469–490.

Ng, B. (1999). Qigong-induced mental disorders: A review. *Australian and New Zealand Journal of Psychiatry, 33*(2), 197–206.

Ng, F. (2007). The interface between religion and psychosis. *Australasian Psychiatry, 15*(1), 62–66.

NiaNia, W., Bush, A., & Epston, D. (2017). *Collaborative and indigenous mental health therapy: Tātaihono—stories of Māori healing and psychiatry.* Routledge.

Noll, R. (1983). Shamanism and schizophrenia: A state-specific approach to the 'schizophrenia metaphor' of shamanic states. *American Ethnologist, 10*(3), 443–459.

Nordgaard, J., Arnfred, S., Handest, P., & Parnas, J. (2008). The diagnostic status of first-rank symptoms. *Schizophrenia Bulletin, 34*(1), 137–154.

Oakland, L., & Berry, K. (2015). 'Lifting the veil': A qualitative analysis of experiences in Hearing Voices Network groups. *Psychosis, 7*(2), 119–129.

O'Callaghan, M. (1982). *A conversation with Dr. John Weir Perry*. Global Vision Corporation. https://web.archive.org/web/20110912000027/http://www.global-vision.org/papers/JWP.pdf

Onions, C. (Ed.) (1966). *The Oxford dictionary of English etymology*. Clarendon Press.

Ortolf, D. (1994). *The classical mystical experience and alexithymia in advanced spiritual practitioners and renewal process psychoses* [Unpublished Doctoral thesis]. United States International University.

Owen, G., & Harland, R. (2007). Editor's introduction: Theme issue on phenomenology and psychiatry for the 21st Century. Taking phenomenology seriously. *Schizophrenia Bulletin, 33*(1), 105–107.

Owen, I. (1994). Introducing an existential-phenomenological approach: Basic phenomenological theory and research: Part I. *Counselling Psychology Quarterly, 7*(3), 261–273.

Owen, M., Craddock, N., & Jablensky, A. (2010). The genetic deconstruction of psychosis. In C. Tamminga, P. Sirovatka, D. Regier & J. van Os (Eds.), *Deconstructing psychosis: Refining the research agenda for DSM-V* (pp. 69–82). American Psychiatric Publishing.

Pahnke, W., & Richards, W. (1966). Implications of LSD and experimental mysticism. *Journal of Religion and Health, 5*(3), 175–208.

Panati, C. (1975, August 26). Laboratories study the paranormal. *Lakeland Ledger*, p. 27.

Pandarakalam, J. (2007). *Aspects of parapsychology relevant to spirituality and psychiatry*. https://web.archive.org/web/20170830064545/http://www.rcpsych.ac.uk/pdf/Parapsychology%20relevant%20to%20Spirituality%20and%20Psychiatry%20James%20Pandarakalam.pdf

Park, R. (1991). *Spiritual emergencies: A quantitative and descriptive examination with an emphasis on Kundalini and the role of ego* [Unpublished Doctoral thesis]. Institute of Transpersonal Psychology.

Pearson, D., Burrow, A., FitzGerald, C., Green, K., Lee, G., & Wise, N. (2001). Auditory hallucinations in normal child populations. *Personality and Individual Differences, 31*(3), 401–407.

Peavy, C. (1974). The secularized Christ in contemporary cinema. *Journal of Popular Film, 3*(2), 139–155.

Peierls, R. (2000). Rudolf Peierls. In P. Davies & J. Brown (Eds.), *The ghost in the atom* (pp. 70–82). Cambridge University Press.

Perceval, J. (1840). *A narrative of the treatment experienced by a gentleman, during a state of mental derangement*. Effingham Wilson.

Perroud, N. (2009). Religion/spirituality and neuropsychiatry. In P. Huguelet & H. Koenig (Eds.), *Religion and spirituality in psychiatry* (pp. 48–64). Cambridge University Press.

Perry, J. (1999). *Trials of the visionary mind: Spiritual emergency and the renewal process*. University of New York Press.

—— (1987). *The self in psychotic process: Its symbolism in schizophrenia*. Spring Publications.

—— (1974). *The far side of madness*. Prentice-Hall.

Peteet, J., Lu, F., & Narrow, W. (2011a). 'Introduction'. In J. Peteet, F. Lu & W. Narrow (Eds.), *Religious and spiritual issues in psychiatric diagnosis: A research agenda for DSM-V* (pp. xvii–xx). American Psychiatric Publishing.

—— (2011b). *Religious and spiritual issues in psychiatric diagnosis: A research agenda for DSM-V*. American Psychiatric Publishing.

Peters, E. (2001). Are delusions on a continuum? The case of religious and delusional beliefs. In I. Clarke (Ed.), *Psychosis and spirituality: Exploring the new frontier* (pp. 191–207). Whurr Publications.

Peters, E., Joseph, S., & Garety, P. (1999). Measurement of delusional ideation in the normal population: Introducing the PDI (Peters et al. Delusions Inventory). *Schizophrenia Bulletin, 25*(3), 553–576.

Petitmengin, C., & Bitbol, M. (2009). The validity of first-person descriptions as authenticity and coherence. *Journal of Consciousness Studies, 16*(10–12), 252–284.

Pfarrer, M. (2012). *What is content analysis?* University of Georgia: Department of Management at the Terry College of Business. https://web.archive.org/web/20131213133606/https://www.terry.uga.edu/management/contentanalysis/

Pfeifer, S. (1994). Belief in demons and exorcism in psychiatric patients in Switzerland. *British Journal of Medical Psychology, 67*(3), 247–258.

Phillips, D. (2009). A quixotic quest? Philosophical issues in assessing the quality of education research. In P. Walters, A. Lareau & S. Ranis (Eds.), *Education research on trial: Policy reform and the call for scientific rigor* (pp. 163–196). Routledge.

Pierre, J. (2001). Faith or delusion?: At the crossroads of religion and psychosis. *Journal of Psychiatric Practice, 7*(3), 163–172.

Pilecki, B., Clegg, J., & McKay, D. (2011). The influence of corporate and political interests on models of illness in the evolution of the DSM. *European Psychiatry, 26*, 194–200.

Plakun, E. (2008). Psychiatry in Tibetan Buddhism: Madness and its cure seen through the lens of religious and national history. *Journal of the American Academy of Psychoanalysis and Dynamic Psychiatry, 36*(3), 415–430.

Podvoll, E. (1979). Psychosis and the mystic path. *Psychoanalytic Review, 66*(4), 571–590.

Posey, T., & Losch, M. (1983). Auditory hallucinations of hearing voices in 375 normal subjects. *Imagination, Cognition and Personality, 3*(2), 99–113.

Powell, A. (2007). *Furthering the spiritual dimension of psychiatry in the United Kingdom.* Spirituality and Psychiatry Special Interest Group. https://web.archive.org/web/20160326034552/http://www.rcpsych.ac.uk/pdf/Andrew%20Powell%20Furthering%20the%20spiritual%20dimension%20of%20psychiatry%20in%20the%20UK.y.pdf

—— (2001). Spirituality and science: A personal view. *Advances in Psychiatric Treatment, 7*(5), 319–321.

Prince, R. (1974). The problem of 'spirit possession' as a treatment for psychiatric disorders. *Ethos, 2*(4), 315–333.

Prince, R., & Savage, C. (1966). Mystical states and the concept of regression. *Psychedelic Review, 8*, 59–75.

Professional Staff of the United States-United Kingdom Cross-National Project. (1974). The diagnosis and psychopathology of schizophrenia in New York and London. *Schizophrenia Bulletin, 1*(11), 80–102.

Pull, C. (2002). Diagnosis of schizophrenia: A review. In M. Maj & N. Sartorius (Eds.), *Schizophrenia—(WPA series: Evidence and experience in psychiatry: Volume 2)* (pp. 1–37). Wiley.

Puthoff, H. (2001). Quantum vacuum energy research and 'metaphysical' processes in the physical world. *Monterey Institute for the Study of Alternative Healing Arts Newsletter, 32–35* (January–December), 40–41.

Raheja, S. (2001). *Examining our spiritual spectacles: Dangers and pitfalls.* Spirituality and Psychiatry Special Interest Group. https://www.rcpsych.ac.uk/docs/default-source/members/sigs/spirituality-spsig/raheja1.pdf?sfvrsn=babe7fd0_2

Raji, O. (2004). *Prayer and Medicine, a healthy alliance? A multi-faith, multi-cultural perspective.* Spirituality and Psychiatry Special Interest Group. https://www.rcpsych.ac.uk/docs/default-source/members/sigs/spirituality-spsig/8-dr-raji-prayer-and-medicine-8-4-04.pdf?sfvrsn=819d24f1_2

Randal, P., & Argyle, N. (2005). *'Spiritual Emergency'—a useful explanatory model?': A literature review and discussion paper.* Spirituality and Psychiatry Special Interest Group. https://www.rcpsych.ac.uk/docs/default-source/members/sigs/spirituality-spsig/patte-randal-and-nick-argyle-spiritual-emergency-1-1-06.pdf?sfvrsn=c9d0331_2

Rao, K. (2005a). Introduction. In K. Rao & S. Marwaha (Eds.), *Towards a spiritual psychology: Essays in Indian psychology* (pp. 1–17). Samvad India Foundation.

—— (2005b). Scope and substance of Indian psychology. In K. Rao & S. Marwaha (Eds.), *Towards a spiritual psychology: Essays in Indian psychology* (pp. 18–40). Samvad India Foundation.

Razzaque, R. (2014). *Breaking down is waking up: The connection between psychological distress and spiritual awakening.* Watkins Publishing.

Read, T. (2011). *Archetype 2012 and our global mid-life crisis.* Spirituality and Psychiatry Special Interest Group. https://www.rcpsych.ac.uk/docs/default-source/members/sigs/spirituality-spsig/2012-archetype-and-global-mid-life-crisis-read-y.pdf?sfvrsn=4ea1295d_2

—— (2004). The invention of 'schizophrenia'. In J. Read, L. Mosher & R. Bentall (Eds.), *Models of madness: Psychological, social and biological approaches to schizophrenia* (pp. 21–34). East Sussex: Brunner-Routledge.

—— (2007). *Transpersonal psychiatry.* Spirituality and Psychiatry Special Interest Group. https://www.rcpsych.ac.uk/docs/default-source/members/sigs/spirituality-spsig/transpersonal-psychiatry-tim-read-editedx.pdf?sfvrsn=a6d4f554_2

Regier, D. (2010). Foreword: Rethinking psychosis in the DSM-V. In C. Tamminga, P. Sirovatka, D. Regier & J. van Os (Eds.), *Deconstructing psychosis: Refining the research agenda for DSM-V* (pp. xv–xix). American Psychiatric Association.

Regner, V. (1998). *Reexamining Christian conversion experiences: Considering kundalini awakenings and spiritual emergencies* [Unpublished Doctoral thesis]. Claremont School of Theology.

Rhys, E. (Ed.) (1912). *'The little flowers' and the life of St. Francis with the 'mirror of perfection'.* J. M. Dent & Sons Ltd.

Robins, E., & Guze, S. (1970). Establishment of diagnostic validity in psychiatric illness: Its application to schizophrenia. *The American Journal of Psychiatry, 126*(7), 983–987.

Robbins, M. (2012). The primordial mind and the psychoses. *Psychosis, 4*(3), 258–268.

—— (2011). *The primordial mind in health and illness: A cross-cultural perspective.* Routledge.

Robbins, B., Higgins, M., Fisher, M., & Over, K. (2011). Conflicts of interest in research on antipsychotic treatment of Pediatric Bipolar Disorder, Temper Dysregulation Disorder, and Attenuated Psychotic Symptoms Syndrome: Exploring the unholy alliance between Big Pharma and psychiatry. *Journal of Psychological Issues in Organizational Culture, 1*(4), 32–49.

Rock, A., Wilson, J., Johnston, L., & Levesque, J. (2008). Ego boundaries, shamanic-like techniques, and subjective experience: An experimental study. *Anthropology of Consciousness, 19*(1), 60–83.

Rogler, L. (1997). Making sense of historical changes in the diagnostic and statistical manual of mental disorders: Five propositions. *Journal of Health and Social Behavior, 38*(1), 9–20.

Romano, J. (1977). Requiem or reveille: Psychiatry's choice. *Bulletin of the New York Academy of Medicine, 53*(9), 787–805.

Romme, M., & Escher, A. (1989). Hearing voices. *Schizophrenia Bulletin, 15*(2), 209–216.

Romme, M., Escher, S., Dillon, J., Corstens, D., & Morris, M. (Eds.) (2009). *Living with voices: 50 stories of recovery.* PCCS Books & Birmingham City University.

Romme, M., Honig, A., Noorthoorn, E., & Escher, A. (1992). Coping with hearing voices: An emancipatory approach. *The British Journal of Psychiatry, 161*(1), 99–103.

Rosenhan, D. (1973). On being sane in insane places. *Science, 179*(4070), 250–258.

Rothman, S. (1982, January 3). Medical notes: Tapping psychic ability. *The Palm Beach Post*, p. 20.

Royal College of Psychiatrists. (2021). *What we do and how.* Royal College of Psychiatrists. https://www.rcpsych.ac.uk/about-us/what-we-do-and-how

Ruiz, P. (1981). Letters to the Editor: More on psychic studies. *The American Journal of Psychiatry, 138*(11), 1515.

Russell, D. (2014). *My mysterious son: A life-changing passage between schizophrenia and shamanism.* Skyhorse Publishing.

Saks, E. (2013, January 25). Successful and schizophrenic. *The New York Times.* http://www.nytimes.com/2013/01/27/opinion/sunday/schizophrenic-not-stupid.html?_r=0

—— (2007). *The centre cannot hold: A memoir of my schizophrenia.* Virago.

Samuel, G. (2010). Possession and self-possession: Towards an integrated mind-body perspective. In B. Schmidt & L. Huskinson (Eds.), *Spirit possession and trance* (pp. 35–52). Continuum International Publishing Group.

Sanderson, A. (2012). *Treatment of patients with delusional states.* Spirituality and Psychiatry Special Interest Group. https://www.rcpsych.ac.uk/docs/default-source/members/sigs/spirituality-spsig/delusional-states-alan-sanderson.pdf?sfvrsn=7ba65569_2

—— (2003). *The case for spirit release.* Spirituality and Psychiatry Special Interest Group. https://www.rcpsych.ac.uk/docs/default-source/members/sigs/spirituality-spsig/sanderson_19_11_03.pdf?sfvrsn=a9662a53_2

Sandweiss, S. (2011). *Spirit and the mind.* Birth Day Publishing Company.

Sannella, L. (1987). *The kundalini experience: Psychosis or transcendence?* Integral Publishing.

Sartorius, N., Shapiro, R., & Jablensky, A. (1974). The international pilot study of schizophrenia. *Schizophrenia Bulletin, 1*(11), 21–34.

Saukko, P. (2003). *Doing research in cultural studies.* SAGE Publications Ltd.

Saver, J., & Rabin, J. (1997). The neural substrates of religious experience. In S. Salloway, P. Malloy & J. Cummings (Eds.), *The neuropsychiatry of limbic and subcortical disorders* (pp. 195–207). American Psychiatric Press, Inc.

Schacht, T. (1985). DSM-III and the politics of truth. *American Psychologist 40*(5), 513–521.

Schaler, J. (1995). Good therapy. *Interpsych Newsletter, 2*(7): August-September. http://www.schaler.net/fifth/goodtherapy.html

Schelling, J. (1942). *Ages of the world*. Columbia University Press.

Schneider, K. (1959). *Clinical psychopathology*. Grune & Stratton.

—— (1946). *Beiträge zur psychiatrie*. George Thieme.

—— (1933). Psychopathie und psychose. *Nervenartz, 7*, 337–344.

Schreber, D. (1988). *Memoirs of my mervous illness*. Harvard University Press.

Schultze-Lutter, F., Ruhrmann, S., & Klosterkötter, J. (2008). Early detection and early intervention in psychosis in Western Europe. *Clinical Neuropsychiatry, 5*(6), 303–315.

Schweitzer, A. (1948 [1913]). *The psychiatric study of Jesus: Exposition and criticism*. The Beacon Press.

Scott, S., Garver, S., Richards, J., & Hathaway, W. (2003). Religious issues in diagnosis: The V-Code and beyond. *Mental Health, Religion and Culture, 6*(2), 161–173.

Scotton, B. (2011). Commentary on 'DSM-IV religious and spiritual problems'. In J. Peteet, F. Lu & W. Narrow (Eds.), *Religious and spiritual issues in psychiatric diagnosis: A research agenda for DSM-V* (pp. 199–201). American Psychiatric Publishing.

Segen, J. (1992). *Concise dictionary of modern medicine*. Parthenon Publishing Group.

Sekida, K. (1985). *Zen training: Methods and philosophy*. Shambala.

Shamdasani, S. (2009). Introduction. In S. Shamdasani (Ed.), *The red book: Liber novus: A reader's edition* (pp. 1–98). W. W. Norton & Co.

Sharfstein, S. (2005, August 19). Big Pharma and American psychiatry: The good, the bad, and the ugly. *Psychiatric News*, https://psychnews.psychiatryonline.org/doi/10.1176/pn.40.16.00400003

—— (1987). Third-party payments, cost containment, and DSM-III. In G. Tischler (Ed.), *Diagnosis and classification in psychiatry: A critical appraisal of DSM-III* (pp. 530–538). Cambridge University Press.

Sharma, A. (2008). *Meditation: The future medication*. Spirituality and Psychiatry Special Interest Group. https://www.rcpsych.ac.uk/docs/default-source/members/sigs/spirituality-spsig/avdesh-sharma-meditation-as-medication2.pdf?sfvrsn=13e6a51_2

Siddle, R., Haddock, G., Tarrier, N., & Faragher, E. (2002). Religious delusions in patients admitted to hospital with schizophrenia. *Social Psychiatry and Psychiatric Epidemiology, 37*(3), 130–138.

Sidgwick, H., Johnson, A., Myers, F., Podmore, F., & Sidgwick, E. (1894). Report on the census of hallucinations' *Proceedings of the Society for Psychical Research, 10*(26), 25–394.

Siegler, M., Osmond, H., & Mann, H. (1969). Laing's models of madness. *The British Journal of Psychiatry, 115*(525), 947–958.

Siglag, M. (1986). *Schizophrenic and mystical experience: Similarities and differences* [Unpublished Doctoral thesis]. University of Detroit.

Silverman, J. (1967). Shamans and acute schizophrenia. *American Anthropologist, 69*(1), 21–31.

Sims, A. (2003). *Mysterious ways: Spirituality and British psychiatry in the 20th century*. Spirituality and Psychiatry Special Interest Group. https://www.rcpsych.ac.uk/docs/default-source/members/sigs/spirituality-spsig/andrew-sims-1-11-03-mysterious-ways—spirituality-and-british-psychiatry-in-the-20th-century.pdf?sfvrsn=40adb83a_4

—— (1997). Commentary on 'Spiritual experience and psychopathology'. *Philosophy, Psychiatry and Psychology, 4*(1), 79–81.

Skodal, A. (2000). Diagnosis and classification of mental disorders. In R. Menninger & J. Nemiah (Eds.), *American psychiatry after World War II (1944–1994)* (pp. 430–456). American Psychiatric Press.

Škodlar, B., Dernovšek, M., & Kocmur, M. (2008). Psychopathology of schizophrenia in Ljubljana (Slovenia) from 1881 to 2000: Changes in the content of delusions in schizophrenia patients related to various sociopolitical, technical and scientific changes. *International Journal of Social Psychiatry, 54*(2), 101–111.

Sommer, I., Daalman, K., Rietkerk, T., Diederen, K., Bakker, S., Wijkstra, J., & Boks, M. (2010). Healthy individuals with auditory verbal hallucinations: Who are they?: Psychiatric assessments of a selected sample of 103 subjects. *Schizophrenia Bulletin, 36*(3), 633–641.

Sourial, S. (2007). *A personal experience of kundalini.* Spirituality and Psychiatry Special Interest Group. https://www.rcpsych.ac.uk/docs/default-source/members/sigs/spirituality-spsig/a-personal-experience-of-kundalini-sarah-sourial-editedx.pdf?sfvrsn=31808fe9_2

Spiegel, A. (2005, January 3). The Dictionary of disorder: How one man revolutionized psychiatry. *The New Yorker: Annals of Medicine,* http://www.newyorker.com/archive/2005/01/03/050103fa_fact?currentPage=al

— (2003, August 18). The man behind psychiatry's diagnostic manual. *National Public Radio: All Things Considered* [Broadcast], https://www.npr.org/templates/story/story.php?storyId=1400925

Spiritual Emergence Network. (n.d.). *A brief history of SEN.* Spiritual Emergence Network. http://www.spiritualemergence.org/a-short-history-of-sen/

Spitzer, R. (2001). Values and assumptions in the development of DSM-III and DSM-III-R: An insider's perspective and a belated response to Sadler, Hulgus, and Agich's 'On values in recent American psychiatric classification'. *The Journal of Nervous and Mental Disease, 189*(6), 351–359.

— (1989). *The development of diagnostic criteria in psychiatry.* Eugene Garfield Citation Classics. http://garfield.library.upenn.edu/classics1989/A1989U310300001.pdf

— (1985). DSM-III and the politics–science dichotomy syndrome: A response to Thomas E. Schacht's 'DSM-III and the politics of truth'. *American Psychologist, 40*(5), 522–526.

— (1984a). A debate on DSM-III—Robert L. Spitzer: First rebuttal. *The American Journal of Psychiatry, 141*(4), 546–547.

— (1984b). A debate on DSM-III—Robert L. Spitzer: Second rebuttal. *The American Journal of Psychiatry, 141*(4), 551–553.

— (1982). Letters to the Editor: Response to Blashfield's 'Feighner et al., invisible colleges, and the Matthew effect'. *Schizophrenia Bulletin, 8*(4), 592.

— (1981). Nonmedical myths and the DSM-III. *APA Monitor, 12*(10), 3, 33.

Spitzer, R., Andreasen, N., & Endicott, J. (1978). Schizophrenia and other psychotic disorders in DSM-III. *Schizophrenia Bulletin, 4*(4), 489–511.

Spitzer, R., & Endicott, J. (1978). Medical and mental disorder: Proposed definition and criteria. In R. Spitzer & D. Klein (Eds.), *Critical issues in psychiatric diagnosis* (pp. 15–39). Raven Press.

Spitzer, R., Endicott, J., & Robins, E. (1978). Research diagnostic criteria: Rationale and reliability. *Archives of General Psychiatry, 35*(6), 773–782.

Spitzer, R., Robins, E., & Endicott, J. (1978). *Research Diagnostic Criteria (RDC) for a selected group of functional disorders*. New York State Psychiatric Unit.

Spitzer, R., Sheehy, M., & Endicott, J. (1977). DSM-III: Guiding principles. In: V. Rakoff, H. Stancer & H. Kedward (Eds.), *Psychiatric diagnosis* (pp. 1–24). Brunner/Mazel.

Spitzer, R., & Williams, J. (1982). The definition and diagnosis of mental disorder. In W. Gove (Ed.), *Deviance and mental illness: Sage annual reviews of studies in deviance, Volume 6* (pp. 15–31). Sage.

Spitzer, R., & Wilson, P. (1969). A guide to the American Psychiatric Association's new diagnostic nomenclature. *The International Journal of Psychiatry, 7*(6), 356–367.

Spirituality and Psychiatry Special Interest Group. (2021). *About us*. Royal College of Psychiatrists. https://www.rcpsych.ac.uk/members/special-interest-groups/spirituality/about-us

—— (2013). *About us: Spirituality and Psychiatry Special Interest Group*. Royal College of Psychiatrists. http://www.rcpsych.ac.uk/workinpsychiatry/specialinterestgroups/spirituality/aboutus.aspx#join

Sri Aurobindo. (2006). *Autobiographical notes and other writings of historical interest*. Sri Aurobindo Ashram Publication Department.

—— (2005). *The life divine*. Sri Aurobindo Ashram Publication Department.

—— (1999). *The synthesis of yoga*. Sri Aurobindo Ashram Publication Department.

—— (1997). *The renaissance in India and other essays on Indian culture*. Sri Aurobindo Ashram Publication Department.

—— (1972). *On Himself*. Site of Sri Aurobindo & The Mother. https://motherandsriaurobindo.in/Sri-Aurobindo/books/sabcl/on-himself/

Standing Bear, L. (1978). *Land of the spotted eagle*. University of Nebraska Press.

Stanghellini, G. (2013). The ethics of incomprehensibility. In G. Stanghellini & T. Fuchs (Eds.), *One century of Karl Jaspers' General Psychopathology* (pp. 166–182). Oxford University Press.

—— (2004). *Disembodied spirits and deanimated bodies: The psychopathology of common sense*. Oxford University Press.

Stanghellini, G., Bolton, D., & Fulford, W. (2013). Person-centered psychopathology of schizophrenia: Building on Karl Jaspers' understanding of patient's attitude toward his illness. *Schizophrenia Bulletin, 39*(2), 287–294.

Star Hawk Lake, T. (1996). *Hawk woman dancing with the moon*. M. Evans & Company.

Steele, C. (1981). Letters to the Editor: Kudos for metapsychiatry. *The American Journal of Psychiatry, 138*(10), 1397–1398.

Stein, D. (1991). Philosophy and the DSM-III. *Comprehensive Psychiatry, 32*(5), 404–415.

Stephen, M. (1997). Cargo cults, cultural creativity, and autonomous imagination. *Ethos, 25*(3), 333–358.

Stephen, M., & Suryani, L. (2000). Shamanism, psychosis and autonomous imagination. *Culture, Medicine and Psychiatry, 24*(1), 5–38.

Stevenson, G. (1937). The psychobiologic unit as a pattern of community function. *Archives of Neurology and Psychiatry, 37*(4), 742–747.

Stifler, K., Greer, J., Sneck, W., & Dovenmuehle, R. (1993). An empirical investigation of the discriminability of reported mystical experiences among religious contemplatives, psychotic inpatients, and normal adults. *Journal for the Scientific Study of Religion, 32*(4), 366–372.

Stoddard, F. (2012). Religious and Spiritual Issues in Psychiatric Diagnosis: A Research Agenda for DSM-V. *The American Journal of Psychiatry, 169*(5), 544–545.

Sturges, S. (1981). Letters to the Editor: Putting psychic studies to the test. *The American Journal of Psychiatry, 138*(3), 396.

Stutchbury, E. (2004). 'The process of cultural translation: Untying the knots that bind'. In M. Blows, Y. Haruki, P. Bankart, J. Blows, M. DelMonte, & S. Srinivasan (Eds.), *The relevance of the wisdom traditions in contemporary society: The challenge to psychology* (pp. 77–97). Eburon Academic Publishers.

Sun Bear, Wabun, & Weinstock, B. (1983), *Sun Bear: The path of power*. Bear Tribe Publishing.

Swami Budhananda. (1971). *Life of Sri Ramakrishna*. Advaita Ashram.

Swedenborg, E. (2010a [1747–1765]). 'piritual Diary (paragraphs 4901–4950)' Sacred-texts. com. http://sacred-texts.com/swd/sd/sd69.htm

—— (2010b [1749–1756]). *Arcana Coelestia (paragraphs 6201–6250)*. Sacred-texts.com. http://sacred-texts.com/swd/ac/ac125.htm

—— (2010c [1749–1756]). *Arcana Coelestia (paragraphs 2451–2500)*. Sacred-texts.com. http://sacred-texts.com/swd/ac/ac050.htm

—— (2009 [1758]). *The last judgment and Babylon destroyed: All the predictions in the Book of Revelation are at this day fulfilled from things heard and seen*. Swedenborg Foundation.

—— (1942 [1763]). *On the divine love; on the divine wisdom*. The Swedenborg Society.

—— (1905 [1758]). *Heaven and its wonders and hell: From things heard and seen*. American Swedenborg Printing And Publishing Society.

—— (1892 [1764]). *Angelic wisdom about the divine providence*. American Swedenborg Printing and Publishing Society.

Szasz, T. (1991). *Ideology and insanity: Essays on the psychiatric dehumanization of man*. Syracuse University Press.

Taitimu, M. (2007). *Ngā whakāwhitinga: Standing at the crossroads: Māori ways of understanding extra-ordinary experiences and schizophrenia* [Unpublished Doctoral thesis]. University of Auckland.

Tamminga, C., Sirovatka, P., Regier D., & van Os J. (Eds.) (2010). *Deconstructing psychosis: Refining the research agenda for DSM-V*. American Psychiatric Publishing.

Task Force on DSM-IV. (1993). *DSM-IV draft criteria: 3/1/93*. American Psychiatric Association.

Teoh, C., & Dass, D. (1973). Spirit possession in an Indian family—a case report. *Singapore Medical Journal, 14*(1), 62–64.

Teodorescu, D. (c2008). ICD-10's limitations to distinguish between psychosis and spiritual emergencies: The need for a new diagnosis in ICD-11 for spiritual or religious problems. *DIN—Spiritual Science*. https://web.archive.org/web/20130326013318/http://din.nu/ICDspirit.htm

The Editor. (1896). Semi-centennial: Proceedings of the American Medico-Psychological Association at the Fiftieth Annual Meeting, held in Philadelphia, May 15–18, 1894. *The British Journal of Psychiatry, 42*, 172–184.

The JHU Gazette. (2005). *Obituary: Jerome Frank, 95, noted psychotherapy researcher*. John Hopkins University. http://www.jhu.edu/gazette/2005/18apr05/18frank.html

Thornton, M. (2005). *I used to be you: A metanoic, refractive, interpersonal phenomenology utilizing the work of Ronald David Laing* [Unpublished Doctoral thesis]. University of Louisiana at Monroe.

Thornton, T., & Schaffner, K. (2011). Philosophy of science perspectives on psychiatry for the person. *International Journal of Person Centered Medicine, 1*(1), 128–130.

Tien, A. (1991). Distribution of hallucinations in the population. *Social Psychiatry and Psychiatric Epidemiology, 26*(6), 287–292.

Torrey, E. (2013). *Surviving schizophrenia: A family manual.* HarperCollins.

Tsuang, M., Stone, W., & Faraone, S. (2000). Toward reformulating the diagnosis of schizophrenia. *The American Journal of Psychiatry, 157*(7), 1041–1050.

Tulku, T. (1984). *Knowledge of freedom.* Dharma Publishing.

—— (1977). *Time, space, and knowledge: A new vision of reality.* Dharma Publishing.

Turkington, D., Spencer, H., Jassal, I., & Cummings, A. (2015). Cognitive behavioural therapy for the treatment of delusional systems. *Psychosis, 7*(1), 48–59.

Turner, R., Lukoff, D., Barnhouse, R., & Lu, F. (1995). Religious or spiritual problem. A culturally sensitive diagnostic category in the DSM-IV. *Journal of Nervous and Mental Disease, 183*(7), 435–444.

Twemlow, S. (1981). Letters to the Editor: Kudos for metapsychiatry. *The American Journal of Psychiatry, 138*(10), 1397.

Underhill, E. (Ed.) (1970). *A book of contemplation the which is called The Cloud of Unknowing, in the which a soul is oned with God.* Stuart & Watkins.

—— (1912). *Mysticism: A study in the nature and development of spiritual consciousness.* Methuen & Co.

Vacariu, G. (2016). *Illusions of human thinking: On concepts of mind, reality, and universe in psychology, neuroscience and physics.* Springer Fachmedien Wiesbaden.

Vaillant, G. (1984). A debate on DSM-III—George E. Vaillant: The disadvantages of DSM-III outweigh its advantages. *The American Journal of Psychiatry, 141*(4), 542–545.

van der Gaag, M., Valmaggia, L., & Smit, F. (2014). The effects of individually tailored formulation-based cognitive behavioural therapy in auditory hallucinations and delusions: a meta-analysis. *Schizophrenia Research, 156*(1), 30–37.

van Dusen, W. (1981). *The natural depth in man.* Swedenborg Foundation Inc.

—— (1974). *The presence of other worlds: The psychological/spiritual findings of Emanuel Swedenborg.* Harper & Rowe.

—— (1970). Hallucinations as the world of spirits. *Psychedelic Review, 11*, 60–69.

van Os, J., Hanssen, M., Bijl, R., & Ravelli, A. (2000). Strauss (1969) revisited: A psychosis continuum in the general population? *Schizophrenia Research, 45*(1), 11–20.

Varga, J. (2011). *Visits to heaven.* ARE Press.

Varma, S. (2005). From the self to the Self: An exposition on personality based on the works of Sri Aurobindo. In K. Rao & S. Marwaha (Eds.), *Towards a spiritual psychology: Essays in Indian psychology* (pp. 169–209). Samvad India Foundation.

Varvoglis, M. (c2009). *What is psi? What isn't?.* Parapsychological Association. http://archived.parapsych.org/what_is_psi_varvoglis.htm

Verhagen, P., & Cook, C. (2010), Epilogue: Proposal for a World Psychiatric Association Consensus or Position Statement on Spirituality and Religion in Psychiatry. In P. Verhagen, H. Van Praag, J. López-Ibor Jr, J. Cox & D. Moussaoui (Eds.), *Religion and psychiatry: Beyond boundaries* (pp. 615–631). Wiley-Blackwell.

Verhagen, P., Van Praag, H., López-Ibor Jr, J., Cox, J., & Moussaoui, D. (Eds.) (2010). *Religion and psychiatry: Beyond boundaries.* Wiley-Blackwell.

Waldram, J., Herring, A., & Young, T. (2006). *Aboriginal health in Canada: Historical, cultural, and epidemiological perspectives*. University of Toronto Press.

Walker, C. (1991). Delusion: What did Jaspers really say? *The British Journal of Psychiatry, 159*(14), 94–103.

Walsh, R. (1997). The psychological health of shamans: A reevaluation. *Journal of the American Academy of Religion, 65*(1), 101–124.

—— (1993). Phenomenological mapping and comparisons of shamanic, Buddhist, yogic, and schizophrenic experiences. *Journal of the American Academy of Religion, 61*(4), 739–769.

Wapnick, K. (1969). Mysticism and schizophrenia. *Journal of Transpersonal Psychology, 1*(2), 49–67.

Ward, C., & Beaubrun, M. (1980). The psychodynamics of demon possession. *Journal for the Scientific Study of Religion, 19*(2), 201–207.

Warner, R. (2004). *Recovery from schizophrenia: Psychiatry and political economy*. Brunner-Routledge.

Warren, I. (1879). *The Parousia: A critical study of the scripture doctrines of Christ's second coming, his reign as king, the resurrection of the dead, and the general judgment*. Hoyt, Fogg, & Donham.

Washburn, M. (2003). *Embodied spirituality in a sacred world*. State University of New York Press.

—— (1988). *The ego and the dynamic ground: A transpersonal theory of human development*. State University of New York Press.

Watkins, J. (2010). *Unshrinking psychosis: Understanding and healing the wounded soul*. Michelle Anderson Publishing.

—— (1998). *Hearing voices: A common human experience*. Hill of Content.

Wernicke, C. (1899). *Über die klassifikation der psychosen: Nach einem in der medicinischen section der vaterländischen gesellschaft zu breslau gegebenen vortag*. Schlettersche Buchhandlung.

Wheelwell, D. (1997). Origins and history of consciousness. *Journal of Consciousness Studies, 4*(5–6), 532–540.

Whitaker, R. (2002). *Mad in America: Bad science, bad medicine, and the enduring mistreatment of the mentally ill*. Basic Books.

Wilber, K. (1984). Introduction: Of shadows and symbols. In K. Wilber (Ed.), *Quantum questions: Mystical writings of the world's greatest physicists* (pp. 3–29). Shambhala Publications.

—— (1975). Psychologia perennis: The spectrum of consciousness. *Journal of Transpersonal Psychology, 7*(2), 105–132.

Williams-Hogan, J. (2005a). Swedenborg, Emanuel. In L. Jones (Ed.), *Encyclopedia of religion* (pp. 8898–8900). Macmillan.

—— (2005b). Swedenborgianism. In L. Jones (Ed.), *Encyclopedia of religion* (pp. 8900–8906). Macmillan.

Wilson, M. (1993). DSM-III and the transformation of American psychiatry: A history. *The American Journal of Psychiatry, 150*(3), 399–410.

Winkelman, M. (2004). Shamanism. In C. Ember & M. Ember (Eds.), *Encyclopedia of medical anthropology: Health and illness in the world's cultures* (pp. 145–154). Kluwer Academic/Plenum Publishers.

Winship, G. (2014). Foreward. In J. Gale, M. Robson & G. Rapsomatioti (Eds.), *Insanity and divinity: Studies in psychosis and spirituality* (pp. xvi–xx). Routledge.

Wu, Y., & Duan, Z. (2015). Analysis on evolution and research focus in psychiatry field. *BMC Psychiatry, 15*(1), 105–120.

Wulff, D. (2000). Mystical experience. In E. Cardeña, S. Lynn & S. Krippner (Eds.), *Varieties of anomalous experience: Examining the scientific evidence* (pp. 397–439). American Psychological Association.

Wykes, T. (2004). Psychological treatment for voices in psychosis. *Cognitive Neuropsychiatry, 9*(1), 25–41.

Wykes, T., Parr, A., & Landau, S. (1999). Group treatment of auditory hallucinations. Exploratory study of effectiveness. *The British Journal of Psychiatry, 175*(2), 180–185.

Yang, C., Lukoff, D., & Lu, F. (2006). Working with spiritual issues of adults in clinical practice. *Psychiatric Annals, 36*(3), 168–174.

Zaehner, R. (1961). *Mysticism sacred and profane: An inquiry into some varieties of praeternatural experiences.* Oxford University Press.

Zung, W. (1975). Operational definitions and diagnoses of depression. *Psychopharmacology Bulletin, 11*(3), 25–27.

INDEX

CPSIA information can be obtained
at www.ICGtesting.com
Printed in the USA
JSHW050751061122
32688JS00001B/1